Assessing and Treating Low Incidence/High Severity Psychological Disorders of Childhood

Stefan C. Dombrowski · Karen L. Gischlar
· Martin Mrazik

Assessing and Treating
Low Incidence/High Severity
Psychological Disorders
of Childhood

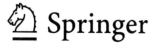 Springer

Stefan C. Dombrowski
Professor & Director, Graduate
Program in School Psychology
Rider University
2083 Lawrenceville Road
Lawrenceville, NJ 08648, USA
sdombrowski@rider.edu

Karen L. Gischlar
Department of Graduate Education,
Leadership and Counseling
Rider University
2083 Lawrenceville Road
Lawrenceville, NJ 08648, USA
kgischlar@rider.edu

Martin Mrazik
Department of Educational Psychology
University of Alberta
6-135 Education North Bldg.
Edmonton, Alberta, Canada
mrazik@ualberta.ca

ISBN 978-1-4419-9969-6   e-ISBN 978-1-4419-9970-2
DOI 10.1007/978-1-4419-9970-2
Springer New York Dordrecht Heidelberg London

Library of Congress Control Number: 2011931527

Printed on acid-free paper

Springer is part of Springer Science+Business Media (www.springer.com)

Acknowledgments

I dedicate this book to my family (Debbie, Maxwell, and Henry), parents (Carl and Mary Lee), and sisters (Laurie, Jennifer, and Melissa). I also thank Rider University for furnishing me with a summer fellowship to work on parts of this project. I appreciate the diligence and expertise of my co-authors, Karen and Marty, in contributing to this book project. I also acknowledge the masterful writing of Fred W. Greer who wrote the chapter on feral children and the editorial assistance of Joanna Harrison-Smith and Robert Carlisle. Finally, I thank Judy Jones and her staff at Springer for their support and encouragement throughout the writing of this book.

SCD

This book is dedicated to my parents, Carol and Bill, and to my niece and nephew, Eryca and Matthew. I appreciate and am grateful for their love and support through all of my professional endeavors. I also thank Stefan and Marty for their partnership and hard work in bringing this book to fruition.

KLG

This book is dedicated to my amazing and supportive family (Marni, Madison, and Mackenzie), parents (Christa and Herbert Reinhart), and brother's family (Peter, Haley, Anca, Lacramioara, Kai, and Benjamin). Thanks for understanding my life-long work. My graduate students, Andrea Krol, Jennifer Gordon, and Ellis Chan, were a dedicated group who devoted countless hours to formulate various chapters into a cohesive piece of scholarly work. Finally, I greatly appreciate my co-authors, Stefan for the leadership and creativity he continues to exemplify as a distinguished scholar, and Karen, for her support and dedication to this project.

MM

Contents

7 Impulse Control Disorders 123
with Jennifer Gordon

Chapter 1
Introduction

All the world is queer save thee and me, and even thou art a little queer.

–Robert Owen (1771–1858)
Welsh Social Reformer

1.1 Introduction

Over the last 20 years, the child psychopathology literature base has burgeoned with much of this research focusing on high prevalence, commonly recognized disorders of childhood such as attention–deficit/hyperactivity disorder (ADHD), autism spectrum, and learning disabilities. There are numerous journal articles and authored/edited books on these widely recognized topics. Both the lay community and the clinical professional have also produced accounts of youth with the conditions noted above. Some of these publications are written by clinical professionals who report on cases throughout their decades of clinical practice; additional books have been written by parents who seek to provide insight into raising and educating youth with a particular disabling condition. All of these sources together – the academic and the anecdotal – foster our understanding of the more prevalent issues in child psychopathology.

1.2 Gap in the Literature

There is considerably less research available on topics that are more extreme and in some cases infrequently observed in the population. These topics include juvenile firesetters, gender identity disorder, feral children, youth gang member, Munchausen by proxy, the gang member, childhood schizophrenia, self-injurious behavior, elective mutism, and impulse control disorders including trichotillomania, kleptomania, and

S.C. Dombrowski et al., *Assessing and Treating Low Incidence/High Severity Psychological Disorders of Childhood*, DOI 10.1007/978-1-4419-9970-2_1, © Springer Science+Business Media, LLC 2011

intermittent explosive disorder. The literature base lacks a source that brings together these extreme conditions of childhood. This book, therefore, fills a gap in the research and clinical literature by providing an overview of the assessment, conceptualization, and treatment literature of more arcane issues in children's mental health. It is recognized that some of the conditions listed in this book (e.g., feral children) do not encumber a distinct diagnostic category and, therefore, may not be technically considered a disorder, but the conditions nonetheless fit our inclusion criteria of being considered high interest and extreme.

Each chapter in this book also highlights important research trends and issues. For instance, the chapter on juvenile firesetters suggests greater need for both public and professional awareness of this costly societal malady that causes hundreds of millions of dollars in annual damage. Other chapters such as gender identity disorder attempt to strike a balance in presentation between two opposing viewpoints on the condition. The tremendous persecution faced by individuals with gender variance suggests need for an element of grace in the face of scientific understanding. The chapter on feral children is fascinating but lacking in empirical support because it represents the rarest of all conditions in our book. The chapter on the youth gang member demonstrates that youth gangs have become a significant concern and reflect the larger social and economic trends in our society. Understanding the forces that draw youth to gangs requires a broad understanding of salient causes and treatments. The chapter on juvenile sexual predators is among the most widely recognized condition discussed in our book. Yet, it is a topic that deserves greater attention including recognition that sexual victimization at the hands of a juvenile causes just as deleterious an outcome as that perpetrated by an adult. The Munchausen by proxy chapter discusses one of the more insidious types of child maltreatment. The research data on this topic are scarce. Verification of the condition is often elusive since perpetrators tend to have a capacity to understand medical and educational systems and either fabricate or directly induce illness in their children. Finally, the chapter on selective mutism discusses a condition of childhood at the extreme end of the anxiety spectrum wherein a youth refuses to communicate verbally outside of familiar venues.

1.3 Chapter Format

The format for each chapter is consistent throughout the book with the following major subsections:

- Overview and historical context
- Description and diagnostic classification
- Etiology and theory
- Assessment
- Treatment
- Future directions and conclusion

When writing each chapter, we included an historical account of the condition/disorder, sometimes noting the topic's portrayal in the cinema, music, and literature of western culture. By reading these historical accounts, the reader may understand that many of these conditions are not distinctly twenty-first century phenomenon, but rather conditions that societies have dealt with for hundreds, if not thousands of years. When discussing the description and diagnostic classification section of each chapter, we reviewed and subsequently discussed the extant research base. Where available, we provided the DSM-IV TR diagnostic criteria. We also included a discussion of the proposed changes for the condition/disorder within the upcoming rendition of the DSM, expected in 2013. Within the theory and etiology section of each chapter, we discussed the literature regarding the interplay of both environmental and biological factors. This sometimes led to a discussion of brain imaging studies, genetic factors, temperament, as well as sociological and environmental factors that contributed to the condition. Also discussed in some chapters were various theoretical models including psychoanalytic, behavioral, attachment, feminist, and sociological. This discussion was not available for all disorders due to limitations in the literature. Our review of assessment methods led to a presentation within each chapter – perhaps redundant, but still essential – of the need for a comprehensive, rather than narrow, evaluation of the child using multiple methods of assessment and sources of information. As part of this discussion, we furnished a brief overview of the available assessment instruments and interview protocols, and in some chapters (e.g., GID) provided an example of actual items from instruments or interview protocols. Our discussion of treatment for all topics was broad-based, but gave the reader a sense of the available literature and treatment approaches that are commonly used. In many cases, a behavioral or cognitive-behavioral component was most widely available and seemed to document effectiveness most clearly. Still, the treatment literature emerging out of the psychodynamic/psychoanalytic perspective yielded numerous case studies where treatment approaches were deemed effective. For all disorders described in this book, the literature was clear in indicating a need for treatment research containing larger sample sizes with longitudinal designs. This is not only a problem that plagues the topics in this book, but also the broader child psychopathology literature base. Lastly, we endeavored to discuss potential future directions for the topic that might be relevant for clinicians and researchers engaged in research or treatment.

1.4   Conclusion

In totality, each topic in this book brings together for the first time an overview of low prevalence, intense, and extreme disorders of childhood. The broader child psychopathology literature base covering higher prevalence conditions is generally well-documented with the exception of longitudinal studies and longer term follow-up. It is due time that the field casts its research gaze more fully and with greater rigor upon the topics addressed in this book. This book portends to spur the interest of the research and clinical community to engage in further exploration.

Chapter 2
Juvenile Firesetters

I hear the alarm at dead of night,
I hear the belts – shouts!
I pass the crowd – I run!
The sight of flames maddens me with pleasure.

–Walt Whitman, Poems of Joy (1860)

2.1 Overview

Approximately 500,000 years ago, human beings learned how to use fire for both constructive and destructive purposes although evolutionary anthropologists trace the manipulation of fire beyond that period with suggestive findings dated as early as 790,000 years ago (Goren-Inbar et al., 2004) and some even surpassing the one million year mark (Brain & Sillen, 1988; Fessler, 2006). The mythology of various cultures attempts to account for fire acquisition among humans. The most prevalent theme emerging out of these myths is that fire was acquired illicitly or secretively. In Greek mythology, for instance, the Titan Prometheus stole fire from the gods and presented it to humankind. Within contemporary western culture, fire is often glamorized as a force of destruction (e.g., Stephan King's Firestarter or Marvel Comic's Pyro from the X-Men) or for its sexual symbolization (e.g., The Door's "Come on baby light my fire"). In only very rare instances, the sensible use of fire is discussed in either the literature or cinema of Western society. This is unfortunate. The firesetting intervention literature suggests that those most in need of guidance on proper fire use – the juvenile firesetter – are the least likely to receive it. Regrettably, a society's glamorization of fire use may serve to reinforce the pathological use of fire among juvenile firesetters who have noted social-cognitive processing deficits that contribute to a misperception and distortion of social and environmental cues (Crick & Dodge, 1994; Crick & Ladd, 1990; Dodge & Coie, 1987; Dodge & Frame, 1982; Dodge, Pettit, McClaskey, & Brown, 1986; Loeber & Dishion, 1984).

S.C. Dombrowski et al., *Assessing and Treating Low Incidence/High Severity Psychological Disorders of Childhood*, DOI 10.1007/978-1-4419-9970-2_2,
© Springer Science+Business Media, LLC 2011

2.2 Historical Context

Information from antiquity suggests that arson has been a problem since the dawn of recorded history. Severe sanctions were often mete out against those who engaged in firesetting. The ancient Romans, for instance, codified criminal penalties for arson. In medieval England, convicted arsonists were banished from the country with one hand and one foot excised. Eighteenth century French Law provided for the death penalty via hanging, decapitation, or burning at the stake (Steinbach, 1986).

The term "pyromania" originated in France and is a derivation of the French expression *monomanie incendiare*. Ray (1838) was the first American writer to discuss individuals with a morbid interest in fire. However, it was not until the fourth edition of his 1838 book that Ray (1844) specifically mentions the term pyromania. Therein, Ray expanded upon prior European writings and argued that pyromania should be viewed as a distinct form of insanity, and even went as far as discussed the need to exculpate responsibility for the behavior (Ray, 1844). In the early nineteenth century, numerous writers, all of whom were male, posited that firesetting was primarily a prepubescent female phenomenon. These writers believed that lower IQ prepubescent females who experienced difficulty in menstruating were the predominant firesetters and their firesetting behavior was related to abnormal psychosexual development (Ray, 1838).

Another theory followed in 1924. Wilhelm Stekel posited that pyromania had a sexual origin and defined it as a developmental disorder caused by impeded or unfulfilled sexual development. In 1932, Freud discussed the importance of a psychoanalytic interpretation: "….in order to possess himself of fire it was necessary for man to renounce his homosexually tinged desire to extinguish it with a stream of urine (p. 405)." Freud indicated that his interpretation was confirmed by an analysis of the Greek myth of Prometheus, the Titan who stole fire from the gods and furnished it to humankind. Noting that Prometheus used a hollow, fennel stalk, Freud suggests that the fennel stalk is a phallic symbol, making the connection between the fennel stalk and the penis tube. Freud also suggested that one needs to "reverse and transform" the exoteric meaning of the myth to discern its esoteric meaning. In other words, man does not harbor fire in his penis tube but rather the capacity to extinguish fire through urination (Freud, 1932). It is interesting to note that this psychoanalytic position (i.e., the connection among fire, sexuality, and urination) dominated psychiatric thinking through the 1970s. It continued to be recommended even up until 1979 that arson suspects be escorted to the bathroom because urination was thought to be a psychological form of sexual gratification for the arsonist.

Helen Yarnell (1940), a psychiatrist at New York's Bellevue Hospital, was the first researcher to investigate children's involvement in firesetting. She supported Freud's psychoanalytic interpretation indicating that firesetting among children is the result of castration-anxiety, enuresis, and a problematic mother–son relationship. It was not until the 1970s that the psychological community experienced a shift away from the more psychoanalytically oriented interpretation to a more cognitive-behavioral conceptualization where firesetting was beginning to be viewed less as a psychoanalytic phenomenon and more as an antisocial one.

2.3 Description and Diagnostic Classification

The first version of the diagnostic and statistical manual (DSM; APA, 1952) classified pyromania as an obsessive-compulsive reaction. The DSM-II (APA, 1968) eliminated pyromania as a diagnostic category. Within the DSM-III (APA, 1980) and DSM-III-R (APA, 1987), pyromania returned as a diagnostic classification under "disorders or impulse not elsewhere classified." Pyromania remains as a diagnostic category in the DSM-IV TR (APA, 2000), but its usefulness as a diagnostic category has been questioned. As of the writing of this book, there are no changes planned for the DSM-V. As a result, clinicians and researchers alike tend to use and develop interventions and assessment tools that discuss the more inclusive category of juvenile firesetting rather than the outdated and low prevalence term pyromania which is scarcely offered as a diagnosis.

Juvenile firesetters are a heterogeneous group, making it difficult to elucidate a psychological typology for the condition. There are several diagnostic categories that more frequently co-occur in youth with firesetting backgrounds (Kolko & Kazdin, 1988; Moore, Thompson-Pope, & Whited, 1996). These include attention-deficit/hyperactive disorder (ADHD), conduct disorder (Kazdin, 1997), oppositional defiant disorder, and disruptive behavior disorder NOS. While recognizing that these are the most prominent co-occurring diagnostic categories, it is important to bear in mind that some children and adolescents involved in firesetting do not meet any diagnostic criteria and those that do meet the aforementioned categories may not be involved in firesetting behavior. Therefore, a typology of juvenile firesetting remains elusive.

The following discussion delineates characteristics of those who might tend to set fires, but should not be viewed in a linear, algorithmic fashion. Because a child manifests some of these characteristics does not mean that child is a firesetter. The converse is true as well. Because a child does not demonstrate one or more of these characteristics does not exclude that child from potential firesetting behavior.

Stadolnik (2000) surveyed mental health professionals who work with juvenile firesetters and listed characteristics of youth who engage in firesetting. Although this survey would have benefited from one of the numerous data reduction techniques, it essentially suggested that youth who fireset display most behaviors that may be described as externalizing including aggression, oppositionality, violence, and impulsivity. Additional characteristics include anger, social isolation, depression, and traumatization. The survey also suggested that youth with access to matches/lighters and who are curious about, but have limited knowledge of, fire are likely to engage in firesetting. Aspects of this survey have been confirmed by other researchers (MacKay et al., 2006; Root, Mackay, Henderson, Del Bove, & Warling, 2008) including in one study on female juvenile firesetters (Hickle & Roe-Sepowitz, 2010).

Further obscuring our understanding of the characteristics of the firesetter generally and the juvenile firesetter specifically, the DSM-IV TR tends to interchangeably use the terms firesetting and pyromania. Unfortunately, limited information is available within the DSM-IV TR on firesetting broadly and juvenile firesetting specifically. The DSM-IV TR notes that pyromania is rare in children and adolescents, but then goes on to state that approximately 40% of arson arrests involve juveniles. Yet, the DSM-IV TR does not contain a diagnostic category for juvenile firesetting. This contradiction suggests dire need for greater understanding of juvenile firesetting behavior and perhaps a reconceptualization of the diagnostic category of pyromania. Unfortunately, as of this writing, the committee of experts charged with revising the DSM-V does not appear to alter dramatically classification of pyromania. A ubiquitous understanding of juvenile firesetting becomes even more imperative when statistics on the immense societal cost are understood. In 2009, intentionally set fires caused more than 12.5 billion dollars in property damage and the loss of 3,010 lives (Karter, 2010).

The DSM-IV TR defines pyromania as follows:

(a) Deliberate and purposeful fire setting on more than one occasion.
(b) Tension or affective arousal before the act.
(c) Fascination with, interest in, curiosity about, or attraction to fire and its situational contexts (e.g., paraphernalia, uses, consequences).
(d) Pleasure, gratification, or relief when setting fires, or when witnessing or participating in their aftermath.
(e) The fire setting is not done for monetary gain, as an expression of sociopolitical ideology, to conceal criminal activity, to express anger or vengeance, to improve one's living condition, in response to a delusion or hallucination, or as a result of impaired judgment (e.g., in dementia, mental retardation, substance intoxication).
(f) The fire setting is not better accounted for by conduct disorder, a manic episode, or antisocial personality disorder. (APA, 2000, p. 671).

2.3.1 DSM-V

As of the writing of this book, the DSM-V working group did not appear to have plans to revise the criteria for pyromania. It is noted that the DSM-IV TR criteria for pyromania is so narrowly defined that a classification of pyromania would elude even the most severe juvenile firesetters. Thus, it seems rather important from both a mental health and a broader societal perspective that the psychiatric community revisit the diagnostic criteria for pyromania in the next rendition of the DSM-V. There appears to be a need for both a change in nomenclature (i.e., juvenile firesetter replace the term pyromania) and a change in criteria to capture a broader array of juvenile firesetters.

2.4   Developmental Course of Fire Behavior: From Fire Interest to Firesetting

Children have a natural curiosity about the world and especially fire. This is positive in most contexts. In the case of fire, this curiosity can be harmful if not downright lethal. Fire is likely one of the most alluring and powerful forces in nature and especially a child's environment. In one study of school-age youth, nearly 45% played with fire (Grolnick, Cole, Laurentis, & Schwartzman, 1990). Fire behavior seems to follow a developmental sequence in children with three distinct, yet progressive, levels that are typically tied to a child's age: fire interest, firestarting, firesetting.

2.4.1   Fire Interest

Most children will become interested in fire between the ages of three and five. Children around this age may begin to ask questions about fire (e.g., why is it hot? why is it orange?) and may even express their interest in fire through their play (Hanson, Mackay, Atkinson, Staley, & Pignatiello, 1995). For instance, they may pretend to be firemen and play with fire trucks. Or, they may pretend to cook food over fire or pretend to light birthday candles. Children's interest in fire should signal a need for education about fire safety. Children in the preschool age period do not have the cognitive capacity to discern the dangers of fire and fail to completely understand that a small fire can escalate to a destructive force in a matter of minutes. It is imperative, therefore, to begin the process of fire safety education during this phase of development.

2.4.2   Firestarting

Gaynor (2002) suggests that, by the time they are 9-years-old, most young boys have experimented with starting fires. Children in the early elementary years process information much more rapidly and begin to use symbolic thinking as well as their imaginations. However, they still are not cognitively sophisticated enough to understand that the small fire that they set in the garbage pail in their bedroom can expand into a conflagration that destroys their home and perhaps even their lives. Children in the early elementary school ages might be given permission to light candles on birthday cakes or start a fire in the fireplace or on the grill, but they should not be given this authority prematurely and without adult supervision and discussion over the perils of fire starting. It is important for caregivers to furnish opportunities for their children to learn how to start fires in a safe and competent manner. Within the child's environment, there will likely be inappropriate models such as an older cousin or younger uncle who plays with ignition sources in a dangerous manner. This type of fireplay is more attractive to the youngster than the

safe, structured use of fire to light candles. As a result, it becomes critically important to discourage inappropriate use of fire and provide a solid education in fire
safety to young children to prevent unsupervised experimentation.

2.4.3 Firesetting

Children entering the latency time period (9–12) attempt to become competent in their
daily activities and gain mastery over their environment. Because of this drive, the
child will experiment (Erikson, 1959). Any youthful experimentation often leads to
mistakes and mishaps. This is the process by which any individual learns and develops
mastery. In the case of firesetting, a trial and error approach to learning can lead to
calamity. The child may have good intentions of helping to start a fire to keep warm,
or to light the torches in the backyard, but due to inability to handle fire, this can
become destructive if not lethal. One other aspect must be understood. It is during the
latency phase that crisis firesetting might emerge. The starting of fires during this
period can lead to a feeling of power and control over the environment.
    By the time a child reaches adolescence, the youth may have a broader under-
standing of fire safety. Youth in adolescence may set fires to attract attention, fit in
or as a cry for help. The adolescent may also set fire because of a need to feel power
or control over his environment (Swaffer & Hollin, 1995). At this stage in development, the adolescent is experiencing significant physical, social, moral, and sexual
change. Compound this change with a chaotic family environment and/or past or
present trauma and this sets the stage for firesetting behavior. The dangers of firesetting are intensified during this phase of development because of the inherently
impulsive and oppositional nature of adolescents who strive for independence and
find firesetting alluring (e.g., it is a crime; it is dangerous; Hanson, Mackay-Soroka,
Staley, & Poulton, 1994). Adolescents also want to fit in and a dare to engage in a
behavior, antisocial, or not, can be a strong impetus for engaging in firesetting.

2.5 Etiological Hypotheses and Theoretical Frameworks

One of the earlier theories regarding the etiology of juvenile firesetting suggested
that firesetting and sexual arousal were intertwined. More recently, scholars have
debunked the perspective that firesetting is related to either deviant sexuality (Geller,
1992) or difficulty making the transition to puberty (Freud, 1932). For instance,
Quinsey, Chaplin, and Upfold (1989) evaluated the penile tumescence of adult
firesetters and nonfiresetters, and found no differences in sexual response to images
of fire presented to either group.
    Several theories of firesetting have been discussed in the literature. One of the
more widely discussed is Fineman's (1980) dynamic-behavioral formulation. This
theory suggests that firesetting is caused by an interaction of historical factors that

Table 2.1 Social-learning model for firesetting behavior conceptual synthesis: A tentative risk model[a]

1. Learning experiences and CUES
    (a) Early modeling (vicarious) experiences
    (b) Early interest and direct experiences
    (c) Availability of adult models and incendiary materials
2. Personal repertoire
    (a) Cognitive components
        • Limited fire-awareness and fire safety skills
    (b) Behavioral components
        • Interpersonal ineffectiveness/skills deficits
        • Antisocial behavior excesses
    (c) Motivational components
3. Parent and family influences and stressors
    (a) Limited supervision and monitoring
    (b) Parental distance and uninvolvement
    (c) Parental pathology and limitations
    (d) Stressful external events

[a]*Note*: From "A Conceptualization of Firesetting in Children and Adolescents," by D. Kolko and A. Kazdin, 1986, *Journal of Abnormal Child Psychology, 14*(1), p. 51. Copyright © 1986 by Kluwer Academic/Plenum Publishers. Reprinted with permission

predispose the firesetter toward maladaptive and antisocial acts, prior environmental factors that have taught and reinforced firesetting as acceptable, and present environmental contingencies that encourage firesetting. Fineman uses his model as part of an assessment process that attempts to evaluate firesetting risk. The dynamic-behavioral theory identifies personality/individual characteristics, family/social circumstances, and immediate environmental factors that are thought to be related to firesetting behavior. Fineman also created an assessment instrument based on his theoretical model.

The second of the more widely discussed models is Kolko and Kazdin's (1986) social-learning model. This theory holds that firesetting behaviors are learned through interaction with peers, family, or other social forces that condone and perhaps even encourage firesetting. Table 2.1 highlights the components of Kolko and Kazdin's model, which they described as tentative subject to further empirical validation.

A review of the literature indicates at least six additional theories regarding the origins of firesetting with the two aforementioned being described in most detail. Putnam and Kirkpatrick (2005) summarize the theories:

- Learning theory. Kolko and Kazdin (1986) indicate that firesetting behavior is learned through involvement with friends, family, or other influences who demonstrate and foster inappropriate fire use.
- Opportunity theory. Cohen and Felson (1979) suggest that firesetters have unrestricted access to fire and use it as an instrument or weapon.
- Expressive trauma theory. Lowenstein (1989) indicates that firesetting is used to vent frustration from victimization from preexisting trauma.

- Stress theory. Lyng (1990) suggests that firesetting serves to release accumulating stress or provides a means to seek danger in an uneventful life. Lyng suggests that juvenile firesetting is often closely related to vandalism, shoplifting, and graffiti among juveniles.
- Power association theory. Sakheim and Osborn (1986) indicate that youth engage in firesetting as a means to attain power over people or the environment.
- Social acceptance theory. Swaffer and Hollin (1995) argue that firesetting is motivated by an attempt to gain acceptance by peers.
- Societal reaction theory. Macht and Mack (1968) contend that firesetters engage in firesetting behavior to obtain a reaction from society via the arrival of the police, media, or fire department.

2.6 Typologies of Firesetting Risk

Classification is an important aspect of science. It allows one to conceptualize and understand a given phenomenon. Profile research has attempted to understand who is at greatest risk for firesetting activity and who might just be of little risk. It is difficult to ascribe a simplified category to an individual person because of the complexity of human behavior. There is not a linear relationship between individual characteristics and behaviors and firesetting activity. The Juvenile Firesetter Intervention Handbook prepared for the The United States Fire Administration Federal Emergency Management Agency by Gaynor (2002) distinguishes levels of firesetting risk: extreme, definite, and little. Generally, curiosity firesetters are considered little risk, crisis and delinquent firesetters, definite risk and pathological firesetters, extreme risk. Although the literature might place a youth in one of the aforementioned categories, it is important to remember that the empirical validation of these categories is minimal at best with most categorization based upon clinician's professional observations and work in the field (e.g., Stadolnik, 2000) or expert consensus opinion (Gaynor). The field direly needs additional empirical investigation using appropriate multivariate analyses.

2.6.1 Curiosity Firesetters (Low Risk)

Curiosity about fire in children is normal, especially at younger developmental levels. Curiosity about firesetting, like most behavior, falls along a continuum. Curiosity firesetting, sometimes referred to as fireplay or nonpathological firesetting, is the most common reason for firesetting. Children seek to learn about or master fire through actual experimentation. Youngsters who play with fire do so to see what happens. For instance, they may play with matches, burn small plastic toys or insects, and watch small pieces of paper burn. There are highly curious youngsters who seem to be fascinated and even obsessed with fire. Curiosity motivated firesetters intuitively tend to be the most dangerous type of firesetter. They tend to play with fire in hidden locations, have poor adult supervision, a lack of working smoke detectors, and a lack of understanding of the dangers of fire. Compared to fires set by other firesetters, there is a higher percentage of fatalities and serious burn injury (Stadolnik, 2000). Gaynor (2002) indicates that the majority of youth involved in curiosity firesetting have little risk for becoming juvenile firesetters if given appropriate intervention. Generally, these individuals tend to be male and younger (below age 7) with relatively normal families, peer relationships, and school functioning.

2.6.2 Crisis Firesetters (Definite Risk)

The juvenile firesetting literature clearly indicates that many youngsters use firesetting either to communicate their distress or in an effort to seek relief from it (Fineman, 1995; Swaffer & Hollin, 1995; Wooden & Berkey, 1984). Youth in this category would be considered definite risk (Gaynor, 2002). For youth in this subset, the intent of firesetting is to bring attention to their pain (Gaynor). Youth who are crisis firesetters are thought to face a host of issues including family turmoil, abuse, neglect, school problems, and other stressful life events (Stadolnik, 2000). Fire safety and prevention programs will not address the primary psychological issues, so psychological, social services and possibly juvenile justice intervention is necessary. In the literature, crisis firesetters have been described as being ineffective, anxious, having difficulty in expressing feelings, and perceiving that their world is out of control. Accordingly, these children use one of the most powerful forces on earth to express themselves. And, they attain a sense of mastery, control, and competence when engaging in firesetting behavior. The fires started by crisis motivated firesetters tend to have a symbolic or communicative function and rarely are intended to hurt others.

2.6.3 Delinquent Firesetting (Definite Risk)

Youngsters in this category display a variety of antisocial personality traits and behavior. There may be the one-incident firesetter who lights a park bench on fire to gain approval of a peer group or the juvenile who sets fire to a couch abutting the kindergarten classroom without regard for the safety and well-being of the children in the classroom. Delinquent firesetters tend to display pervasive oppositional and conduct disorders, often violating the rules of authority figures and society. It is commonly accepted within the firesetting literature that antisocial behavioral is significantly associated with juvenile firesetting (MacKay et al., 2006); however, other smaller-scale studies suggest that the association may not be as strong (e.g., Pollinger, Samuels, & Stadolnik, 2005). Kolko and Kazdin (1986) suggest, further, that this conceptualization is more complex, infused with not only high levels of anger but also anxiety (Forehand, Wierson, Frame, Kempton, & Armistead, 1991; Gale, 1999). Delinquent youth, compared to the troubled youth subset, tend to engage in more aggressive, antisocial, and criminal behavior (Gaynor, 2002). These youth tend to be male, impulsive, and angry (Koson, 1982). They may also have engaged in other antisocial activities such as substance abuse, petty theft, and vandalism. These youth make no attempt to extinguish the fire and little or no remorse or guilt is felt. School truancy is common. There tends to be little fear of consequences or punishment. They would be considered definite risk for firesetting activity (Gaynor).

2.6.4   Pathological Firesetting (Extreme Risk)

This is the rarest form of firesetting. This group includes youth with severe psychopathology and serious emotional and behavioral disturbance that includes active psychosis and delusional thinking. These youth have often faced extremely traumatic backgrounds and may even be motivated by the sensory stimulation of fire (e.g., sight, sound, smell). Perhaps even a diagnosis of pyromania is indicated, although even most of the pathologically motivated firesetting subset would not meet the criteria for a diagnosis of pyromania (Gaynor, 2002; Stadolnik, 2000). Gaynor indicates that less than 1% of firesetting children and adolescents fall into the extreme risk category. Pathological firesetters often have significant deficits in the cognitive, social, and emotional domains (Barron, Hassiotis, & Banes, 2004). They have been subjected to environments characterized by domestic violence, physical and sexual abuse, and parental substance abuse (Root et al., 2008). Gaynor indicates that children and adolescents in the extreme risk group are beyond the help of most fire safety and prevention programs, often requiring institutionalization because of dangerousness to themselves or others.

2.7   Assessment and Evaluation

Evaluation of the level of firesetting risk is essential prior to placement in a firesetting treatment program. There are several structured and semistructured interviews that may be used to determine the level of firesetting risk (Slavkin, 2007). Norm-referenced firesetting assessment instruments with appropriate reliability, validity, and standardization procedures are unavailable, but sorely needed. Instead, several firesetting risk interview forms are used, some of which are available for public use within the Juvenile Firesetter Intervention Handbook (Gaynor, 2002).

Regardless of which assessment method is ultimately used, one of the most important aspects of any firesetting risk evaluation is to determine a youth's firesetting history (e.g., first fire; one fire in a series of fires). A good starting point in the evaluation of juvenile firesetters is to gather pertinent background information. With a confirmed firesetting case, the clinician should obtain a copy of the report written by the fire department describing how the fire was started, how it was extinguished, and the probable cause and origin of the fire. If the fire was serious enough to involve an arson investigator, then the clinical specialist can work in partnership with the arson investigator to gather facts about the case. In most cases, however, an arson investigator is not involved and the clinician is left to sort out the reason for the fire (Stadolnik, 2000). Unfortunately, the clinician requires expertise in fire science to test the veracity of a child's or parent's statement. Without a basic understanding of how fires start, grow, and spread, it is difficult to discern whether the child's story is indeed credible.

There are essentially two approaches to gathering information on a child's firesetting behavior. The first is more structured and involved rating forms and the second is more narrative in nature and involves a semistructured interview (Slavkin, 2007). Kolko and Kazdin (1988) developed an instrument called the firesetting history screen (FHS) that query about incidents in two time frames – within the past 12 months and more than 12 months ago. The FHS provides for yes/no response. Sample questions include (1) Does the child like fire? (2) Does the child play with matches? (3) Did the child burn anything or set anything on fire? (4) How many times did the child set a fire? Both parents and children are rated on the same form. Although dated, one of the strengths of the form is its brevity and high agreement between child and parent ratings. Kolko and Kazdin (1991) also developed a longer firesetting measure that is administered to parents. The firesetting incident analysis (FIA) consists of 50 questions that address four domains: characteristics of the firesetting incident (e.g., how materials were obtained, site of fire); ratings of the behavioral and emotional correlates that were present two weeks prior to the incident (e.g., aggression, oppositionality, depression); child's motives for the fire (e.g., curiosity, anger, attention); and consequences following the fire (e.g., family disciplinary, financial, legal).

Additional firesetting instruments are available including the Juvenile Firesetter Child and Family Risk Surveys and the Comprehensive FireRisk Evaluation (Fineman, 1996), both semistructured narrative forms are available in the Juvenile Firesetter Intervention Handbook (Gaynor, 2002). Both forms involve a more semistructured approach to the evaluation process, although they can be tabulated to estimate firesetting risk. Like any of the available firesetting instruments, both of these are not formal, standardized instruments with norms categorized by age or gender. The field is in need of more formal assessment instruments, but likely the difficulty with determining a profile or typology of the firesetter hinders the creation of a standardized instrument. One recent study by Gallagher-Duffy, Mackay, Duffy, Sullivan-Thomas, and Peterson-Badali (2009) investigated a measure of emotional arousal to fire-related stimuli. This study found that a fire-specific pictorial Stroop task might be a useful addition to the clinical interview as a potential measure of adolescents' cognitive processing bias for fire-related stimuli.

Each firesetting interview will allow the clinician to determine the level of firesetting risk. If it is determined that there is an extreme risk of firesetting, then the youth should be placed in immediate treatment within a residential setting that specializes in the treatment of juvenile firesetters.

2.8 Prevention and Intervention

The *empirical* literature on intervention and prevention options for juvenile firesetting is sparse, but increasing. Prevention options are typically education-oriented.
These programs focus on fire safety education and emphasize the need for appropriate adult modeling and supervision of incendiary devices in the home (Pinsonneault,
2002). We are not aware of any such programs that have been empirically evaluated.
Fire services personnel are typically the contact point for primary prevention and
fire safety education (Winget & Whitman, 1973). Accordingly, fire services have
the most advanced fire safety prevention and intervention programs. There are
numerous programs available for download cost free (http://www.sfm.state.or.us,
http://www.sosfires.com, http://www.usfa.fewma.gov). Fire service personnel have
also been involved in screening of potential juvenile firesetters since fire service
personnel are typically first responders. The screening instruments available to
fire service personnel (see Gaynor, 2002) have been criticized as lacking appropriate
psychometric characteristics and should be used with caution because of unknown
reliability and validity information. Further, fire service personnel, while having
expertise in fire safety education and prevention, do not have expertise in psychological assessment and often overlook the needs of firesetting youth who receive
elevated ratings of psychopathology on screening instruments and are in need of
psychological intervention although they may not require intensive firesetting intervention (Pierce & Hardesty, 1997). As a result, there is need for collaboration
between psychologists with expertise in the psychological assessment of children
and fire service personnel. It also suggests a critical need for objective firesetting
screener instruments and rating scales that have appropriate psychometric characteristics (e.g., norming, reliability, validity).

Much of the intervention literature involves single case studies, some of which
involve a multidisciplinary approach to treatment (e.g., family therapy, individual
therapy, pharmacological, juvenile justice, fire service and law enforcement, social
services; Kolko, 1999, 2001; Kolko, Herschell, & Scharf, 2006; Sharp, Blaakman,
Cole, & Cole, 2005). Although reduced firesetting has been found in these single
case studies, they typically do not include controlled designs or follow-up data.
Another problem that plagues the field overall is the lack of a widely utilized,
empirically guided approach to treatment for firesetting. This does not mean that
treatments are unavailable. They are available particularly through fire service protection. However, these treatment programs have not been formally subjected to
empirical scrutiny. With that caveat, most treatment approaches emphasize four
important goals and recommend the use of a multidisciplinary approach to treatment that includes fire service personal and mental health professionals (Kolko
et al., 2008):

1. Eliminate the firesetting behavior.
2. Target and eliminate family characteristics and environmental factors that support
   firesetting behavior.

3. Attempt to improve social, emotional, and academic functioning.
4. Emphasize fire safety and fire knowledge.

Because of this need for diversity of treatment and collaboration among various constituencies, mental health professionals who provide services to juvenile firesetters must have capacity to collaborate with fire service, law enforcement, educational professionals, and the juvenile justice system (Kolko, 1999; Stadolnik, 2000). Mental health professionals also must increase understanding of the culture of fire services and law enforcement and be willing to share power in the treatment relationship.

2.8.1 Fire Service Collaboration

The involvement of fire service personnel is an important component of treatment (Kolko, 2001). Fire service agencies have had in place for a long period of time established treatment programs. Stadolnik (2000) states that the mental health professional needs to relinquish a degree of autonomy in clinical decision-making because of the need to collaborate with fire service personnel who have firesetting intervention programs that emphasize fire safety education, a component best addressed by fire service personnel. Likely, a barrier for the collaborative efforts of mental health professionals attempting to treat juvenile firesetters is the distinctly different cultures of the fire services community and that of the mental health profession. Stadolnik contends that there is a level of cultural difference, if not incompatibility, within each group that can hamper productive collaboration. To increase collaborative efforts, mental health professionals should seek to understand the motivations, values, and ideals of fire services personnel. Further, mental health professionals would benefit from a greater respect for and appreciation of the tremendous emotional pressures faced by fire service personnel which might involve chronic exposure to traumatic events such as extractions from burning buildings and cars, fire fatalities, and severe burn injuries. This exposure to trauma year after year may lead to a cognitive, affective, and interpersonal style that may be quite different from the style offered by the mental health professionals (Stadolnik). Fire fighters, as with police officers, often establish a close bond through their work experience – a brotherhood – that cannot be readily understood by people working outside of fire service and law enforcement. This makes it important for mental health professionals to work as part of a team where the mental health professional offers an important, but not necessarily preeminent perspective on intervention (Zipper & Wilcox, 2005). One component, with limited empirical validation, is the common community practice of a firefighter visit to the home of youth's who have been involved in firesetting (Kolko, 1988). One study that investigated firefighter home visitation demonstrated that it was effective in reducing the number of fires set by children, but less effective than the combination of fire safety education and cognitive-behavior treatment (Kolko, 2001).

2.9 Treatment Modalities

2.9.1 Fire Safety Education

The provision of fire safety education skills is considered a mandatory component of treatment, regardless of the severity of the firesetting behavior (Cole, Grolnick, & Schwartzman, 1999; Cook, Hersch, Gaynor, & Roehl, 1989; Cox-Jones, Lubetsky, Fultz, & Kolko, 1990; Kolko et al., 2006; Raines & Foy, 1994). Numerous publications are available, particularly from the National Fire Protection Association, with structured fire safety education curriculums (see http://www.nfpa.org/catalog/ for a publication listing for preschool age children through adolescence). However, only a few outcome studies, most of which investigated a combination of cognitive-behavioral treatments and fire safety education, have been reported in the literature (Adler, Nunn, Northam, Lebnan, & Ross, 1994; Kolko, 2001). Youth who only have a curiosity about fire are best served by being furnished with information about the dangers of fire and specific safety skills (e.g., stop, drop, roll). There are numerous fire safety programs available for this purpose. At the preschool age level, BIC Corporation's Play Safe! Be Safe! © is a fire safety educational program designed for classroom use (Cole et al., 2006). In this program, children learn the preventative behavior of telling a grown up if they find matches or lighters; they also learn the following fire safety behaviors: (1) go to a firefighter; (2) stop, drop, and roll; and (3) crawl low under smoke. The program includes a 22 min video tape, discussion cards, a teacher's manual, and a game that reinforces learning objectives. Cole et al. report that 1 month after implementation of Play Safe! Be Safe! children showed greater knowledge and capacity to perform fire safety skills than a comparison group. In another fire safety education program administered during a residential treatment program found that only 1 of 35 children had set another fire 1 year after FSE treatment (DeSalvatore & Hornstein, 1991). At the preschool through eighth grade level the National Fire Protection Association has a classroom-based prevention program called Risk Watch. Material may be downloaded from the National Fire Protection Association website at http://www.nfpa.org. Teachers are furnished with a curriculum, necessary materials, and guided instructions. Youth who are involved in antisocial firesetting behavior that involves the juvenile justice system should be held accountable for successful completion of a fire safety education program with consequences for noncompliance with the program. Within this subtype, some type of rubric (e.g., a pretest–posttest measure) for compliance and knowledge acquisition should be an important aspect of the program.

2.10 Psychological Intervention

2.10.1 Psychotherapy

Individual approaches have used the behavioral techniques of response cost, contingent reinforcement, and punishment in the intervention of firesetting youth (Adler et al., 1994; Kolko et al., 2006). The effectiveness of these approaches has been documented primarily through case reports, limiting the generality of their effectiveness. Some of the older firesetting intervention literature reports the use of negative practice (e.g., repeatedly lighting matches) as a means to satiate and extinguish firesetting behavior (Holland, 1969; Kolko, 1983). However, the effectiveness of satiation strategies has been called to question (Cole, Grolnick, & Schwartman, 1993) and even rejected (Sharp et al., 2005). Cognitive-behavioral strategies have also been discussed in the literature (Campbell & Elliot, 1996; Kolko et al.). One cognitive approach requires that youth openly explore in a safe therapeutic environment the feelings and cognitions that appeared concurrent with each firesetting event. The goal is to replace the maladaptive cognitions with a set of alternative responses. Bumpass, Fagelman, and Brix (1983) describe a visual graphing approach for use with firesetting youth and parents to help identify triggering events, making it easier to determine targets for intervention. In the Bumpass et al. (1983) study, events are plotted on one axis while feelings and thoughts are plotted on the other axis to assist in understanding the relationship between firesetting and cognitions or feelings that might have preceded or occurred simultaneous with the incidents. Other therapeutic approaches that have been utilized include behavioral rehearsal, didactic discussion, and role play. Still other programs, within either an individual and group therapeutic context, emphasize strategies for social skills deficits and peer relationship difficulties, both of which are commonly experienced by juvenile firesetters. These programs tend to utilize assertiveness training and reframing of thoughts and feelings that precipitated angry outbursts at peers (Koles & Jenson, 1985). Kolko (2001) utilized cognitive-behavioral treatment and fire safety education and found that among 38 children randomly assigned to CBT or fire safety education CBT decreased the frequency of firesetting, the proportion of children playing with matches, and overall deviant fire activities. Since most of the studies involve single case studies or small sample sizes, there is a dire need for larger sample, prospective studies with treatment protocols that allow for empirical validation. Unfortunately, the subset of clinicians who treat juvenile firesetters is small and researchers who investigate this subset is even smaller, so both the clinical and research literature base is sparse.

2.10.2   Family Therapy

Firesetting youth often come from families that experience higher levels of stress, marital discord, reduced problem-solving capabilities, and authoritarian discipline styles (Fineman, 1995; Gale, 1999; Kolko & Kazdin, 1990). These families tend to be chaotic, disorganized, and can only provide minimal supervision for children (Kolko, 2001). Parenting styles of caregivers of juvenile firesetters tend to be either extremely authoritarian or extremely lax. Caregivers may use harsh, abusive punishment techniques. On the other hand, certain parents may allow their child to continue to engage in dangerous firesetting or other antisocial behaviors unsupervised and without regard for the safety of others. There is another dimension that must be considered when treating juvenile firesetters. Because of the high prevalence of child maltreatment in this group, mental health professionals must be well-versed in mandated child abuse reporting statues of their respective states (Dombrowski, Ahia, & McQuillan, 2003). From a family systems perspective, the cycle of chaotic, and even abusive family styles transmits to subsequent generations. Thus, many of the caregivers of juvenile firesetters have themselves been raised in chaotic and abusive families, leaving them without appropriate parenting skills. Appropriate parent training programs become an essential component of intervention for juvenile firesetters. However, there limited available literature on outcomes of family therapy suggests either a high dropout rate or a loss of therapeutic gains upon termination of family therapy (Kolko).

2.10.3   Hospitalization and Residential Treatment Facilities

Although common practice when a youth is a danger to himself or others, the use of inpatient hospitalization or placement in a residential treatment center has received scant attention in the firesetting literature (Kolko & Kazdin, 1988; Pollinger et al., 2005). One of the paradoxes of both hospital and residential placements is the policy to prohibit or put up impediments to youth with a firesetting history. Notwithstanding this situation, one program for compulsive firesetters placed in a hospital setting utilized a behavioral approach that attempted to determine the antecedents and furnish the youth with functionally equivalent alternative behaviors (Geffen, 1991 as cited in Stadolnik, 2000). When a child is considered to be dangerous and unpredictable, posing a significant risk to self or others, then a more structured setting is needed that can monitor the youth and offer appropriate services. Professionals facilitating this placement should ensure that the facility has expertise in treating youth with firesetting behavior.

2.10.4   Psychopharmacology

Although pharmacological intervention is frequently used with juvenile firesetters, there is a paucity of research that investigates the effectiveness of psychotropic medication for this population. Since psychotropic medication is often one facet of a multicomponent approach to treatment of youth with antisocial and impulse-control disorders, it makes sense that psychotropic medication might be an important treatment modality. Psychotropic medication has proven effective in treating children with both internalizing and externalizing disorders, so it makes sense that, when used in the context of a multicomponent treatment, medication for juvenile firesetters may be beneficial for ameliorating symptoms that contribute to firesetting behavior. However, research regarding the treatment effectiveness for firesetting youth is generally unavailable.

2.11   Recidivism

Because of the dangers of firesetting, one of the biggest questions involves recidivism. Unfortunately, the literature on recidivism and prognostic factors is sparse (Cox-Jones et al., 1990; Kolko, Day, Bridge, & Kazdin, 2001). One study (e.g., Kolko et al., 2006) reported that several factors may contribute to continued firesetting behavior posttreatment. This includes a high frequency of matchplay, fire setting incidents and greater involvement in fire-related acts such as hiding matches/lighters and pulling of fire alarms. Also there tends to be greater curiosity about and interest in fire. Youth who are more likely to repeat firesetting experience higher externalizing behavior problems. This same study found that neither exposure to a fire model such as an uncle or older brother, nor level of family dysfunction was related to recidivism. Additional research is necessary before these associations should be considered confirmed.

2.12   Future Directions

Although increased attention has been paid to the problem of juvenile firesetting, there still needs to be much greater awareness among laypeople, practitioners and researchers alike. The cost to society of firesetting is enormous and greater assessment, prevention and intervention tools are direly needed. Before addressing the specific assessment, prevention and intervention tools that are needed, we would like to discuss other possible recommendations that would set the stage for greater intervention. It is recommended that a statewide and perhaps even a nationwide database be established to track the characteristics of youth who engage in firesetting. An analogous database system is available for children who are maltreated (NDACAN). Perhaps this database system could serve as a model for juvenile firesetters? This database system would also then allow researchers to address questions such as actual costs, recidivism, and typological characteristics of the firesetter.

Unfortunately, juvenile firesetting has not received the attention of the research community as say populations with ADHD, although juvenile firesetting poses considerable cost to society. The research community has not systematically evaluated the thousands of intervention programs that are available (Kolko, 2001). The field would benefit tremendously from dissemination of treatment protocols that have been manualized and empirically validated. In particular, there is need to evaluate the longer term effectiveness of treatment programs some months to years after a youth has completed it. Related to this, there are numerous assessment instruments and interview approaches that are available. However, most of these suffer from poor psychometric properties with unknown reliability and validity. The field would benefit from the creation of an assessment instrument that has psychometric properties comparable to personality and behavioral rating scales presently available. Third, the field would benefit from additional research regarding the motivational, behavioral, and emotional characteristics of youth who set fires (Kolko et al., 2001). Much of what we know emanates from case reports and anecdotal evidence. Fourth, smoking cessation programs are critical and may also have a secondary health benefit to juvenile firesetters. It would also potentially remove an ignition source that is often readily available and perhaps overlooked by those involved in the developmental well-being of youth who fireset. And, treatment facilities (e.g., group homes; residential treatment facilities) should be trained in the management of firesetting behavior and should have sprinkler systems installed. Because of the complexity of working with youth who set fires, it might be prudent to also establish credentialing standards for various personnel who work with youth who set fires. Fire service personnel already have credentialing efforts in place. Perhaps mental health or social work professionals who treat juvenile firesetters should be required to undergo similar credentialing. This might make sense for child protective services workers who make home visits. This way the worker will be better able to recognize the signs of fireplay in the home (e.g., cigarette burns; scorched walls or floors). We have made strides in understanding how to properly assess and treat juvenile firesetters, but research is still in its infancy in this area.

References

Adler, R., Nunn, R., Northam, E., Lebnan, V., & Ross, R. (1994). Secondary prevention of childhood firesetting. *Journal of the American Academy of Child and Adolescent Psychiatry, 33,* 1194–1202.

American Psychiatric Association. (1952). *Diagnostic and statistical manual of mental disorders.* Washington, DC: Author.

American Psychiatric Association. (1968). *Diagnostic and statistical manual of mental disorders* (2nd ed.). Washington, DC: Author.

American Psychiatric Association. (1980). *Diagnostic and statistical manual of mental disorders* (3rd ed.). Washington, DC: Author.

American Psychiatric Association. (1987). *Diagnostic and statistical manual of mental disorders* (3rd ed. rev.). Washington, DC: Author.

American Psychiatric Association. (2000). *Diagnostic and statistical manual of mental disorders – Text revision* (4th ed. rev.). Washington, DC: Author.

Barron, P., Hassiotis, A., & Banes, J. (2004). Offenders with intellectual disability: AA prospective, comparative study. *Journal of Intellectual Disability Research, 48*(1), 69–76.

Brain, C. K., & Sillen, A. (1988). Evidence from the Swartkrans cave for the earliest use of fire. *Nature, 336*(6198), 464–466.

Bumpass, E., Fagelman, F., & Brix, R. (1983). Intervention with children who set fires. *American Journal of Psychotherapy, 37*, 328–345.

Campbell, C., & Elliot, E. (1996). *Skills curriculum for intervening with firesetters (Ages 13–18)*. Salem, OR: Office of State Fire Marshal.

Cohen, L. E., & Felson, M. (1979). Social change and crime rate trends: A routine activity approach. *American Sociological Review, 44*, 588–608.

Cole, R., Crandall, R., Kourofsky, C. E., Sharp, D., Blaakman, S. W., & Cole, E. (2006). *Juvenile firesetting: A community guide to prevention & intervention*. Pittsford, NY: Fireproof Children/Prevention First.

Cole, R., Grolnick, W., & Schwartman, P. (1993). Fire setting. In R. Ammerman, C. Last, & M. Hersen (Eds.), *Handbook of prescriptive treatments for children and adolescents* (293–307). Boston: Allyn & Bacon.

Cole, R., Grolnick, W., & Schwartzman, P. (1999). Fire setting. In R. T. Ammerman, M. Hersen, & C. G. Last (Eds.), *Handbook of prescriptive treatments for children and adolescents* (293–307). Boston: Allyn & Bacon.

Cook, R., Hersch, R., Gaynor, J., & Roehl, J. (1989). *The national juvenile firesetter/arson control and prevention program: Assessment report, executive summary*. Washington, DC: Institute for Social Analysis.

Cox-Jones, C., Lubetsky, M., Fultz, S. A., & Kolko, D. J. (1990). Inpatient treatment of young recidivist firesetter. *Journal of the American Academy of Child Psychiatry, 29*, 936–941.

Crick, N. R., & Dodge, K. A. (1994). A review and reformulation of social information-processing mechanisms in children's social adjustment. *Psychological Bulletin, 115*, 74–101.

Crick, N. R., & Ladd, G. W. (1990). Children's perceptions of the outcomes of aggressive strategies: Do the ends justify being mean? *Developmental Psychology, 26*, 612–620.

DeSalvatore, G., & Hornstein, R. (1991). Juvenile firesetting: Assessment and treatment in psychiatric hospitalization and residential placement. *Child and Youth Care Forum, 20*, 103–114.

Dodge, K. A., & Coie, J. D. (1987). Social information-processing factors in reactive and proactive aggression in children's peer groups. *Journal of Personality and Social Psychology, 53*, 1146–1158.

Dodge, K. A., & Frame, C. L. (1982). Social cognitive biases and deficits in aggressive boys. *Child Development, 53*, 620–635.

Dodge, K. A., Pettit, G. S., McClaskey, C. L., & Brown, M. M. (1986). Social competence in children. *Monographs of the Society for Research in Child Development, 51* (2, Serial No. 213).

Dombrowski, S. C., Ahia, C. E., & McQuillan, K. (2003). Protecting children through mandated child abuse reporting. *The Educational Forum, 67*(2), 76–85.

Erikson, E. H. (1959). *Identity and the life cycle*. New York: International Universities Press.

Fessler, D. M. T. (2006). A burning desire: Steps toward an evolutionary psychology of fire learning. *Journal of Cognition and Culture, 6*(3–4), 429–451.

Fineman, K. (1980). Firesetting in children and adolescents. *The Psychiatric Clinics of North America, 3*, 483–500.

Fineman, K. (1995). A model for the qualitative analysis of child and adult fire deviant behavior. *American Journal of Forensic Psychology, 13*, 31–60.

Fineman, K. (1996). *Comprehensive fire risk assessment*. Published in Poage et al. (1997). Colorado Juvenile Firesetter Prevention Program: Training Seminar Vol. 1. Denver, CO: Colorado Division of Fire Safety.

Forehand, R., Wierson, M., Frame, C., Kempton, T., & Armistead, L. (1991). Juvenile firesetting: A unique syndrome or an advanced level of antisocial behavior? *Behavior Research and Therapy, 29*, 125–128.

Freud, S. (1932). The acquisition of power over fire. *The International Journal of Psychoanalysis, 13*, 405–410.

Gale, C. M. (1999). *A survey of incarcerated male juveniles with a history of fire misuse*. Portland, OR: Morrison Center.

Gallagher-Duffy, J., Mackay, S., Duffy, J., Sullivan-Thomas, M., & Peterson-Badali, M. (2009). The pictorial fire stroop: A measure of processing bias for fire-related stimuli. *Adolescent Psychopathology, 37*(8), 1165–1176.

Gaynor, J. (Ed.). (2002). *Juvenile firesetter intervention handbook.* Emittsburg, MD: United States Fire Administration. Retrieved from http://www.usfa.dhs.gov/downloads/pdf/publications/fa-210.pdf.

Geffen, M. (1991). *Juvenile firesetting.* Denver, CO: Juvenile Firesetters Conference.

Geller, J. (1992). Pathological firesetting in adults. *International Journal of Law and Psychiatry, 15,* 283–302.

Goren-Inbar, N., Alperson, N., Kislev, M. E., Simchoni, O., Melamed, Y., Ben-Nun, A., et al. (2004). Evidence of hominin control of fire at Gesher Benot Ya'aqov, Israel. *Science, 304*(5671), 725–727.

Grolnick, W. S., Cole, R. E., Laurentis, L., & Schwartzman, P. (1990). Playing with fire: A developmental assessment of children's fire understanding and experience. *Journal of Clinical Psychology, 19,* 126–135.

Hanson, M., Mackay, S., Atkinson, L., Staley, S., & Pignatiello, A. (1995). Firesetting during the preschool period: Assessment and intervention issues. *Canadian Journal of Psychiatry, 40,* 299–303.

Hanson, M., Mackay-Soroka, S., Staley, S., & Poulton, L. (1994). Delinquent firesetters: A comparative study of delinquency and firesetting histories. *Canadian Journal of Psychiatry, 39,* 230–232.

Hickle, K. E., & Roe-Sepowitz, D. E. (2010). Female juvenile arsonists: An exploratory look at characteristics and solo and group arson offences. *Legal and Criminological Psychology, 15*(2), 285–399.

Holland, C. J. (1969). Elimination by the parents of fire setting behaviors in a seven year old boy. *Behavioral Research Therapy, 7,* 135–137.

Karter, M. J. (2010). *Fire loss in the United States 2009.* National Fire Protection Association Fire Analysis and Research Division. Quincy, MA: National Fire Protection Association.

Kazdin, A. (1997). Practitioner review: Psychological treatments for conduct disorder in children. *Journal of Child Psychology and Psychiatry, 38,* 161–178.

Koles, M., & Jenson, W. (1985). Comprehensive treatment of chronic fire setting in a severely disordered boy. *Journal of Behavior Therapy and Experimental Psychiatry, 16,* 81–85.

Kolko, D. (1983). Multicomponent parental treatment of chronic fire setting in a severely disordered boy. *Journal of Behavior Therapy and Experimental Psychiatry, 16,* 81–85.

Kolko, D. J. (1988). Community interventions for childhood firesetters: A comparison of two national programs. *Hospital & Community Psychiatry, 39,* 973–979.

Kolko, D. (1999). Firesetting in children and youth. In V. Van Hasselt & M. Hersen (Eds.), *Handbook of psychological approaches with violent offenders: Contemporary strategies and issues* (pp. 95–115). New York: Kluwar Academic/Plenum.

Kolko, D. J. (2001). Efficacy of cognitive-behavioral treatment and fire safety education for firesetting children: Initial and follow-up outcomes. *Journal of Child Psychology and Psychiatry, and Allied Disciplines, 42,* 359–369.

Kolko, D. J., Day, B. T., Bridge, J., & Kazdin, A. E. (2001). Two-year prediction of children's firesetting in clinically-referred and non-referred samples. *Journal of Child Psychology and Psychiatry and Allied Disciplines, 42,* 371–380.

Kolko, D. J., Herschell, A. D., & Scharf, D. M. (2006). Education and treatment for boys who set fires: Specificity, moderators and predictors or recidivism. *Journal of Emotional and Behavioral Disorders, 14,* 227–239.

Kolko, D., & Kazdin, A. (1986). A conceptualization of firesetting in children and adolescents. *Journal of Abnormal Child Psychology, 14,* 49–61.

Kolko, D., & Kazdin, A. (1988). Prevalence of firesetting and related behaviors among child psychiatric patients. *Journal of Consulting and Clinical Psychology, 56,* 628–630.

Kolko, D., & Kazdin, A. (1990). Matchplay and firesetting in children: Relationship to parent, marital, and family dysfunction. *Journal of Clinical Child Psychology, 19,* 229–238.

Kolko, D. J., & Kazdin, A. E. (1991). Motives of childhood firesetters: Firesetting characteristics and psychological correlates. *Journal of Child Psychology and Psychiatry, 32,* 535–550.

Kolko, D. J., Schark, D. M., Herschell, A. D., Wilcox, D. K., Okulitch, J., & Pinsonneault, I. (2008). A survey of juvenile firesetter intervention programs in North America. *Psychology Journal, 26*(4), 41–66.

Koson, D. F. (1982). Forensic psychiatric examinations: Competency. *Journal of Forensic Science, 27,* 119–124.

Loeber, R., & Dishion, T. (1984). Boys who fight at home and school: Family conditions influencing cross-setting consistency. *Journal of Consulting and Clinical Psychology, 52*, 759–768.

Lowenstein, L. (1989). The etiology, diagnosis, and treatment of the fire-setting behavior of children. *Child Psychiatry and Human Development, 19*, 186–194.

Lyng, S. (1990). Edgework: A social psychological analysis of voluntary risk-taking. *The American Journal of Sociology, 95*, 851–886.

Macht, L., & Mack, J. (1968). The firesetter syndrome. *Psychiatry, 31*, 277–288.

Mackay, S., Henderson, J., Del Bove, G., Marton, P., Warling, D., & Root, C. (2006). Fire interest and antisociality as risk factors in the severity and persistence of juvenile firesetting. *Journal of the American Academy of Child and Adolescent Psychiatry, 45*(9), 1077–1084.

Moore, J., Thompson-Pope, K., & Whited, R. (1996). MMPI-A profiles of adolescent boys with a history of firesetting. *Journal of Personality Assessment, 67*, 116–126.

Pierce, J., & Hardesty, V. (1997). Non-referral of psychopathological child firesetters to mental health services. *Journal of Clinical Psychology, 53*, 349–350.

Pinsonneault, I. (2002). Developmental perspectives on children and fire. In D. J. Kolko (Ed.), *Handbook on firesetting in children and youth* (pp. 15–31). New York: Kluwer/Academic.

Pollinger, J., Samuels, L., & Stadolnik, R. (2005). A comparative study of the behavioral, personality, and fire history characteristics of residential and outpatient adolescents (ages 12–17) with firesetting behaviors. *Adolescence, 40*(158), 345–353.

Putnam, C. T., & Kirkpatrick, J. T. (2005). Juvenile firesetting: A research overview. *Juvenile Justice Bulletin.* Retrieved August 11, 2010 from http://www.ncjrs.gov.

Quinsey, V., Chaplin, T., & Upfold, D. (1989). Arsonists and sexual arousal to fire setting: Correlation unsupported. *Journal of Behavioral Therapy and Experimental Psychiatry, 20*, 203–209.

Raines, J., & Foy, C. (1994). Extinguishing the fires within: Treating juvenile firesetters. *The Journal of Contemporary Human Services, 75*, 595–606.

Ray, I. (1838). *A treatise on the medical jurisprudence of insanity.* Boston: C. C. Thomas and J. Brown.

Ray, I. (1844). *A treatise on the medical jurisprudence of insanity* (4th ed.). Boston: Little Brown & Co.

Root, C., Mackay, S., Henderson, J., Del Bove, G., & Warling, D. (2008). The link between maltreatment and juvenile firesetting: Correlates and underlying mechanisms. *Child Abuse & Neglect, 32*(2), 161–176.

Sakheim, G., & Osborn, E. (1986). A psychological profile of juvenile firesetters in residential treatment: A replication study. *Child Welfare, 65*(5), 495–502.

Sharp, D., Blaakman, S., Cole, E., & Cole, R. (2005). Evidence-based multidisciplinary strategies for working with children who set fires. *Journal of American Psychiatric Nurses, Association, 11*, 329–337.

Slavkin, M. L. (2007). Juvenile firesetting. In M. Hersen (Ed.), *Handbook of clinical interviewing with children* (pp. 384–403). Oaks, CA: Sage.

Stadolnik, R. F. (2000). *Drawn to the flame: Assessment and treatment of juvenile firesetting behavior.* Sarasota, FL: Practitioner's Resource Series.

Steinbach, G. (1986). Les differentes conceptions du droit en matiere d'incendie et les generalites criminologiques sur les incendiarires. *Neuropsychiatric de l'Enfance et de l'Adolescence, 34*, 33–38.

Swaffer, T., & Hollin, C. (1995). Adolescent firesetting? Why do they say they do it? *Journal of Adolescence, 18*(5), 619–623.

Winget, C., & Whitman, R. (1973). Coping with problems: Attitudes towards children who set fires. *The American Journal of Psychiatry, 130*, 442–445.

Wooden, W., & Berkey, M. (1984). *Children and arson: America's middle class nightmare.* New York: Plenum.

Yarnell, H. (1940). Firesetting in children. *The American Journal of Orthopsychiatry, 10*, 272–287.

Zipper, P., & Wilcox, D. K. (2005). Juvenile arson: The importance of early intervention. *FBI Law Enforcement Bulletin*, 1–9.

Chapter 3
Gender Identity Disorder

> *Look at this stuff*
> *Isn't it neat?*
> *Wouldn't you think my collection's complete?*
> *Wouldn't you think I'm the girl*
> *The girl who has everything?*
>
> –Ariel, Disney's Little Mermaid

3.1 Overview

History is replete with accounts of individuals who consider themselves a different gender from which their genitalia indicates. In some societies, these individuals were revered and even granted shamanic duties. In others, most recently contemporary Eurocentric cultures, individuals with gender incongruence have been the subject of scorn if not downright brutality. One has only to view movies such as Neil Jordan's *The Crying Game* (1992) or Kimberly Peirce's *Boys Don't Cry* (1999) to view animosity toward individuals with gender incongruence. The Belgian movie (available in English subtitle) *Ma Vie En Rose* (1997) furnishes insight into the trials and extreme tribulations of a child and her family who try to navigate closed-minded societies that reject anything other than binary gender identity.

Although these movies give insight into societal reaction toward individuals with gender incongruence, they do not portray the extreme hurdles faced by youth with gender variance. Such youth face considerable social ostracism, if not aggression, an extremely high rate of suicide, and high rates of psychopathology including depression and substance use (Bradley, 1990; Zucker & Bradley, 1995). Most diagnostic systems pathologize individuals with gender incongruence; however, advocates for the transgender community indicate that any individual who faces such chronic scorn, ridicule and ostracism would develop a mental health issue. The transgender community as well as clinical and research professionals, therefore, argue that any

S.C. Dombrowski et al., *Assessing and Treating Low Incidence/High Severity Psychological Disorders of Childhood*, DOI 10.1007/978-1-4419-9970-2_3,
© Springer Science+Business Media, LLC 2011

[handwritten annotations in margins:] *proven by study that showed improveme[nt] in grades*

[left margin handwritten:] here, cite study of multiple sex chromosomes

psychopathology associated with GID tends to be exogenously, rather than endogenously, induced (Gottschalk, 2003; Winters, 2008). Most cultures, with few exceptions such as a northern province in India, view gender dichotomously. Ironically, although there is a sizeable amount of research literature available on the topic of GID in children, what is available is based on small sample sizes or single case reports.

There are generally two approaches to the treatment of youth with gender identity disorder. The accommodation approach suggests that children and their families are to be supported as the child develops and perhaps transitions to his or her preferred gender identity (Gottschalk, 2003). This approach is supported by the transgender community, with recognition that gender is fluid and individuals may sometimes switch back and forth between preferred gender roles (Fraser, 2009). Intervention is provided to families whereby they are helped to accept, support, guide, and love their child as the child transitions (Bockting, 2008; Lev, 2004; Meyer et al., 2001). The other approach recommends behavioral and cognitive-behavioral intervention for preadolescent youth to reinforce gender-typical behavior and ignore gender nonconforming behavior. Each camp views the others treatment approach as potentially unethical (Winters, 2008; Zucker & Bradley, 1995).

3.2   Controversy: Whether a Disorder and Whither to Treat?

Considerable controversy and often contentious debate surrounds whether GID is a disorder and deserves treatment (Blanchard & Steiner, 1990; Gottschalk, 2003; Hausman, 2003; Langer & Martin, 2004; Richardson, 1999; Winters, 2008). Numerous psychologists as well as the transgender community are categorically opposed to the notion that gender variance is a disorder (Ault & Brzuzy, 2009; Winters). On the other hand, several researchers, including Kenneth Zucker of the Gender Identity Clinic within the Centre for Addiction and Mental Health in Toronto, contend that gender incongruence is a treatable disorder if intervention is provided sufficiently early and prior to adolescence. What follows is a brief discussion of both perspectives on classification and treatment with a description of the DSM-IV TR criteria delineated thereafter.

3.2.1   Perspective 1: Accommodation

Several researchers and transgender advocacy groups (Gottschalk, 2003; Langer & Martin, 2004; Mass, 1990; Sedgwick, 1991) hold that gender incongruence is not a disorder and that psychiatric nosologies inappropriately pathologize individuals with gender variance when instead the dysphoria is related to social rejection and dissatisfaction with genitalia and overall physical development. This perspective also maintains that the DSM reinforces binary, stereotypical gender roles (e.g., to be male is to be loud, boisterous, active, and aggressive; to be female is to be meek, nurturing, vulnerable, and sensitive). The accommodation perspective contends that the DSM does not account for the spectrum of gender variations and inappropriately forces gender into a simple dichotomy (Bockting & Coleman, 2007; Fraser, 2009). Other researchers have even argued that the classification GID is a back door way to pathologize homosexuality since gender dysphoria is highly correlated with same-sex interest (Burke, 1996; Mass, 1990).

Those who embrace the accommodation perspective maintain that not only society, but also the psychiatric community needs to be more accepting and accommodating of gender variations. This perspective suggests that the dysphoria experienced by individuals with gender incongruence is largely environmentally induced and based upon society's intolerance for gender variation. As support for this position, the accommodation camp suggests that the DSM is less tolerant of boys with gender nonconforming behavior than girls (Mass, 1990). Also, society views "sissy-like" behavior worse than it does tomboy behavior (Green, 1987; Minter, 1999). The accommodation perspective contends that the treatment of youth with gender incongruence is akin to the practice of reparative therapy for individuals who are gay and is therefore unethical (Pleak, 1999). Langer and Martin (2004) contend that such treatment "bears striking resemblance to conversion therapy for homosexuality," which is considered unethical by most psychiatric and psychological groups in North America including the American Psychological Association and the National Association of Social Workers. Langer and Martin indicate that the "history of efforts to change the gender identities of children is no less disturbing than those directed toward changing sexual orientation, especially because of the young age and vulnerability of those involved" (p. 19). Those from this perspective therefore eschew both labeling and treatment in favor of working with the families and communities to love and support their children as they accommodate to their preferred gender identity (Ehrensaft, 2007). Individuals from the accommodation perspective also suggest that inclusion of GID in the DSM serves to perpetuate stigmatization, harm self-esteem, destroy human dignity, and place individuals with gender incongruence at risk for emotional or physical abuse from the broader society (Winters, 2008).

3.2.2 Perspective 2: Psychological Intervention

The second perspective maintains that gender incongruence is a disorder since the condition causes distress and impairs social, academic, and vocational functioning. This perspective is supported to a large degree by Kenneth Zucker of the Centre for Addiction and Mental Health in Toronto and other researchers (e.g., Blanchard, 1989; Coates & Person, 1985; Coates, Friedman, & Wolfe, 1991; Green, 1976; Magee & Miller, 1992) who argue that rates of psychopathology are high among individuals with GID and point to increased rates of suicidality, depression, and substance abuse (Zucker & Bradley, 1995) as a rationale for intervention. These researchers suggest that psychopathology is also high in families of children with GID (Bates, Skilbeck, Smith, & Bentler, 1974; Coates, 1990). Treatment of children diagnosed with GID is undertaken to reduce experience of social ostracism and its psychopathological sequelae (Zucker, 2006; Zucker & Bradley). Zucker and Bradley contend that to accommodate to a child's desire to be the opposite gender is inappropriate if not unethical. Zucker explains that the desire of a child to change his or her gender is similar to a child who wants to change his or her skin color:

> I would argue that it is as legitimate to want to make youngsters comfortable with their gender identity (to make it correspond to the physical reality of their biological sex) as it is to make youngsters comfortable with their ethnic identity (to make it correspond to the physical reality of the color of their skin) (p. 550).

In this scenario, treatment should focus on helping the child accept his or her gender that matches biological sex (in a child who does not have an intersex condition). Zucker and Bradley (1995) explain that the stress and extreme measures necessary to align the preferred gender identity with biological sex provides sufficient rationale for attempting to prevent children from accommodating and even transitioning to a transgender lifestyle. Zucker and Bradley note that intervention for gender dysphoria can effectively alter a child's desire to be the opposite gender and is therefore protective, not harmful. Zucker and Bradley also note that intervention has no bearing on sexual orientation and do not recommend treatment for youth with gender dysphoria who have attained adolescence, contending that the window of opportunity for the treatment of gender identity is early childhood (Zucker, 2001, 2005).

Zucker (2006) and Zucker and Bradley (1995) note that if gender is a social construction, then it makes sense that it is malleable and amenable to behavioral shaping. Zucker and Bradley discuss numerous studies that provide shorter-term (usually 1 year or less) treatment follow-up. These studies found that treatment for gender incongruence was helpful, not harmful, to youth's development because treatment helped to mitigate feelings of gender dysphoria. This contrasts with Burke (1996) who discussed several cases where children experienced distress and even more intensely disrupted family relationships subsequent to treatment for GID. These divergent outcomes suggest a critical need for long-term follow-up to determine effectiveness of treatment. Part of this follow-up should include an assessment of youth who were treated for gender dysphoria to discern whether treatment adversely impacted their mental status.

3.3   Description, Prevalence, and Diagnostic Classification

Although a person may be born with a specific genitalia that person may identify with the opposite gender. That same person may even switch gender identities, at one point identifying as male and at another as female. An in-depth investigation of whether gender is socially constructed or biologically determined is beyond the scope of this chapter, but it is important to point out that there is a distinction between gender identity and biological sex.

3.3.1   Prevalence

The worldwide, lifetime prevalence of GID is estimated at 0.001–0.002% (Roberto, 1983). However, in countries that tend to be more open to gender variation, the lifetime prevalence is higher. In the Netherlands, a country that permits gender transitioning as young as age 16, the prevalence of gender identity disorder appears to be higher. Male-to-female gender identity disorder is found in about 1 per 12,000 of people and female-to-male gender identity disorder is seen in 1 per 30,000 (Bakker, Van Kesteren, Gooren, & Bezemer, 1993). The DSM-IV TR reports that there are no recent epidemiological data on the prevalence of GID. The DSM-IV TR reports that roughly 1 per 30,000 adult males and 1 per 100,000 adult females seek sex-reassignment surgery (APA, 2000).

3.3.2   DSM-IV TR Diagnostic Criteria

The American Psychiatric Association's DSM-IV TR (2000) indicates that individuals receive a classification of GID when they manifest the following:

- A. Strong and persistent cross-gender identification (not merely a desire for any perceived cultural advantages of being the other sex). In children, the disturbance is manifested by four (or more) of the following:

  1. Repeatedly stated desire to be, or insistence that he or she is, the other sex.
  2. In boys, preference for cross-dressing or simulating female attire; in girls, insistence on wearing only stereotypical masculine clothing.
  3. Strong and persistent preferences for cross-sex roles in make-believe play or persistent fantasies of being the other sex.
  4. Intense desire to participate in the stereotypical games and pastimes of the other sex.
  5. Strong preference for playmates of the other sex.

- B. Persistent discomfort with his or her sex or sense of inappropriateness in the gender role of that sex.
- C. The disturbance is not concurrent with a physical intersex condition.
- D. The disturbance causes clinically significant distress or impairment in social, occupational, or other important areas of functioning.

3.3.3   Description

Zucker and colleagues (e.g., Zucker, 2005, 2006; Zucker & Bradley, 1995) contend that children with GID display behaviors that intensely identify with the opposite sex including identity statements, dress-up play, toy play, role play, peer relations, motoric and speech characteristics, statements about sexual anatomy, and involvement in rough-and-tumble play. This reflects not only a desire to act like the opposite sex, but a genuine belief that the child *is* the opposite sex. The typical age of onset of most behaviors is between two and four. Zucker and Bradley indicate that a clinic referral occurs when parents begin to feel that the child's behaviors no longer represent a phase out of which they will outgrow (Stoller, 1967). The following is a more in-depth discussion of the characteristics of youth who have been observed by Zucker and Bradley to receive a classification of GID.

3.3.3.1 Identity Statements

During the preschool years, the chronic desire to be the opposite gender is a common reason for referral to treatment (Zucker & Bradley, 1995). In some children, this statement may be a mistake of gender labeling, a defensive remark, or an interest in role playing the opposite gender. In other children, the statement reflects a genuine desire to become the opposite sex. Still, other children do not make identity statements but their behavior and play points to identification with the opposite gender. By middle childhood, Zucker and Bradley indicate that the open wish to be the opposite sex remits, though there are some children with severe gender dysphoria who may continue to state their wish to be the opposite gender and who wonder how they could change their sex. It is unclear whether the desire actually remits or if the child becomes conditioned not to make desire known.

3.3.3.2 Cross-Dressing

Cross-dressing is considered one of the more obvious signs of cross-gender identification. Green (1976) reported that cross-dressing begins between ages 2 and 4 and by age 6; 94% of boys were involved in cross-dressing. In some cases, boys are obsessed by the need to cross-dress, insisting either during preschool or when they come home from school that they need to wear female attire. Even in nondirective and accepting parents, there may be discomfort with the child's cross-dressing behavior which results in limit setting. This limit setting in turn sometimes results in covert attempts at cross-dressing when no one is around. By late childhood, Zucker and Bradley (1995) report that the interest in cross-dressing may be transformed into a preoccupation with the appearance of female movie stars. Although most boys wear stereotypically conventional male clothing, Zucker and Bradley indicate that boys with gender dysphoria may prefer colors that are stereotypically female such as pink or purple. Other boys may even refuse to wear shirts with superheroes such as Power Rangers.

According to Zucker and Bradley (1995), girls with gender incongruence may reject feminine clothing. They may prefer more comfortable, masculine attire such as jeans or sweatpants. When required to wear feminine attire, such as a dress or skirt, some girls will vehemently protest. Still other girls will demand that their hair be cut short, presenting them as a boy.

3.3.3.3   Toy and Role Play

Boys with gender dysphoria may show little interest in toys and roles that are stereotypically masculine. Instead, Zucker and Bradley (1995) note that boys prefer feminine toys and interests. For instance, boys might be fascinated with the Little Mermaid, Snow White, Barbie, Tinker Bell, or Sleeping Beauty. Girls engage in role play with male figures, including being a father or a male character from movies or books. Girls' toy interest and activities are stereotypically masculine. They might be preoccupied with violent and aggressive fantasy play, eschewing stereotypically feminine, nurturing play.

3.3.3.4   Peer Relations

Zucker and Bradley (1995) explain that boys display a preference for affiliation with girls. This preference is enduring, demonstrated in older boys, but these boys tend to become isolated socially when boys and girls engage in segregation of the sexes throughout the early to late elementary school years (Leaper, 1994; Maccoby & Jacklin, 1987). A small percentage of the boys lack close friends with either sex and suffer poor peer relations. In early childhood, these boys experience less teasing from girls than other boys regarding feminine interests and activities. Boys will attempt to avoid rough-and-tumble play, fearing that they might get hurt (Pellegrini, 1989). Others may have social-cognitive processing problems in which they cannot distinguish play fighting from intent to harm and therefore avoid play fighting (Costabile et al., 1991). Females with gender dysphoria generally experience less ostracism and may suffer less peer rejection, at least through childhood (APA, 2000). This is perhaps explained by society's greater tolerance for cross-gender peer relations and play in girls than boys.

3.4   Developmental Course

The psychological literature base, particularly the psychoanalytic literature, attempts to describe the etiology and developmental course of GID. This model posits that a combination of factors contribute to GID, including a specific traumatic event in the life of the child during a sensitive period of development between the ages of 12 and 18 months. This traumatic event might include maternal miscarriage, rape, or another event that is perceived by the child to be traumatic (Marantz & Coates, 1991). Second, the literature points to a dysfunctional family environment including parental separation or divorce (Coates & Person, 1985; Rekers & Swihart, 1989) and parental over protectiveness (Bates et al., 1974). Case reports (e.g., Green, 1987) out of the psychoanalytical literature indicate that mothers often experience high degrees of depression and anxiety. Some of these mothers are so chronically depressed that they do not attend to the basic needs of their children. Third, the

temperamental literature base suggests that highly inhibited, sensitive, and emotionally reactive boys have the temperamental disposition for GID if other factors also
contribute. These boys also suffer extreme separation anxiety, which may play an
important role in the development of GID (Coates & Person). In addition, boys with
GID generally avoid rough-and-tumble play and are inclined to female activities
and playmates. The developmental course of GID is difficult to empirically validate.
What is known is that most children, especially boys, who experience gender
dysphoria do not go on to experience full-fledged GID. Rather, these children upon
attaining adolescence are satisfied with their gender. The literature is consistent in
reporting that a subset of gender dysphoric children, particularly males, may experience a homosexual or bisexual orientation (Baily, Dunne, & Martin, 2000; Brown,
1957, 1958; Freud, 1965; Green, 1987; Zuger, 1988, 1989). But, this still remains
controversial (Zucker, 2008). Those who continue to experience gender dysphoria
as they move into adolescence and beyond might seek out gender reassignment or
engage in cross-dressing behavior. The proportion of youth who actually seek out
gender reassignment is unknown. Of those who seek gender reassignment, there is
a very small subset that regrets the decision and may experience gender dysphoria
after sex reassignment (Bentler, 1976; Olsson & Möller, 2006). However, anecdotal
reports from one source that contained interviews with hundreds of individuals who
transitioned suggested improved mental status following transition (Winters, 2008).
In totality, the research base is deficient regarding and individual's mental status and
happiness quotient following transition.

3.5 Relationship Between Gender Atypicality and Homosexuality

In some publications that furnish an overview of GID, there is sometimes a side
discussion regarding the association with homosexuality. Selected studies have
linked gender atypical behavior in boys with later homosexuality (Baily et al.,
2000; Brown, 1957, 1958; Freud, 1965; Green, 1987; Green & Money, 1960;
Zuger, 1988, 1989). Scant attention has been paid to this issue in girls. In fact, there
are no prospective studies examining the association between gender-atypical
behavior in girls and later sexual orientation. The few retrospective studies available suggest a more equivocal relationship between gender atypicality and later
sexual orientation in females. Phillips and Over (1995) and Bem (1996) indicate
that 60% of heterosexual women were tomboys when compared with 77% of
lesbian and bisexual women. Both studies suggested that a high number of heterosexual as well as homosexual women engaged in gender nonconforming activities
in childhood. In several other studies, more lesbian than heterosexual women
recalled being a tomboy or engaging in gender-atypical behavior (Bell, Weinberg,
& Hammersmith, 1981; Dunne, Bailey, Kirk, & Martin, 2000; Saghir & Robins,
1973). Gottschalk (2003) contends that when considering that being a tomboy is
one childhood experience that is most often spoken of as a biological basis for

lesbianism, the high number of heterosexual women who report gender nonconformity makes such conclusions questionable.

This conclusion contrasts with that of researchers who investigate the relationship between gender atypicality and homosexuality in boys. Some researchers (e.g., Minter, 1999; Pleak, 1999; Zuger, 1988) believe that effeminate behavior in boys is a precursor to later homosexuality. Corbett (1998) suggests that gender-atypical behavior might be part of the normal course of development for some prehomosexual children. Pleak contends that therapeutic intervention should focus, therefore, on supporting children's development to become healthy gay adults since the evidence about capacity to alter sexual orientation is scant, if not unavailable (Duberman, 2002; Kopay & Young, 2001; Zucker, 2006; Zucker & Bradley, 1995).

3.6 Etiological Hypotheses and Theoretical Frameworks

Individuals studying gender identity disorder and sexual orientation have invested considerable time attempting to identify the etiology of gender incongruence and related psychosexual conditions. Researchers investigating underlying etiology tend to examine specific hypotheses in attempt to indicate that gender variation is predominantly biologically based, psychologically based or environmentally induced. Still others adopt a more integrative perspective and advocate a biopsychosocial model.

3.6.1 Biological Correlates

The following discussion will discuss the literature to date regarding any possible biological linkage to GID. Topics thought to hold most relevance include behavioral genetics, molecular genetics, and prenatal development.

3.6.1.1 Prenatal Sex Hormones

Since the seminal article by Phoeniz, Goy, Gerall, and Young (1959) on the influence of sex hormones on the development of sexual behavior in animals, there has been considerable discussion regarding the relationship of prenatal sex hormones in the influence of human sexual orientation and behavior. Phoeniz et al. (1959) injected pregnant guinea pigs with testosterone propionate throughout gestation and found that female offspring developed masculinized external genitalia that were indistinguishable from normal male controls. These females were also more likely to show mounting behavior, a male-typical sex behavior. Phoeniz et al. concluded that prenatal hormones influence both sexual reproductive tissues and mating behavior. This line of research prompted researchers to focus their attention on the possible role of prenatal hormones in influencing human gender identity.

However, the extrapolation of animal models to gender identity is difficult. There is no analog in the animal kingdom whereby animals seek to identify with the opposite gender. There seem to be better animal analogs for gender role behaviors such as rough-and-tumble play, aggression, and parenting. And, animal models do not account for the cultural and historical variability in meaning-making that humans apply to sexuality and gender (male/female/transgender/gender fluid) or sexuality (homosexual/heterosexual/bisexual). In totality, youngsters with gender incongruence do not show signs of physical hermaphroditism or hormonal anomaly. However, the possibility of a feminization or masculization of the brain during prenatal development through the influence of hormones has been discussed as one biologically plausible mechanism and should be investigated further (Martin & Dombrowski, 2008). Perhaps also useful might be brain imagining studies to determine whether there are structural differences in the brains of individuals with GID.

3.6.1.2 Behavior Genetics

Researchers in the behavioral genetics arena have turned their gaze toward homosexuality and GID (Plomin, 1994). Through an exploration of family history and the twin study method, the two approaches used by behavioral genetic researchers, the relationship with GID has been investigated. Early studies revealed little evidence for familiarity. Most siblings reported in Green (1987) were not concordant for GID. And, most case reports of monozygotic and dizygotic twins have not revealed a linkage with GID (Chazan, 1995). The range reported for concordance in MZ twins is 25–71% with DZ twin studies reporting lower rates around 39% (Bailey & Pillard, 1991; Whitam, Diamond, & Martin, 1993). However, a more recent, larger-scale retrospective study (e.g., Baily et al., 2000) of 1,891 adult twins reported a significantly heritable pattern for both men and women, with a stronger heritability estimate in men (.50–.57) than in women (.37–.40). This study, though retrospective, is consistent with that of Coolidge et al. (2002) who reported on the heritability of 314 twins (aged 4–17 years) in the first nonretrospective study to date. These authors reported that "although a model including only shared and nonshared environmental effects could not be rejected, the best fitting model indicated that GID was highly heritable" (p. 256). These authors concluded that GID, therefore, has a large biological component which has significant implications for treatment of the condition.

3.6.1.3 Molecular Genetics

There is a paucity of molecular genetic research regarding the relationship with GID. Because of this unavailability and the possible linkage between gender dysphoria and homosexuality, we discuss the potential molecular genetic basis of homosexuality. Some research has pointed to the relationship between the X chromosome (inherited from the mother) and homosexuality. Hamer, Hu, Magnuson,

Hu, and Pattatucci (1993) studied 114 families of homosexual men and noted increased rates of homosexuality in maternal male relatives. Specifically, markers have been found on the Xq28 subtelomeric region of the X chromosome. Yet, additional replication is needed because of limited molecular genetic studies.

3.6.2   Social-Cultural Context

Bem's Developmental Theory of "exotic become erotic" discusses a context in which a gender nonconforming child experiences heightened arousal in the presence of children they see different (Bem, 1996, 2000). For example, the inhibited, highly sensitive boy who engages in female typical play is taunted and labeled a sissy for his gender nonconformity. Bem contends that this boy experiences autonomic arousal and then associates that arousal with romantic attraction. Gottschalk (2003) argues that gender nonconforming boys are not interested in rough-and-tumble play and gender nonconforming girls prefer more active play. Gottschalk argues that gender categorization is socially constructed. Moreover, Gottschalk suggests that some boys may just be simply interested in more artistic or passive pursuits and this should not suggest a particular disorder. A feminist explanation further suggests that gender is a social construction and note that boys and girls engage in gender-atypical behaviors. The feminist perspective suggests that gender nonconformity in either sex may or may not lead to gender dysphoria. It is one thing not to conform to typical gender roles. It is a whole other issue to want to alter physical appearance to become another gender. Zucker (2009) notes that the important philosophical and empirical question is whether one can determine a distinction between variance and disorder.

practical implications

3.7   DSM-V TR: Change in Label and Revised Criteria?

There portends to be a change in the label used to describe individuals with gender variance (see http://www.dsm5.org/ProposedRevisions/Pages/proposedrevision. aspx?rid=192). Within the upcoming DSM-V, American Psychiatric Association leaders are proposing to rename the condition to "gender dysphoria." This change in nomenclature follows years of criticism by individuals from the transgender community who believe that the term GID is pejorative (Hausman, 2003; Winters, 2008). Instead, the transgender community prefers a less stigmatizing medical diagnosis that allows for the possibility of third-party payment for gender transition treatment and recognizes that the associated psychosocial problems are not related to a mental disease but rather to dissatisfaction with outward physical appearance. Individuals from the transgender community have argued for years that the DSM-IV TR and prior editions have inappropriately mislabeled gender variations as a disorder and that this mislabeling jeopardizes the health, dignity, and safety of the gender variant community (de Cuypere, Knudson, & Bockting, 2009;

Vance et al., 2010). More discussions are apparently planned regarding whether GID will be reconceptualized for the next rendition of the DSM (Zucker, 2009). As of the writing of this book, it appears that the term "gender dysphoria" may very well supplant the term gender identity disorder in the next rendition of the DSM (Meyer-Bahlburg, 2009).

3.7.1 Proposed DSM-V Diagnostic Criteria

3.7.1.1 Gender Dysphoria (in Children)

A. A marked incongruence between one's experienced/expressed gender and assigned gender, of at least 6 months duration, as manifested by at least six of the following indicators (including A1):

1. A strong desire to be of the other gender or an insistence that he or she is the other gender (or some alternative gender different from one's assigned gender).
2. In boys, a strong preference for cross-dressing or simulating female attire; in girls, a strong preference for wearing only typical masculine clothing and a strong resistance to the wearing of typical feminine clothing.
3. A strong preference for cross-gender roles in make-believe or fantasy play.
4. A strong preference for the toys, games, or activities typical of the other gender.
5. A strong preference for playmates of the other gender.
6. In boys, a strong rejection of typically masculine toys, games, and activities and a strong avoidance of rough-and-tumble play; in girls, a strong rejection of typically feminine toys, games, and activities.
7. A strong dislike of one's sexual anatomy.
8. A strong desire for the primary and/or secondary sex characteristics that match one's experienced gender.

B. The condition is associated with clinically significant distress or impairment in social, occupational, or other important areas of functioning, or with a significantly increased risk of suffering, such as distress or disability.

Subtypes

With a disorder of sex development
Without a disorder of sex development

3.7.1.2 Gender Dysphoria (in Adolescents or Adults)

A. A marked incongruence between one's experienced/expressed gender and assigned gender, of at least 6 months duration, as manifested by two or more of the following indicators:

1. A marked incongruence between one's experienced/expressed gender and primary and/or secondary sex characteristics (or, in young adolescents, the anticipated secondary sex characteristics).

2. A strong desire to be rid of one's primary and/or secondary sex characteristics because of a marked incongruence with one's experienced/expressed gender (or, in young adolescents, a desire to prevent the development of the anticipated secondary sex characteristics).
3. A strong desire for the primary and/or secondary sex characteristics of the other gender.
4. A strong desire to be of the other gender (or some alternative gender different from one's assigned gender).
5. A strong desire to be treated as the other gender (or some alternative gender different from one's assigned gender).
6. A strong conviction that one has the typical feelings and reactions of the other gender (or some alternative gender different from one's assigned gender).

B. The condition is associated with clinically significant distress or impairment in social, occupational, or other important areas of functioning, or with a significantly increased risk of suffering, such as distress or disability.

Subtypes

With a disorder of sex development
Without a disorder of sex development

Specifier

Post-transition, i.e., the individual has transitioned to full-time living in the desired gender (with or without legalization of gender change) and has undergone (or is undergoing) at least one cross-sex medical procedure or treatment regimen, namely, regular cross-sex hormone treatment or gender reassignment surgery confirming the desired gender (e.g., penectomy, vaginoplasty in a natal male, mastectomy, phalloplasty in a natal female).

3.8 Assessment

The availability of psychometrically valid and reliable instruments for the assessment of youth with gender incongruence is a considerable problem for the field. This poses to hamper appropriate evaluation of the condition and leave the clinician to rely upon more subjective clinical judgment. There are several assessment instruments and approaches available to assist in the evaluation of youth with gender incongruence, but these instruments tend to be primarily qualitative in nature, involving rating forms, structured and semistructured observations of children's play as well as interviews of parents and children. Please see Tables 3.1 and 3.2 below for an example of a rating forms and interview questions. Bear in mind that these questionnaires would be inappropriate for individuals with an intersex condition.

One parent report instrument, a modified version of Elizabeth and Green's (1984) gender identity questionnaire (GIQ), is available. Johnson et al. (2004) revised and factor analyzed the 16-item instrument and found that the instrument

Table 3.1 Clinical rating form for the core behavioral features of gender identity disorder of childhood

1. Identity statements
   - Child frequently states the wish to be of the opposite sex or that he or she is a member of the opposite sex (e.g., "I want to be a girl, I am a girl," or "I want to grow up to be a Mommy, not a Daddy")
   - Child occasionally states the wish to be of the opposite sex
   - Child rarely states the wish to be of the opposite sex
   - Child does not state the wish to be of the opposite sex
2. Anatomical dysphoria
   - Child frequently states a dislike of his or her sexual anatomy (e.g., "I don't like my penis"; "I want a penis, not a vagina") or demonstrates this behaviorally (e.g., in a boy, sitting to urinate to simulate having female genitalia; in a girl, standing to urinate to simulate having male genitalia)
   - Child occasionally states a dislike of his or her sexual anatomy or demonstrates this behaviorally
   - Child rarely states a dislike or his or her sexual anatomy or demonstrates this behaviorally
   - Child never states a dislike of his or her sexual anatomy or demonstrates this behaviorally
3. Cross-dressing
   - Child frequently cross dresses (e.g., in boys, use of mother's clothes, such as dresses, high-heeled shoes, jewelry, and makeup; simulation of long hair with towels)
   - In girls, refusal to wear culturally typical feminine clothing and use of clothing, such as boy's pants and shirts, to simulate a masculine appearance; often desire hair to be very short, in accordance with masculine convention
   - Child occasionally cross dresses
   - Child rarely cross dresses
   - Child never cross dresses
4. Toy and role play
   - Child prefers to play with toys and to engage in roles stereotypically associated with the opposite sex (e.g., in boys, a preference for female dolls, such as Barbie or Gem, role play as a female, emulation of female superheroes; drawings invariably are of women. In girls, a preference for male dolls, such as GI Joe or male transformers, role play as a male, emulation of male superheroes; drawings invariably are of men)
   - Child plays with toys and engages in roles that are both stereotypically masculine and feminine
   - Child avoids toys and roles that are stereotypically associated with his or her sex but does not engage in toy or role play associated with the opposite sex
   - Child prefers neutral activities (e.g., drawing, making music) and does not engage in either same-sex or cross-sex toy or role play
   - Child prefers to play with toys and to engage in roles stereotypically associated with own sex
5. Peer relations
   - Child prefers to play with opposite-sex peers
   - Child is a loner or is rejected
   - Child plays with both same-sex and opposite-sex peers
   - Child prefers to play with same-sex peers
6. Mannerisms
   - Child frequently displays motoric movements and speech characteristics that are associated with the opposite sex, whether in "natural" or "exaggerated" form (e.g., in boys, this includes hand movements, hip control, elevated pitch and lisp; in girls, this includes low voice projection)
   - Child occasionally displays motoric movements and speech characteristics that are associated with the opposite sex

(continued)

Table 3.1 (continued)

- Child rarely displays motoric movements and speech characteristics that are associated with the opposite sex
- Child never displays motoric movements and speech characteristics that are associated with the opposite sex
7. Rough-and-tumble play
   - In boys, there is an aversion to rough-and-tumble play or participation in group sports, such as hockey, football, and soccer. There is often a concern regarding physical injury. In girls, there is a strong attraction to rough-and-tumble play and group sports, particularly with boys
   - In boys, there is no interest in rough-and-tumble play or participation in group sports, but the accompanying fear is not present
   - In boys, there is an interest in rough-and-tumble play or participation in group sports. In girls, such interests are not dependent on a male peer group, but, rather are expressed in more typical ways (e.g., mixed-sex teams, all-girl teams)

From Zucker (1992, pp. 327–328). Copyright 1992 by Lawrence Erlbaum Associates, Inc. Reprinted with permission

Table 3.2 Interview for gender identity

1. Are you a ___ (boy/girl)?
2. Do you want to be a ___ (boy/girl)?
3. Do you feel more like a ___ (boy/girl)? Probe, where appropriate
4. Is it better to be a ___ (boy/girl)? Probe, where appropriate
5. When you dream at night, do you ever dream that you are a ___ (boy/girl)? Probe, where appropriate
6. Are there any good things about being a ___ (boy/girl)? Probe, where appropriate

demonstrated adequate psychometric properties with 14 of the 16 items loading on a single factor (>.30). The GIQ may be used alongside observation of play and clinical interviews to evaluate youth with GID. Another instrument, the gender identity interview for children (GIIC), is a 12-item screening instrument that might be useful in the assessment of children with GID (Wallien et al., 2009). Projective measures including the Rorschach (Tuber & Coates, 1985) and the Draw-a-Person (Zucker, Finegan, Doering, & Bradley, 1984) test have also been used to assist in the evaluation of youth. However, the clinician needs to consider the psychometric limitations of the Rorschach and other projective measures in detecting underlying conditions in youth including gender incongruence (Kamphaus & Frick, 2010). In totality, multiple methods and modes of assessment that utilize clinical judgment including knowledge of the literature base, assessment instruments, clinical interviews of caregivers and children, and observation of children's play is an appropriate method of assessing for GID, should the clinician decide to assess for the condition.

3.9   Prevention and Intervention

The literature regarding the treatment of adolescents with GID is scant and mostly anecdotal or descriptive (Bradley, 1990; Davenport & Harrison, 1977; Kronberg, Tyano, Apter, & Wijsenbeek, 1981; Westhead, Olson, & Meyer, 1990). Those from both the accommodation perspective and the psychological intervention perspective indicate that the course of treatment for GID in adolescence and beyond is to allow the youth to accommodate to his or her preferred gender identity and consider the nuances of gender reassignment, if sought (Lothstein, 1982; Zucker, 2006). Working with adult clients with gender dysphoria is beyond the scope of this chapter, but should only be undertaken by therapists with knowledge of the condition and how to treat it. The common therapeutic issues such as counter transference, establishment of a therapeutic alliance, as well as working through a surgical solution to gender dysphoria are just a few of the issues with which a therapist must deal (Zucker & Bradley, 1995).

There are essentially two approaches to the treatment of gender incongruence in children. Both approaches are controversial and require additional empirical validation. The first approach, the therapeutic approach, has been in existence since the 1970s. This approach, first advocated by Rekers and colleagues when working with boys with gender dysphoria consists of extinguishing or punishing selected feminine behaviors (e.g., playing with female dolls or jewelry) and rewarding masculine behaviors (e.g., playing with a Nerf rifle or water gun) (Winkler, 1977; Wolfe, 1979). The rationale for this treatment approach has been justified based upon several factors. First, cross-gender identified children experience extreme social ostracism (Zucker, 2001, 2005, 2006; Zucker & Bradley, 1995) particularly from peers. Boys seem to be rejected at an earlier age. Social ostracism for cross-gender identified individuals often results in social isolation and concomitant behavioral and emotional difficulties. Those from this perspective argue that reducing cross-gender identification may not only alleviate short-term distress by allowing the child to mix with same-sex peers, but also may mitigate or prevent longer-term psychological sequelae. Of course, this approach raises considerable questions and concerns about how cultures define "masculine" and "feminine" behaviors and seems to marginalize all but a narrow definition of masculinity and femininity.

A second view holds that gender dysphoria is secondary to underlying psychopathology in the child and his or her family. Di Ceglie (1995) suggests that cross-gender identification in youth should receive clinical attention at the level of both the child and family (Newman, 1976). For instance, Coates and others (e.g., Bleiberg, Jackson, & Ross, 1986) suggests that separation anxiety is a core symptoms of GID so alleviation of separation anxiety should be a primary treatment goal. A more recent twin study did not find an association between GID and separation anxiety (Coolidge et al., 2002).

A third rationale for treatment of gender incongruence is to prevent later onset of GID in adulthood which sometimes leads to painful operations and other medical measures to align an adult's external genitalia and physiognomy with his or her perceived gender identity (Blanchard & Steiner, 1990).

3.10 Treatment Modalities

3.10.1 Behavior Therapy

There are numerous, older case reports of the use of behavior therapy for the treatment of GID in children (Dowrick, 1983; Hay, Barlow, & Hay, 1981; Rekers & Lovaas, 1974; Rekers, Lovaas, & Low, 1974; Rekers & Mead, 1979; Rekers, Willis, Yates, Rosen, & Low, 1977). Classic behaviorism posits that children learn gender-typed behaviors much as they learn any other behaviors. Gender behaviors, therefore, can be shaped by rewarding some and ignoring or even punishing others. Targets of intervention within behavioral therapy include several cross-gender behaviors including toy and dress-up play, role playing, exclusive affiliation with the opposite sex, and mannerisms. In essence, the child is permitted to engage in gender stereotypical behavior but discoursed to engage in cross-gender behavior. Some treatments have also focused on attempting to improve poor athletic abilities in boys. Most of the case reports focused primarily on overt behaviors and did not target cognitive attributions such as fantasy play or thoughts about wanting to be of the opposite sex. Another type of intervention (e.g., Rekers & Lovaas) that has been used involves differential reinforcement of sex-typed play. For instance, the therapist establishes baseline measures regarding the child's play. A parent or another person is introduced to the session and instructed to attend to the child's same-sex play by looking, smiling, and furnishing verbal praise. The adult is also instructed to ignore cross-gender play by looking away or pretending to do something else. Rekers et al. (1974) note that differential reinforcement of other behavior using social attention has two limitations. First, it was reported that some of the children reverted to the cross-gender play patterns in the adult's absence or in other environments. Second, the generality of the behavior to other settings was limited. There seems to be some evidence that behavior therapy has at a minimum short-term effects on sex-typed behavior of children with GID. Rekers and colleague in follow-up studies from 5 months to over 3 years after treatment reported maintenance of reductions in cross-sex behavior after treatment. These results have been criticized from several angles. Can the behavioral improvement be attributable solely to behavioral therapy without a control group? Second, were the participants selected for inclusion in the study different in some way from other children with GID (e.g., more motivated parents, lower comorbid psychopathology)? Finally, we do not have much empirical data on the long-term outcome of behavior therapy with children with gender incongruence. Rekers (1985) has only provided anecdotal data in one study of 50 children followed-up when he reported changes in gender identity. Second, Rekers, Kilgus, and Rosen (1990) suggested that 29 boys treated by behavior therapy techniques 51 months later experience reduction in cross-gender behavior and that therapy accounted for 20% of the change variance. To date, there are no adolescent follow-up of these same children in regard to their gender identity or perception of participation in behavioral treatment.

3.10.2 *Psychoanalysis*

There are numerous, older case reports of clinicians with a psychoanalytic orientation treating cross-gender identified children with psychoanalytic therapy (Bleiberg et al., 1986; Greenson, 1966; Karush, 1993; Siegel, 1991, Silverman, 1990). The psychoanalytic position states that cross-gender behavior starts in the preoedipal years. Targets for intervention include the mother–child relationship. There is the presumption that a real or perceived loss of the mother preceded the emergence of feminine behaviors. This loss is thought to wound the child resulting in a defensive reaction where the child resorts to fetish type behavioral enactments of gender representations. The goal of therapy is to help the child work through the loss of the attachment figure which should in turn alleviate the desire to engage in cross-gender behavior. Several articles (e.g., Coates & Person, 1985; Coates et al., 1991) reported that psychological loss or withdrawal of the mother during a sensitive time period for gender identity formation resulted in psychological and behavioral sequelae including separation anxiety, and feminine behavior for boys consistent with those who actually lost their mothers. Conversely, some psychoanalytical therapists (e.g., Loeb & Shane, 1982; Stoller, 1965, 1985) suggest that feminine identification is caused not by excessive distance from the mother but extreme closeness to her. In this view, the task will be to help the boy separate or individuate from the mother.

Paternal involvement in GID has received research attention. In many case reports, the father has been described as either physically absent or emotionally peripheral. This made it difficult for the father to diffuse distortions in the mother–son relationship. If the father is absent or uninvolved, the target of therapy will be to help the child obtain a more complete view of men and maleness and work through the negative impact of the father's psychopathology. As part of this process, the psychoanalytic position might suggest a male therapist to allow for transference phenomenon including idealization and identification that can help facilitate a masculine identification.

Finally, one other psychoanalytic perspective holds that parental attitudes toward masculinity and femininity could impact a child's gender development. Stoller (1965) argued that mothers of feminine boys hold males and masculinity in disdain and had their own gender identity conflicts in childhood. The son of this mother believes that his mother will reject him if he portrays himself as masculine but that he can preserve his relationship with her if he is feminine. From another angle, there appears to be parental tolerance and even encouragement of cross-gender behavior (Loeb & Shane, 1982; Lothstein, 1988). To counter, the psychoanalytic perspective would hold that both parents should encourage a sex-typed gender identity.

The therapeutic approach of Green, Newman, and Stoller (1972) is one that deserves comment since it seems to encapsulate much of the psychoanalytic position. These authors suggested four overarching goals for therapy. First, the child should develop a trusting relationship with his male therapist. Second, the parent's should increase their concern about their son's cross-gender behavior. Third, the father should increase his role in the child's life. Fourth, the parents should be sensitized to the dynamics of their own relationship in order to alter the mother–son over closeness and the father's peripheral role in the family. As part of this therapeutic process, the child is taught that being masculine is good and signs of masculinity are given approval.

3.10.3   Group Therapy

Several older studies have discussed the treatment of cross-gender identified boys via group therapy. Green and Fuller's (1973) study involved seven boys ranging in age from 4 to 9 years old. A male therapist facilitated weekly sessions on a playground where gender-typical behaviors were reinforced and gender atypical behaviors were admonished. Anecdotal reports from the authors, but no further data, suggested a decrease in feminine behavior and an increase in masculine behavior. Group therapy with boys between 8 and 13 was employed by Bates, Skillbeck, Smith, and Bentler (1975). Feminine behavior was not discouraged, rather therapist modeling of gender-typical behaviors was utilized along with involvement of the father to enhance the father–son relationship. Bates et al. (1975) reported less cross-dressing behavior, improved social skills development for play with boys, and increased masculine interests and abilities. Meyer-Bahlburg (1993) produced another study in which parents of boys with GID were to arrange consistent play dates for their sons with other boys. The goal was to have the boys with GID associate with other non threatening boys who could serve as a role model for more gender-typical play and activities. Detailed outcome data were lacking although the authors reported a reduction in cross-gender behavior.

3.10.4   Effectiveness of Psychotherapy

Case reports suggest that psychotherapy may have a short-term effect on improving sex-type play and cross-gender identification. However, case reports did not assign children with GID to a control group so shorter-term outcomes appear difficult to analyze. Long-term, randomized, and well-controlled follow-up studies into adolescence are nonexistent. Anecdotal evidence presented by several authors of psychotherapy case reports indicated positive effects of therapy on gender identity and transsexual behavior (Zucker, 1985). Still, longer-term follow-up studies are generally unavailable.

3.10.5   Transition to Preferred Gender

Case accounts, also highlighted in popular media outlets, furnish insight into the process by which a child transitions to his or her preferred gender. This approach requires individual and family therapy as well as advocacy on the part of the caregivers to request school-based accommodation for the child (Lev, 2004). The first step involves supporting the child's desire to present as the preferred gender while at home. The next step will involve a coming out process to the public (Bockting & Coleman, 2007). The parent will need to be assured that certain cross-gendered rights are afforded within the school (e.g., allowance for boys to wear dresses and stereotypically female jewelry; allowance to change clothing and use the restroom in the nurse's office). After consulting with school personnel, the child may be permitted to come to school as his or her preferred gender. Bullying and ridicule is a problem faced by any child, let alone a child with gender variance. Therefore, the family of the child with gender incongruence will need to be constantly vigilant, perhaps assuming an advocacy role, regarding school policies toward children who identify with the opposite gender (Fraser, 2009). One of the greatest steps that can and should be taken is to approach both the school psychologist and the principal to ensure that antibullying, antihate crime policies have been established. If not, then it is essential that the parent enlist the support of the school psychologist and the school counselor to establish such policies.

As the child moves closer to adolescence, medication intervention may become necessary to suppress puberty (Ettner, Monstrey, & Eyler, 2007). As the youth moves through adolescence and approaches the age of majority, the option of hormonal therapy and surgical intervention for sex reassignment should be discussed as options for transitioning (Ettner et al., 2007). As part of this process, the adolescent should be involved in counseling to ensure the youth is indeed ready for and interested in transitioning. Regardless of the adolescent's level of functioning, guidance and support will be critical as the adolescent adopts a particular gender role (Cohen-Kettenis & van Goozen, 1997; Fraser, 2009; Lev, 2004).

3.11 Conclusion and Future Directions

Because of the intense suffering and social stigmatization faced by individuals with gender identity disorder, it is imperative to conduct studies regarding possible neurological, genetic, and biological underpinnings of gender variance. There is need for long-term treatment outcome studies with larger sample sizes. What appears in the literature to date is still primarily based upon studies that have small sample sizes with limited follow-up. The majority of psychological treatment outcome studies are now also 10 years old or older. And, there is an absolute dearth of available outcome research regarding gender transitioning. This research is critically needed.

Because individuals in the transgender community face considerable persecution, the negative impact on their well-being needs to be considered in the face of scientific contributions. If it is found, indeed, that intervention for youth with GID is harmful and akin to reparative therapy for individuals with a homosexual orientation, then treatment should be immediately stopped and a position paper advanced by all major psychiatric/psychological groups. Zucker and colleagues (e.g., Zucker, 2006; Zucker & Bradley, 1995) contend that after a certain age (age 12 or so), treatment is ineffective and can have an adverse impact on social-emotional development.

On the other hand, Zucker and colleagues indicate that intervention can divert a youth from gender dysphoria if the youth receives intervention in early childhood (before age 12). Thus, Zucker and colleagues contend that there appears to be a critical period – a period of gender identity plasticity (Zucker) – by which intervention for gender dysphoria might be tenable.

Instruments for the evaluation of gender identity are needed. Perhaps these instruments can assist researchers in more fully understanding gender variance and allow for conclusions to be based more on empirical data than on case reports emanating from books, presentations at scholarly societies, and unpublished manuscripts. If clinicians decide to intervene with youth, Zucker and colleagues caution that the window of opportunity appears to be prior to about age 12. After that age, Zucker (2006) contends that intervention should focus on assisting a youth transition to his or her to preferred gender and helping families work through and understand this process. When intervention occurs for children with gender dysphoria, appropriate follow-up protocols across several stages of development including the perspective of the youth regarding how the intervention impacted them should be put in place. In so doing, it is similarly important to be mindful of the perspective of the transgender community who support the view that intervention for gender dysphoria amounts to reparative therapy, is psychologically harmful, and should be eschewed (Fraser, 2009). The merits of both perspectives should be entertained by any serious scholar or practitioner seeking to conduct research on or treat children with gender dysphoria. The stakes are critically high. This is a politically hot topic because of the intense discrimination faced by those who are ultimately affected. Winters (2008) described the scientific debate metaphorically as one between an etymologist and a butterfly who is pinned upon the board by the etymologist studying the butterfly. Although just a scientific exercise for the etymologist, the detached investigation by the scientist has an impact on the subject which can be quite harmful, if not lethal. To date, unfortunately, the available scientific literature is limited. And, that which is available from the psychological treatment camp is increasingly dated. The prospect for future generations of researchers to establish well-controlled studies with long-term follow-up may be dimmed by groups opposed to intervention for youth with gender dysphoria citing a linkage to reparative therapy. Therefore, perhaps the field should focus its efforts on possible biological linkages to gender variation. Large size, prospective twin studies like that of Coolidge, Thede, and Young (2002) is a promising avenue of research that may help to uncover the biological and genetic underpinnings of GID. In fact, Coolidge et al. concluded within their study – but perhaps prematurely so because their model was just outside the level of statistical significance – that gender identity may be more a matter of biology than a matter of choice.

When conducting research regarding GID, an element of grace may be necessary to temper scientific conclusions that are highly nuanced and therefore easily misinterpreted by broader society, some of whom already foster an intolerance for diversity of any sort, particularly that of non traditional gender construction. Above all, the scientific community must strike a balance between social responsibility and scientific evaluation.

References

American Psychiatric Association. (2000). *Diagnostic and statistical manual of mental disorders – Text revision* (4th ed. rev). Washington, DC: Author.

Ault, A., & Brzuzy, S. (2009). Removing gender identity disorder from the Diagnostic and Statistical Manual of Mental Disorders: A call for action. *Social Work, 54*, 187–189.

Bailey, J. M., & Pillard, R. C. (1991). A genetic study of male sexual orientation. *Archives of General Psychiatry, 48*, 1089–1096.

Baily, J. M., Dunne, M. P., & Martin, N. G. (2000). Genetic and environmental influences on sexual orientation and its correlates in an Australian twin sample. *Journal of Personality and Social Psychology, 78*, 524–536.

Bakker, A., Van Kesteren, P. M., Gooren, L. J., & Bezemer, P. D. (1993). The prevalence of transsexualism in the Netherlands. *Acta Psychiatrica Scandinavica, 87*, 237–238.

Bates, J. E., Skilbeck, W. M., Smith, K. V. R., & Bentler, P. M. (1974). Gender role abnormalities in boys: An analysis of clinical ratings. *Journal of Abnormal Child Psychology, 2*, 1–16.

Bates, J. E., Skillbeck, W. M., Smith, K. V. R., & Bentler, P. M. (1975). Intervention with families of gender-disturbed boys. *The American Journal of Orthopsychiatry, 45*, 150–157.

Bell, A. P., Weinberg, M. S., & Hammersmith, S. K. (1981). *Sexual preference, It's development in men and women*. Bloomington, IN: Indiana University Press.

Bem, D. (1996). Exotic becomes erotic: A developmental theory of sexual orientation. *Psychological Review, 103*, 320–335.

Bem, D. (2000). Exotic becomes erotic: Interpreting the biological correlates of sexual orientation. *Archives of Sexual Behavior, 26*(6), 531–548.

Bentler, P. M. (1976). A typology of transsexualism: Gender identity theory and data. *Archives of Sexual Behavior, 5*, 567–584.

Blanchard, R. (1989). The classification and labeling of nonhomosexual gender dysphorias. *Archives of Sexual Behavior, 18*, 315–334.

Blanchard, R., & Steiner, B. W. (1990). *Clinical management of gender identity disorders in children and adults*. Washington, DC: American Psychiatric Press.

Bleiberg, E., Jackson, L., & Ross, J. L. (1986). Gender identity disorder and object loss. *Journal of the American Academy of Child Psychiatry, 25*, 58–67.

Bockting, W. O. (2008). Psychotherapy and the real-life experience: From gender dichotomy to gender diversity. *Sexologies, 17*, 211–224.

Bockting, W. O., & Coleman, E. (2007). Developmental stages of the transgender coming-out process. In R. Ettner, S. Monstrey, & A. Eyler (Eds.), *Principles of transgender medicine and surgery* (pp. 185–208). New York: Haworth Press.

Bradley, S. J. (1990). Gender dysphorias in childhood and adolescence. In B. D. Garfinkel, G. A. Carlson, & E. B. Weller (Eds.), *Psychiatric disorders in children and adolescents* (pp. 121–134). Philadelphia: W. B. Saunders.

Brown, D. G. (1957). The development of sex-role inversion and homosexuality. *The Journal of Pediatrics, 50*, 613–619.

Brown, D. G. (1958). Inversion and homosexuality. *The American Journal of Orthopsychiatry, 28*, 424–429.

Burke, P. (1996). *Gender shock: Exploding the myths of male and female*. New York: Bantam Doubleday Dell Publishing.

Chazan, S. E. (1995). *The simultaneous treatment of parent and child*. New York: Basic Books.

Coates, S. (1990). Ontogenesis of boyhood gender identity disorder. *The Journal of the American Academy of Psychoanalysis, 18*, 414–438.

Coates, S., Friedman, R. C., & Wolfe, S. (1991). The etiology of boyhood gender identity disorder: A model for integrating temperament, development, and psychodynamics. *Psychoanalytic Dialogues, 1*, 481–523.

Coates, S., & Person, E. S. (1985). Extreme boyhood femininity: Isolated behavior or pervasive disorder? *Journal of the American Academy of Child Psychiatry, 24*, 702–709.

Cohen-Kettenis, P. T., & van Goozen, S. H. M. (1997). Sex reassignment of adolescent transsexuals: A follow-up study. *Journal of the American Academy of Child and Adolescent Psychiatry, 36,* 263–271.

Coolidge, F. L., Thede, L. L., & Young, S. E. (2002). The heritability of gender identity disorder in a child and adolescent twin sample. *Behavior Genetics, 32,* 251–257.

Corbett, K. (1998). Cross-gendered identification and homosexual boyhood: Toward a more complex theory of gender. *The American Journal of Orthopsychiatry, 68,* 352–360.

Costabile, A., Smith, P. K., Matheson, L., Aston, J., Hunter, T., & Boulton, M. (1991). Cross-national comparison of how children distinguish serious and playful fighting. *Developmental Psychology, 27,* 881–887.

Davenport, C. W., & Harrison, S. I. (1977). Gender identity change in a female adolescent transsexual. *Archives of Sexual Behavior, 6,* 327–341.

de Cuypere, G., Knudson, G., & Bockting, W. O. (2009). *WPATH's consensus statement on gender dysphoria and the DSM-V.* Symposium presented at The World Professional Association for Transgender Health, XXI Biennial Symposium, Oslo, Norway.

Di Ceglie, D. (1995). Gender identity disorders in children and adolescents. *British Journal of Hospital Medicine, 53,* 251–256.

Dowrick, P. W. (1983). Video training of alternatives to cross-gender identity behaviors in a 4-year-old boy. *Child and Family Behavior Therapy, 5,* 59–65.

Duberman, M. (2002). *Cures: A gay man's odyssey.* Cambridge, MA: Westview.

Dunne, M. P., Bailey, J. M., Kirk, K. M., & Martin, N. G. (2000). The subtlety of sex-atypicality. *Archives of Sexual Behavior, 29,* 549–565.

Ehrensaft, D. (2007). Raising girlyboys: A parent's perspective. *Studies in Gender and Sexuality, 8,* 269–292.

Elizabeth, P. H., & Green, R. (1984). Childhood sex-role behaviors: Similarities and differences in twins. *Acta Geneticae Medicae et Gemellologiae, 33,* 173–179.

Ettner, R., Monstrey, S., Eyler, A. E. (2007). Principles of Transgender Medicine and Surgery. Binghamton, NY: Haworth Press.

Fraser, L. (2009). Psychotherapy in the World Professional Association for Transgender Health's Standards of Care: Background and recommendations. *International Journal of Transgenderism, 11,* 110–126.

Freud, A. (1965). *Normality & pathology in childhood: Assessments of development.* Madison, CT: International Universities Press.

Gottschalk, L. (2003). Same-sex sexuality and childhood gender non-conformity: A spurious connection. *Journal of Gender Studies, 12,* 35–50.

Green, R. (1976). One-hundred ten feminine and masculine boys: Behavioral contrasts and demographic similarities. *Archives of Sexual Behavior, 5,* 425–446.

Green, R. (1987). *The "sissy boy syndrome" and the development of homosexuality.* New Haven, CT: Yale University Press.

Green, R., & Fuller, M. (1973). Group therapy with feminine boys and their parents. *International Journal of Group Psychotherapy, 23,* 54–68.

Green, R., & Money, J. (1960). Incongruous gender role: nongenital manifestations in prepubertal boys. *The Journal of Nervous and Mental Disease, 131,* 160–168.

Green, R., Newman, L. E., & Stoller, R. J. (1972). Treatment of boyhood transsexualism: An interim report of four years' experience. *Archives of General Psychiatry, 26,* 213–217.

Greenson, R. (1966). A transvestite boy and a hypothesis. *The International Journal of Psychoanalysis, 47,* 396–403.

Hamer, D. H., Hu, S., Magnuson, V. L., Hu, N., & Pattatucci, A. M. L. (1993). A linkage between DNA markers on the X chromosome and male sexual orientation. *Science, 261,* 321–327.

Hausman, K. (2003). Controversy continues to grow over DSM's GID diagnosis. *Psychiatric News, 38,* 25.

Hay, W. M., Barlow, D. H., & Hay, L. R. (1981). Treatment of stereotypic cross-gender motor behavior using covert modeling in a boy with gender identity confusion. *Journal of Consulting and Clinical Psychology, 49,* 388–394.

Johnson, L. L., Bradley, S. J., Birkenfeld-Adams, A. S., Tadzins Kuksis, M. A., Maing, D. M., Mitchell, J. N., et al. (2004). A parent-report gender identity questionnaire for children. *Archives of Sexual Behavior, 33*, 105–116.

Kamphaus, R. W., & Frick, P. J. (2010). *Clinical assessment of child and adolescent personality and behavior* (3rd ed.). New York: Springer.

Karush, R. K. (1993). Sam: A child analysis. *Journal of Clinical Psychoanalysis, 2*, 43–62.

Kopay, D., & Young, P. D. (2001). *David Kopay story*. Los Angeles: Advocate Books.

Kronberg, J., Tyano, S., Apter, A., & Wijsenbeek, H. (1981). Treatment of transsexualism in adolescence. *Journal of Adolescence, 4*, 177–185.

Langer, S. J., & Martin, J. I. (2004). How dresses can make you mentally ill: Examining gender identity disorder in children. *Child and Adolescent Social Work Journal, 21*, 5–23.

Leaper, C. (1994). *Childhood gender segregation: Causes and consequences*. San Francisco: Jossey-Bass.

Lev, A. (2004). *Transgender emergence: Therapeutic guidelines for working with gender-variant people and their families*. New York: Haworth Clinical Practice.

Loeb, L., & Shane, N. (1982). The resolution of a transsexual with in a five-year-old boy. *Journal of the American Psychoanalytic Association, 30*, 419–434.

Lothstein, L. M. (1982). Sex reassignment surgery: Historical, bioethical, and theoretical issues. *The American Journal of Psychiatry, 139*, 417–426.

Lothstein, L. M. (1988). Self object failure with gender identity. In A. Goldberg (Ed.), *Frontiers in self psychology* (Vol. 3, pp. 213–235). Hillsdale, NJ: Analytic.

Maccoby, E. E., & Jacklin, C. N. (1987). Gender segregation in childhood. *Advances in Child Development and Behavior, 20*, 239–287.

Magee, M., & Miller, D. (1992). She foreswore her womanhood: psychoanalytic views of female homosexuality. *Clinical Social Work Journal, 20*, 67–85.

Marantz, S., & Coates, S. (1991). Mothers of boys with gender identity disorder: A comparison of matched controls. *Journal of the American Academy of Child and Adolescent Psychiatry, 30*, 310–315.

Martin, R. P., & Dombrowski, S. C. (2008). *Prenatal exposures: Psychological and educational consequences for children*. New York: Springer.

Mass, L. (1990). *Dialogues of the sexual revolution*. New York: Haworth Press.

Meyer, W., Bockting, W., Cohen-Kettenis, P., Coleman, E., DiCeglie, D., Devor, H., et al. (2001). The standards of care for gender identity disorder, sixth version. *Journal of Psychological Human Sex, 13*, 1–30.

Meyer-Bahlburg, H. F. L. (1993). *Gender identity disorder in young boys: A treatment protocol*. Paper presented at the XIII International Symposium on Gender Dysphoria, New York.

Meyer-Bahlburg, H. F. L. (2009). Variants of gender differentiation in somatic disorders of sex development: Recommendations for Version 7 of the World Professional Association for Transgendered Health's Standards of Care. *International Journal of Transgenderism, 11*, 226–237.

Minter, S. (1999). Diagnosis and treatment of gender identity disorder in children. In M. Rottnek (Ed.), *Sissies and Tomboys: Gender nonconformity and homosexual childhood*. New York: New York University Press.

Newman, L. E. (1976). Treatment for the parents of feminine boys. *The American Journal of Psychiatry, 133*, 683–687.

Olsson, S. E., & Möller, A. (2006). Regret after sex reassignment surgery in a male-to-female transsexual: A long-term follow-up. *Archives of Sexual Behavior, 35*, 501–506.

Pellegrini, A. D. (1989). What is a category? The case of rough-and-tumble play. *Ethology and Sociobiology, 10*, 331–341.

Phillips, G., & Over, R. (1995). Differences between heterosexual, bisexual and lesbian women in recalled childhood experiences. *Archives of Sexual Behavior, 24*, 1–20.

Phoeniz, C. H., Goy, R. W., Gerall, A. A., & Young, W. C. (1959). Organizing action of prenatally administered testosterone propionate on the tissues mediating mating behavior in the female guinea pig. *Endocrinology, 65*, 369–382.

Pleak, R. (1999). Ethical issues in diagnosing and treating gender-dysphoric children and adolescents. In M. Rottenek (Ed.), *Sissies and Tomboys: Gender nonconformity and homosexual childhood.* New York: New York University Press.

Plomin, R. (1994). *Genetics and experience: The interplay between nature and nurture.* Thousand Oaks, CA: Sage.

Rekers, G. A. (1985). Gender identity problems. In P. A. Bornstein & A. E. Kazdin (Eds.), *Handbook of clinical behavior therapy with children* (pp. 658–699). Homewood, Il: Dorsey.

Rekers, G. A., Kilgus, M., & Rosen, A. C. (1990). Long-term effects of treatment for gender identity disorder of childhood. *Journal of Psychology and Human Sexuality, 3,* 121–153.

Rekers, G. A., & Lovaas, O. I. (1974). Behavioral treatment of deviant sex-role behaviors in a male child. *Journal of Applied Behavior Analysis, 7,* 173–190.

Rekers, G. A., Lovaas, O. I., & Low, B. (1974). The behavioral treatment of a transsexual preadolescent boy. *Journal of Abnormal Child Psychology, 2,* 99–116.

Rekers, G. A., & Mead, S. (1979). Early intervention for female sexual identity disturbance: Self-monitoring of play behavior. *Journal of Abnormal Child Psychology, 7,* 405–423.

Rekers, G. A., & Swihart, J. J. (1989). The association of gender identity disorder with parental separation. *Psychological Reports, 65,* 1272–1274.

Rekers, G. A., Willis, T. J., Yates, C. E., Rosen, A. C., & Low, B. P. (1977). Assessment of childhood gender behavior change. *Journal of Child Psychology and Psychiatry, 18,* 53–65.

Richardson, J. (1999). Response: Finding the disorder in gender identity disorder. *Harvard Review of Psychiatry, 7,* 43–50.

Roberto, G. (1983). Issues in diagnosis and treatment of transsexualism. *Archives of Sexual Behavior, 12,* 445–473.

Saghir, M., & Robins, E. (1973). *Male and female homosexuality: A companion investigation.* New York: New York University Press.

Sedgwick, E. K. (1991). *Epistemology of the closet.* Berkeley, CA: University of California Press.

Siegel, E. V. (1991). *Middle-class waifs: The psychodynamic treatment of affectively disturbed children.* Hillsdale, NJ: Analytic.

Silverman, M. A. (1990). The prehomosexual boy in treatment. In C. W. Socarides & V. D. Volkan (Eds.), *The homosexualities: Reality, fantasy, and the arts* (pp. 177–197). Madison, CT: International Universities Press.

Stoller, R. J. (1965). The mother's contribution to infantile transvestic behavior. *The International Journal of Psychoanalysis, 47,* 384–395.

Stoller, R. J. (1967). It's only a phase: Femininity in boys. *Journal of the American Medical Association, 201,* 314–315.

Stoller, R. J. (1985). *Presentations of gender.* New Haven, CT: Yale University Press.

Tuber, S., & Coates, S. (1985). Interpersonal phenomena in the Rorschach's of extremely feminine boys. *Pyschoanalytic Psychology, 2,* 251–265.

Vance, S. R., Cohen-Kettenis, P. T., Drescher, J., Meyer-Bahlburg, H. F. L., Pfafflin, F., & Zucker, K. J. (2010). Opinions about the DSM gender identity disorder diagnosis: Results from an international survey administered to organizations concerned with the welfare of transgender people. *International Journal of Transgenderism, 12*(1), 1–14.

Wallien, M. S. C., Quilty, L. C., Steensma, T. D., Singh, D., Lambert, S. L., Leroux, A., et al. (2009). Cross-national replication of the Gender Identity Interview for Children. *Journal of Personality Assessment.* doi:10.1080/00223890903228463.

Westhead, V. A., Olson, S. J., & Meyer, J. K. (1990). Gender identity disorders in adolescence. In M. Sugar (Ed.), *Adolescent sexuality* (pp. 87–107). New York: Norton.

Whitam, F. L., Diamond, M., & Martin, J. (1993). Homosexual orientation in twins: A report on 61 pairs and three triplet sets. *Archives of Sexual Behavior, 22,* 187–206.

Winkler, R. C. (1977). What types of sex-role behavior should behavior modification promote? *Journal of Applied Behavior Analysis, 10,* 549–552.

Winters, K. (2008). *Gender madness in American psychiatry: Essays from the struggle for dignity.* Dillon, CO: GID Reform Advocates.

Wolfe, B. E. (1979). Behavioral treatment of childhood gender disorders: A conceptual and empirical critique. *Behavior Modification, 3*, 550–575.

Zucker, B. (1985). Cross-gender-identified children. In B. W. Steiner (Ed.), *Gender dysphoria: Development, research, management* (pp. 75–174). New York: Plenum.

Zucker, K. J. (1992). Gender identity disorder. In S. R. Hooper, G. W. Hynd, & R. E. Mattison (Eds.), *Child psychopathology: Diagnostic criteria and clinical assessment* (pp. 305–342). Hillsdale, NJ: Erlbaum.

Zucker, K. J. (2001). Gender identity disorder in children and adolescents. In G. O. Gabbard (Ed.), *Treatments of psychiatric disorders* (3rd ed., pp. 2069–2094). Washington, DC: American Psychiatric Press.

Zucker, K. J. (2005). Gender identity disorder in children and adolescents. *Annual Review of Clinical Psychology, 1*, 467–492.

Zucker, K. J. (2006). Commentary on Langer and Martin's (2004) "How dresses can make you mentally ill: Examining gender identity disorder in children". *Child and Adolescent Social Work Journal, 23*, 533–555.

Zucker, K. J. (2008). On the "natural history" of gender identity disorder in children [Editorial]. *Journal of the American Academy of Child and Adolescent Psychiatry, 47*, 1361–1363.

Zucker, K. J. (2009). The DSM diagnostic criteria for gender identity disorder in children. *Archives of Sexual Behavior*. doi:10.1007/s10508-009-9540-4.

Zucker, K. J., & Bradley, S. J. (1995). *Gender identity disorder and psychosexual problems in children and adolescents*. New York: Guilford.

Zucker, K. J., Finegan, J. K., Doering, R. W., & Bradley, S. J. (1984). Two subgroups of gender-problem children. *Archives of Sexual Behavior, 13*, 27–39.

Zuger, B. (1988). Early effeminate behavior in boys: Outcome and significance for homosexuality. *The Journal of Nervous and Mental Disease, 172*, 90–97.

Zuger, B. (1989). Homosexuality in families of boys with early effeminate behavior: An epidemiological study. *Archives of Sexual Behavior, 18*, 155–166.

Chapter 4
Munchhausen Syndrome by Proxy

*Your reality, sir, is lies and balderdash and I'm delighted to say
that I have no grasp of it whatsoever.*

–The Adventures of Baron Munchausen (1988)

Conrad was 7 years old when he died from pneumonia after months on a life support
system. Over the course of his young life, Conrad had been treated for epilepsy and had
been admitted to the hospital on numerous occasions for tests and treatments. Eventually,
evidence mounted that suggested that his mother had fabricated the symptoms of
epilepsy and that she had induced illness by giving Conrad antiepilepsy medications.
She was sentenced to 10 years in prison for child cruelty (Horwath & Tidbury, 2009).

4.1 Overview

In 1951, Asher described Munchhausen's syndrome, a condition in which a person
self-induces, feigns, or aggravates an illness or injury to gain attention and medical
treatment. Some individuals seek to be hospitalized and even submit to invasive,
unnecessary procedures. Asher chose the term "Munchhausen's syndrome" to
describe the disorder because he likened the stories told by these individuals to the
dramatic and untruthful stories that the famous Baron von Munchhausen, a German
military man, told about himself (Patterson, 1988). Decades later in 1977, Meadow
coined the term "Munchhausen syndrome by proxy" (MSBP) to describe a form of
child abuse in which a caretaker induces or deliberately exaggerates an illness in a
child for attention-seeking purposes. MSBP is a form of abuse that is associated
with deleterious outcomes, including high mortality, morbidity, family disruption,
and increased chance of harm to siblings of the abused child (Klepper, Heringhaus,
Wurthmann, & Voit, 2008). Although it is a rare disorder, it is an important one to
recognize, given the often times devastating effects. This chapter reviews the history of MSBP, criteria for identification, potential treatments, and suggested future
directions for research.

S.C. Dombrowski et al., *Assessing and Treating Low Incidence/High Severity
Psychological Disorders of Childhood*, DOI 10.1007/978-1-4419-9970-2_4,
© Springer Science+Business Media, LLC 2011

4.2   Historical Context

Baron Karl Friedrich Hieronymus von Munchhausen was born in Germany in 1720 and joined the Russian cavalry as a young man. Upon his retirement, he would regale people with stories of his travels, sometimes exaggerating to a ridiculous point. There is no evidence to suggest that the baron, or his listeners, took his tales seriously. However, in 1785, Rudolf Eric Raspe anonymously published a book of 17 of these stories, *Baron von Munchhausen's Narrative of His Marvellous* (sic) *Travels and Campaigns in Russia.* The initial printing sold poorly, so the second edition was expanded, illustrated with woodcuts, and translated into German. The book in its second printing became very popular and caused Baron von Munchhausen to become an instant, albeit reluctant, celebrity. Tourists began to trespass on his estate and invade his privacy and as a result, the baron initiated legal action against the author of the book. However, Raspe had published anonymously and, thus, the lawsuit proved fruitless. Shortly before his death at age 77, the Baron granted an interview to the father of the editor of the sixth German edition of the book and expressed his disdain and resentfulness for the author (Patterson, 1988).

During the mid-20th century, Asher wrote a paper for *The Lancet* in which he described adult patients who frequented doctor offices and hospitals with factitious somatic complaints. Asher recognized a pattern among these patients that included both presenting with increasingly dramatic symptoms and demanding painful diagnostic procedures and treatments. In the initial paper, he made a distinction between the organ systems involved in presentation: (a) abdominal symptoms, with repeated complaints and sometimes numerous surgeries that resulted in scarring ("grill stomach"); (b) hemorrhagic symptoms with frequent bleeding; and (c) neurological symptoms which included seizures, headaches, fainting, or paralysis (Heubrock, 2001). Asher selected the term "Munchausen syndrome" (anglicized from the original German spelling) because of the similarity of the wanderings from doctor to doctor and fabrications of illness observed in these patients to the stories attributed to Baron von Munchhausen. It should be noted that the similarity ends there – the baron was never reported to have submitted himself to the medical treatments that patients identified with the syndrome that bears his name do (Howe, Jordan, & Lockert, 1983).

More than 25 years after Asher published his work, Meadow coined the term "Munchausen by proxy" when he reported a form of child abuse in which mothers deliberately induced physical symptoms of illness in their offspring (Gross, 2008). Although the term has been used to describe abuse in adults (e.g., with couples and among health care workers who have abused people under their care), the term "Munchausen syndrome by proxy" generally is reserved for parents who induce illness in their children. In most cases, it is the mother who perpetrates the abuse (Bande & García-Alba, 2008). Meadow's original paper published in *The Lancet* in 1977 related the cases of two mothers who made their children ill over a period of years before being detected. In the first case, the parent continually provided false information in regard to her daughter's symptoms, tampered with urine specimens to alter the results, and interfered with observations by hospital staff. The mother's behavior resulted in numerous anesthetic, surgical, and radiological procedures for the girl. In the second case, the mother intermittently administered toxic doses of salt to her child, which led to myriad medical tests and procedures before the child eventually died (Meadow, 1977). Since this initial publication, numerous cases of MSBP have been detailed in the literature.

4.3 Description and Diagnostic Classification

Since its first usage in 1977, the term MSBP has been used variably from both pediatric and psychiatric perspectives, with missed and mistaken diagnoses resulting. Rosenberg (2003) suggested that formal diagnostic criteria are needed because the disorder can have deleterious effects for both the child and his/her family. First, MSBP can have harmful, and even deadly, results for its child victims. The child may be harmed as a direct result of the actions of the caregiver, or by unnecessary treatments and medical procedures resulting from the fabrication of illness (Bools, Neale, & Meadow, 1994). Once the disorder is diagnosed, the likelihood of successful intervention is poor, if the child remains with the family. Risk of further abuse of the patient and abuse of siblings is high for those not placed in protective custody (Klepper et al., 2008). It also has been suggested that as children grow older, there is a tendency for them to participate in the deception and to believe themselves ill or disabled (Meadow, 1985). Second, misdiagnosis of MSBP can tear a family apart and also result in litigation. Formalization of diagnostic criteria could help to ameliorate or remedy the effects of inconclusive diagnoses (Rosenberg, 2003). However, definitive diagnosis can be difficult because symptoms are unspecific and many times include multiple organ systems (Klepper et al.).

4.3.1 Factitious Disorder by Proxy and Pediatric Condition Falsification

The American Professional Society on the Abuse of Children (APSAC) formed a multidisciplinary work group in the late 1990s whose task was to define the constellation of behaviors that describe MSBP (Ayoub & Alexander, 1998; Siegel & Fischer, 2001). As a result of their work, the task force suggested that MSBP be conceptualized as two separate diagnostic entities. First, the parent who perpetrates the abuse warrants a diagnosis of *factitious disorder by proxy* (FDBP), a psychiatric condition characterized by the falsification of child illness to meet self-serving needs. Second, the child who is subjected to the behaviors of the parent is a victim of *pediatric condition falsification* (PCF). The APSAC introduced these terms to differentiate the abuse a child suffers from MSBP from other forms of abuse (Ayoub & Alexander; Siegel & Fischer).

PCF abuse covers a vast range of inappropriate health-seeking behaviors (Siegel & Fischer, 2001). At one end of the spectrum is classic PCF, which includes exaggeration, fabrication, or simulation of symptoms. At the opposite end of the MSBP spectrum is extreme PCF, which encompasses the direct production of illness, the most lethal type of behavior associated with the disorder. PCF is also considered when parents falsely present a child with behavioral and neurological symptoms, including attention deficit hyperactivity disorder, Tourette's syndrome, or seizures, and also when parents coach a child to fake symptoms of mental illness (Ayoub & Alexander, 1998; Siegel & Fischer). It should be noted that not all cases of PCF abuse necessarily involve a perpetrator who meets criteria for a diagnosis of FDBP. For example, a parent may feel overwhelmed and exaggerate her child's symptoms to gain support. Likewise, a parent might lie about a child's illness to gain custody or to keep the child dependent. The child is still considered to be a victim of PCF in these instances, but the parent should not be diagnosed with FDBP (Siegel & Fischer).

The APSAC task group (Ayoub & Alexander, 1998) listed a number of conditions that may warrant identification as PCF, but that should not be considered FDBP. These conditions include: (a) a parent who abuses his/her child directly, then lies about it (e.g., the parent who tries to suffocate her child to get him to stop crying); (b) the child who fails to thrive because the parent is too overwhelmed to care for the child properly; (c) the parent who falsifies symptoms to get help caring for her child because she is overwhelmed; (d) the overanxious or distressed parent who exaggerates symptoms in order to receive attention for her child when she feels that he/she is not receiving proper care; (e) the child who presents with illness that results in missed school time when the parent's primary motivation is to keep the child at home and dependent; and (f) the parent who is psychotic and presents her child for medical attention (Ayoub & Alexander). Although these circumstances do not warrant classification as MSBP (or FDBP), they are serious issues that warrant intervention.

4.3.2   Warning Signs

A few years after publishing his seminal work in *The Lancet*, Meadow (1985) proposed a list of warning signs for MSBP that are still used in the field and by researchers today. He suggested that the following signals should alert a physician to the possible presence of the disorder: (a) the child's illness is unexplained, prolonged, or extraordinary; (b) the symptoms are incongruous and only observed when the perpetrator is present; (c) attempted treatments have proven ineffective; (d) the child is alleged by the caretaker to be allergic to a wide variety of foods and drugs; (e) the mother does not appear to be as worried about the child's illness as doctors and nurses; (f) the mother is constantly with the child in the hospital, not even leaving for brief outings; (g) the mother has formed unusually close relationships with medical staff; (h) a sudden unexplained infant death has occurred in the family; and (i) the family includes many individuals alleged to have serious medical conditions. Meadow indicated that when any of the warning signs suggest MSBP, every effort should be made to establish with certainty that fabrication of illness is taking place to afford intervention and avoid catastrophe for the child.

4.3.3 Rosenberg's Diagnostic Criteria

Rosenberg (2003) proposed a set of indicators that, when observed, may suggest MSBP: (a) the child is presented on a frequent basis for medical care; and (b) there appears to be tampering with the child and/or his medical situation and the child has a condition that cannot be adequately explained medically. Finally, Rosenberg indicated that MSBP can definitely be ruled out when the following criteria are met: (a) the child has been presented for medical care repeatedly; and (b) the illness has been wholly and credibly accounted for in some other way. However, Rosenberg stressed that knowledge of a case changes with time, as more testing and reports become available. Thus, the degree of medical certainty surrounding a diagnosis of MSBP may heighten or diminish as more evidence is collected and reviewed. In addition, it should be noted that there are no standard medical terms to define the degree of certainty of diagnosis. For example, one doctor could refer to a diagnosis as a *possible diagnosis*, whereas another could use terms such as *provisional diagnosis* or *working diagnosis*. Although this approach may work well with other medical diagnoses, it is not ideal for situations involving child abuse because of the legal implications (Rosenberg).

4.3.4 The Diagnostic and Statistical Manual of Mental Disorders

Although MSBP does not appear by name in the *Diagnostic and Statistical Manual of Mental Disorders-IV-Text Revision* (DSM-IV TR; American Psychiatric Association [APA], 2000), the manual does include an entry for factitious disorder by proxy (FDBP) and these terms are often used interchangeably in the literature (Mart, 2004). In the manual, FDBP is included in the appendix as a proposal for a category for which more research is needed. Because it is not an official category, research criteria for the disorder are included: (a) intentional production or feigning of physical or psychological symptoms in a person who is under the perpetrator's care; (b) the motivation for the individual's behavior is to assume the sick role by proxy; (c) external incentives, such as economic gain, are not present; and (d) the behavior is not better explained by another mental disorder (APA, 2000). FDBP must be distinguished from a general medical condition, physical or sexual abuse that is not motivated by the goal of assuming the sick role, and malingering, which involves external gain. If criteria are met, the perpetrator can be assumed to have FDBP and, when appropriate, the child can be given a diagnosis of physical abuse of child. In the case of a child who collaborates with the adult in the production of symptoms, that child may also be assigned a diagnosis of factitious disorder (APA). A search of the APA's DSM-V Development Web site (http://www.dsm5.org/Pages/

Default.aspx) did not produce information regarding the inclusion of FDBP in the forthcoming edition, suggesting it will be omitted.

4.4 Prevalence

MSBP lacks diagnostic precision, a controlled research base, and agreement among health care professionals, which renders it an elusive, unclear, and debatable entity (Bütz, Evans, & Webber-Dereszynski, 2009), making actual prevalence rates difficult to document (Schreier & Libow, 1993). However, Shaw, Dayal, Hartman, and DeMaso (2008) reported that annual prevalence likely ranges from 0.4 to 2 cases per 100,000. In a definitional paper, the APSAC extrapolated results from a British study and suggested an even higher incident rate, a minimum of 600 new cases annually in the USA alone (Ayoub & Alexander, 1998). According to the APSAC, the occurrence of MSBP is not as rare as previously believed and there are many cases that go undetected because of the covert nature of the disorder and the lack of public awareness (Ayoub & Alexander).

In her review of 117 cases, Rosenberg (1987) reported that the mean age for children affected by the disorder was 40 months, with equal prevalence in male and female children. The majority of children involved are younger than 5 years, but there are documented cases of MSBP in which the child was older. The presentation in older children and adolescents appears to be similar to that of younger children, but older children are more apt to participate in the deceit with their parents than are their younger counterparts (Shaw et al., 2008). Other statistics indicate that the mortality rate for MSBP is approximately 10%, with a rate as high as 33% in cases involving poisoning or suffocation (Shaw et al.).

Although fathers and other caretakers can be involved in MSBP, the majority of perpetrators, more than 90%, is female (Shaw et al., 2008). Not surprisingly, 14–30% of these women have professional medical training and/or are employed in a health-care setting. Often, these mothers are described as model clients, who interact in an exemplary fashion with both their children and medical staff. However, over time, these same parents are reported to react with inappropriate affect, such as excitement, when discussing their children's symptoms. Many mothers who engage in MSBP report previous psychiatric treatment, commonly for depression or a personality disorder, and/or a history of factitious or somatoform disorders (Shaw et al.).

4.5 Etiological Hypotheses and Theoretical Frameworks

Most etiological theories of MSBP include psychopathology or mental illness in the perpetrator. However, there is no single factor or psychopathology to explain the cause of the disorder. Rather, the etiology most likely lies in an interaction between psychological, sociological, and biological factors (Shaw et al., 2008). Plassmann (1994) suggested that mothers who are affected by MSBP tend toward self-injury or physical self-manipulation because they experience their own bodies and their children's bodies as interchangeable entities. Their histories usually include psychopathology, indications of personality disorders, and childhood abuse. The MSBP behaviors are viewed as the mother's attempt to ward off psychotic and suicidal crises and when she is confronted with her deceitful behavior, the chance for psychotic or suicidal behaviors increases greatly. Confrontation can also cause the mother to suffer from personal illness, often factitious in nature (Plassmann).

It has been posited that parents may engage in the behaviors associated with MSBP because they need the attention or recognition that accompanies the role of parent to the sick child (Shaw et al., 2008). It may be that mothers who perpetrate this type of abuse find a sense of purpose and safety in the middle of the disastrous situation they have personally caused. Commonly, these women report depression and feelings of isolation and loneliness (Rosenberg, 1987), which may be the impetus for attention-seeking behaviors. From a psychodynamic perspective, MSBP may be a reaction to a traumatic loss early in the mother's life, such as maternal rejection, that has caused her to seek close relationships with doctors and other staff. A doctor may inadvertently reinforce this type of relationship due to the doctor's inability to accept the difficulty she is having in resolving the child's clinical presentation (Shaw et al.). It also has been suggested that the parent may be responding to a need to manipulate or deceive authority figures, such as medical personnel. Whatever the mother's motivation, the bond that she forms with doctors and nurses is usually intense and crosses the typical boundaries in the professional and parent relationship (Shaw et al.).

4.5.1   Maternal Psychological and Psychiatric Histories

One study examined the attachment representations in mothers who were identified as having factitious illness by proxy (Adshead & Bluglass, 2005). Attachment theory suggests that mothers who fabricate or induce illness in their children have insecure mental representations of care-giving and eliciting relationships and that unresolved issues related to childhood illness or loss fuel the behaviors associated with MSBP. To examine this theory, Adshead and Bluglass assessed the attachment representations in 85 mothers who had been referred because they had engaged in abnormal illness behaviors by proxy or because there were reasonable grounds for child protective intervention. Participants underwent a clinical psychiatric interview during which the Adult Attachment Interview was administered. This interview, which has documented validity and reliability, gathers an account of the respondent's early care experiences (Adshead & Bluglass).

Results were obtained for 67 cases. Attachment data indicated that 85% of the participants were rated as insecure. Patterns of insecurity that were uncovered included insecure-dismissing, insecure-enmeshed, and insecure-cannot classify (Adshead & Bluglass, 2005). The insecure-dismissing parent was described as one who dismisses distress at times of illness, fear, or loss, which may indicate a lack of empathy for another's pain. In this study, 46% of the mothers were identified as this type.

The second type, insecure-enmeshed, was described as the mother who finds it difficult to view herself as a separate person from her family of origin. The enmeshment is with the attachment figures of childhood; in many cases, the individual acted as a caregiver for her own parent as a child. The results indicated that 12% of the mothers in the study fit this category. Those mothers who had a highly disorganized attachment narrative upon assessment were termed as insecure-cannot classify. These mothers may have provided an incoherent interview or a narrative that indicated mixed states of dismissing and enmeshed attachment. Twenty-seven percent of the mothers in the study were not classifiable as either of the two aforementioned types. Finally, 60% of participants related unresolved psychological distress surrounding trauma or loss in childhood (Adshead & Bluglass). Adshead and Bluglass concluded that the study demonstrated that mothers who fabricate and/or induce illness in their offspring have highly disorganized thoughts about caring and being cared for in their own childhoods. This finding has implications for treatment and prevention packages. Rather than viewing the parent's behavior in MSBP as mental illness or a crime to be punished, this view would suggest that the mother has attachment issues from childhood that could be explored through a psychodynamic approach.

Bools et al. (1994) examined the psychiatric histories of mothers in 56 families from across the UK in which there had been fabrication of illness in a child. The authors used hospital notes and, in some cases, general practitioner files to glean information about individual cases. In 19 of the 56 cases, a maternal interview was conducted, which included historical questions about childhood and the administration of two standard psychiatric scales, the *Clinical Interview Schedule* (CIS) and the *Personality Assessment Schedule* (PAS). The CIS was used to assess current mental status and the PAS was administered to gather information about the mother's personality traits (Bools et al.). When lifetime problems of the mother were considered, results indicated that for the 47 mothers for whom there were case note data available, 26 had reported a history of self-harm, 10 had reported substance abuse, and 34 had reported a somatizing disorder. In regard to the somatizing disorder, 15 of the 19 mothers interviewed reported such behaviors as pulling out hair and claiming that it was the result of a disease, claiming to be a diabetic, and fabricating stories about kidney stones and hematemesis (Bools et al.). Finally, of the 19 mothers interviewed, 15 reported emotional abuse or neglect, 4 reported physical abuse, and 5 reported sexual abuse (4 within the family and 1 outside the family) during childhood (Bools et al.).

Although there were limitations to Bools' et al. (1994) study, including the small sample size and reliance on case notes and self-report, the findings suggested that there may be historical events or psychiatric symptoms in the mother that could predict the behaviors associated with MSBP. However, as the authors noted, a detailed evaluation should include assessment of the family functioning, and not just symptoms or behaviors displayed by the mother. It has been suggested that the disorder is systemic and occurs when a mother with an existing somatoform or factitious disorder joins an enmeshed family with a history of exploitation of children (Bools et al.). Although there is no research to support this hypothesis, it seems reasonable to believe that MSBP is the result of dysfunction within the system and that blame most likely should not be placed solely on the mother.

4.5.2 Characteristics of Perpetrators

Libow and Schreier (1986) suggested dividing the behaviors associated with MSBP into three subcategories, "active inducers," "doctor addicts," and "help seekers." Within this framework, active inducers are considered to be prototypical, whereas help seekers may not truly meet the criteria for MSBP. When confronted, perpetrators in the first two subgroups continue to deny their behavior. Conversely, help seekers generally express relief and begin to cooperate when confronted. Those people falling in the third subcategory often share feelings of depression and anxiety when their help-seeking behaviors are brought to light (Libow & Schreier). Consideration of this sort of categorical framework has strong implications for practice. Because active inducers and doctor addicts continue to deny behavior when confronted, medical personnel need to be more persistent in uncovering the true cause of a child's illness.

4.5.3 The Parent/Professional Relationship

Another framework for categorizing parental behaviors in MSBP was suggested by Eminson and Postlethwaite (1992). These authors indicated that because the disorder primarily involves parent consultation with medical professionals, it is also important to consider the professional's behavior in the relationship. Within this proposed framework, the behavior of the parent is considered along two dimensions. First, the appropriateness of the parent's desire to consult should be evaluated. Consultation behaviors should be considered along a continuum from "normal" behavior to "outside of normal" behavior. Commonly, parents and health care professionals are in agreement about the need to consult. However, the normal range of behavior, which lies in the middle of the spectrum, also includes parents who might exhibit more anxiety than the doctor; these parents may be frequent visitors to the doctor's office and may request medications more often than other parents. Conversely, there are also parents who display less anxiety than the doctor, which may cause them to present their children for treatment later in the course of an illness than other parents might. This behavior also can be considered within the normal range (Eminson & Postlethwaite).

At one end of the continuum are the behaviors that comprise MSBP. This pole is characterized by a gross discrepancy between parental and professional views, wherein the parent seeks medical attention despite the professional opinion that it is unnecessary (Eminson & Postlethwaite, 1992). The difference between the parent's desire and the doctor's view becomes so great that the parent causes illness in the child to force the doctor to investigate and treat. A step back from MSBP to normal behavior are the parents who invent or exaggerate symptoms to get the doctor's attention, but who do not evoke symptoms. Between this group and the group considered to exhibit normal behaviors is the group of parents who insist on specialized treatment or who give intrusive attention to every detail of the treatment regimen.

This group of parents does not invent or exaggerate symptoms, but dwells upon existing symptoms and makes the rounds through medical specialists (Eminson & Postlethwaite).

Finally, at the opposite end of the continuum are the parents who neglect their children's health, ignoring professional recommendations for care (Eminson & Postlethwaite, 1992). These parents do not attend to their ill children and ignore presenting symptoms. A step back from this pole toward normal behavior includes the group of parents who present their children for treatment late in the course of illness, or who sporadically attend to treatment regimens. According to Eminson and Postlethwaite, pediatricians serving communities probably see more parents falling at this end of the spectrum than do their professional counterparts working in hospitals.

4.5.4   Factors Affecting the Parent/Child Relationship

Eminson and Postlethwaite (1992) caution that it is important to consider other factors that may impact the parent–child dyad. These variables may be found within the child, parent, wider family, and society and can affect a parent's consultation behavior and her ability to distinguish her child's needs from her own. Factors within the child that may impact the relationship between him and his mother include: (a) his tendency to experience somatic symptoms and his temperament (e.g., anxious or depressive behaviors); (b) his history of illness, including serious illness; and (c) his learning that symptoms of illness gain attention from his parent better than other behaviors (Eminson & Postlethwaite). This discussion is not intended to suggest that the child causes his parent to engage in the behaviors associated with MSBP or that he is any way responsible for the actions of his parent. Rather, the implication is that when a professional considers a diagnosis of MSBP, he/she should investigate myriad factors, including the behavior and health history of the child victim.

In addition to factors within the child, the health care professional should also consider factors within the parent, beyond those previously discussed (Eminson & Postlethwaite, 1992). For example, a parent may have low intellectual ability or be inexperienced, which could cause her to misinterpret symptoms in her child or the actions of medical staff. Further, the mother may be affected by mental health problems or social circumstances, including difficulties with a partner, finances, or on the job, that potentially could impact her behavior. Finally, a doctor should consider the mother's own history and early experiences. Psychodynamically, it is believed that if a person had her needs met in childhood, she will be more able to meet her own child's needs. Although more research in this area is needed, there is anecdotal evidence to suggest that mothers adopt the pattern of behaviors associated with MSBP as a result of a combination of early experiences, inherent personality traits, and unfulfilling personal relationships (Eminson & Postlethwaite).

Beyond the child–parent dyad, Eminson and Postlethwaite (1992) suggest factors within the larger family system that should be considered when contemplating a diagnosis of MSBP. First, the professional should observe family history for the general tendency to somatize. If the behavior is common within the larger system, it could be that the parent and child are predisposed or have learned the behaviors within the family. Second, the professional should consider the family's culture before making a judgment. Different cultural groups have been shown to vary in the frequency with which they visit doctor's offices and seek help for symptoms (Eminson & Postlethwaite). A doctor should be well-versed in working with patients and caregivers from diverse cultural backgrounds and should be willing to consider individual differences in diagnosing and judging behavior.

Finally, when considering whether behaviors warrant identification as MSBP, the professional should examine current factors within the larger society that may be impacting the parent and child (Eminson & Postlethwaite, 1992). For example, an outbreak in a serious illness, such as meningitis, may cause a mother to behave in a more anxious way concerning her child's health than she typically would. Most likely, myriad factors across individuals and systems interact to alter the likelihood of the parent–child dyad to consult for, ignore, or seek intervention for symptoms (Eminson & Postlethwaite). The challenge then for the healthcare provider is to collect and analyze data from a number of sources, with the intent of intervening in such a way that is most beneficial for the child.

4.6   Presentation of MSBP in Medical and Educational Contexts

4.6.1   The Medical Context

It is important to note that a parent may feign illness in a child for external incentives, including economic gain, escape from a difficult life situation, or to gain custody of the child. However, these motivations are not primary to MSBP. Although they may be present, external incentives are secondary to the psychological and/or social reinforcers, such as attention, that are suspected to be primary to the disorder (Ayoub & Alexander, 1998). Furthermore, the diagnosis of MSBP excludes those cases of physical abuse only, sexual abuse only, and failure to thrive only. Rather, the diagnosis is made only when symptoms have been induced or fabricated for the attention or other gratification that it brings the adult perpetrator, who is typically the mother (Sheridan, 2003).

Ayoub and Alexander (1998) stated that MSBP most commonly involves falsification of physical symptoms. The two most common methods of producing physical symptoms are suffocation and poisoning with medications. Symptoms can be induced across organ systems and include: (a) respiratory manifestations, such as asthma and cystic fibrosis; (b) gastrointestinal manifestations, including vomiting and chronic diarrhea; (c) hematological manifestations, such as anemia; (d) infection and fever; (e) dermatological manifestations, including vesiculations from burns and lacerations; (f) allergies; (g) ophthalmic manifestations, such as keratitis and recurrent conjunctivitis; (h) renal manifestations, including hematuria and bateriuria; and (i) neurological manifestations, such as seizures and disorders of consciousness (Shaw et al., 2008). In some cases, rather than directly harming the child, the parent alters laboratory specimens to produce the appearance of illness. For example, a parent may add blood to urine or stool samples or substitute a diabetic parent's urine for a child's specimen to suggest the presence of an illness (Shaw et al.).

4.6.2 The Educational Context

In addition to fabricating physical symptoms in her child, a parent might falsify psychological and developmental symptoms. These include symptoms of Tourette's syndrome, bipolar disorder, posttraumatic stress disorder, psychosis (Ayoub & Alexander, 1998), learning disability, neuromotor dysfunction, and pervasive developmental disorder (Shaw et al., 2008). Although symptoms of these disorders could be brought to the attention of health care providers, it is plausible to concede that an educational professional also might encounter a parent who has falsified a disorder in her child. In fact, Ayoub, Schreier, and Keller (2002) reported nine cases of what they termed "educational condition falsification" in which students had been erroneously diagnosed with attention deficit hyperactivity disorder, a learning disability, or a behavior disorder. These authors contended that as with MSBP where physical symptoms have been fabricated, mothers also may fabricate or exaggerate learning problems in their children that frequently escalate over time (Ayoub et al., 2002). As in MSBP, a primary function of fabricating a learning problem might be the attention that it brings the mother. Furthermore, Jennens (2009) suggested that this sort of deceit might keep the child dependent and living in the home.

Of the nine cases encountered, Ayoub et al. (2002) presented case studies for two families. The first family, the Joneses, had three children, Harry, Mary, and Susie. Harry had behavioral difficulties that persisted through his entry into the first grade, when he was evaluated and found to be eligible for special education services; he was subsequently placed in a self-contained special education classroom for children with behavior problems. His mother fought against this placement, stating that her son was "just different." However, when Harry was eventually diagnosed with Asperger's Syndrome, his mother became an expert on the subject and fought to have her son placed in a special school that she had identified. Harry was placed in that school, but the authors of the case study believed that this experience may have caused Mrs. Jones to become preoccupied with the educational performance of her two younger children (Ayoub et al.).

Although her middle daughter Mary was quiet and polite at school, Mrs. Jones described the child as "wild" at home and referred her for a special education evaluation when she was in the second grade (Ayoub et al., 2002). When the evaluation did not reveal any problems, her mother insisted that Mary had a "sequencing problem" that the school missed and that the child also had ADHD. There were no behavior problems evident in school, but Mary was placed on Ritalin. When it came to her youngest child, Susie, Mrs. Jones began to speak of medical problems when the child was only an infant. It should be noted that Susie was a half-sister to Harry and Mary. The family lived with Susie's father, but he never attended meetings for the two older children and only attended sporadically for his daughter. When Mr. Jones did attend, he sat quietly and let his wife do the talking (Ayoub et al.).

Mrs. Jones had started seeking services for Susie upon her entrance into kindergarten because of serious health problems, which had never been documented for the school (Ayoub et al., 2002). Rather, Mrs. Jones insisted that Susie had "episodes" and that she was concerned that her child had a learning disability and needed a special education placement. The family's pediatrician was also the school's doctor and he confirmed that, despite numerous tests, Susie did not have a valid, diagnosable illness. Both the doctor and school personnel noted many discrepancies in Mrs. Jones' reporting. Unfortunately, despite no diagnoses or educational testing to suggest a learning problem, Susie was placed in the same special education school as her brother, against the wishes of school personnel who believed that Mrs. Jones was making her daughter "more disabled" than the school evaluation team believed her to be (Ayoub et al.).

The second family in the case study report by Ayoub et al. (2002) was composed of a single mother and her son, Carlo. When he was in the first grade, Carlo's mother insisted that he should be evaluated at school for special education placement because he had ADHD. The results of this initial evaluation indicated that Carlo had mild ADHD and some problems with written language and math; his intelligence was reported as being within the average range of functioning. At the end of first grade, Carlo was evaluated again at the insistence of his mother, who argued that her son had superior intelligence, but that he was handicapped by severe ADHD. After this second evaluation, Carlo was referred for individual academic support services for a brief period at school each day (Ayoub et al.).

Over the course of the next few years, Carlo's mother became a self-proclaimed expert in ADHD, reading many books and attending parent support groups 3–5 times per week, sometimes as far away as 10 miles from her home (Ayoub et al., 2002). She also began to appear at school several times weekly, insisting that she should be permitted to sit in Carlo's classroom and observe. She was disruptive in the classroom and oftentimes antagonistic toward her son's teacher. With time, Carlo began to miss school and when he was there, presented with increasingly erratic, unfocused behavior. Carlo would claim that he had not taken his medication, but when calls were made home, his mother insisted that he had, in fact, taken it and that his dosage needed to be increased. His mother continued to take Carlo for independent psychopharmacological assessments (Ayoub et al.).

Throughout the ensuing years, Carlo's mother requested many different evaluations. She also enrolled as a part-time student at the local community college to study psychology. During this time, conflicts between the parent and school personnel increased and Carlo's behavior became more erratic; he became withdrawn and aggressive. By the time he entered the fourth grade, Carlo was quite distressed. He was eventually admitted to the hospital that year for psychiatric care, but was dismissed early when his mother disagreed with hospital staff over her compliance

with hospital procedures. He was discharged on clonopine and when he was rehos-
pitalized within a month of discharge, child protective services were called. Carlo
was eventually placed in foster care and his mother was permitted to see him twice
per month. At the time the case study was published, Carlo was in a general education fourth grade class, where he was making good progress, earning A's and B's
(Ayoub et al., 2002). These two cases demonstrate that MSBP can manifest in the
educational setting, as well as the medical arena, with parents fabricating school and
learning problems for their own benefit.

Wilde (2004) suggested that the causative factors in educational Munchausen
syndrome by proxy (EMSBP) are similar to those found in MSBP. The parent, usually the mother, has a need for attention that she meets through fabricating educational needs or diagnoses within her child. Commonly, the parent who has EMSBP
has a child who is eligible for special education and related services. As a nature of
policy and procedure, these parents tend to have more knowledge and influence than
parents whose children are in general education classrooms. Parents of children in
special education programs have the right to request individualized education program (IEP) meetings at any time and the school must honor that request. Through
an IEP meeting, the parent has the opportunity to engage school personnel in any
number of issues (Wilde), including requests for additional evaluations and for
accommodations and modifications to the curriculum and program.

One indicator of EMSBP might be when a parent describes problems that have
not been observed by school personnel (Wilde, 2004). For example, a parent may
report that her child has great difficulty in attending to task, whereas his teacher
reports appropriate attending skills. A second indicator of EMSBP would be the
parent who has an intense interest in educational disorders. Like the parent with
MSBP who commonly has medical training, the parent with EMSBP might have
educational training, or might profess a desire to work in a school setting with children with disabilities. Finally, the parental relationship could be an indicator of
EMSBP. Often, the mother appears to be overly attentive and concerned with the
child's progress, while the father fails to participate in the process (Wilde). Although
there is not a strong research base to confirm the presence of EMSBP, it is important
for educators to be aware that there are parents who feign educational problems in
their children solely for the associated attention. This type of behavior can draw the
educator's attention from other important tasks, such as intervening with children
who need help and consulting with other teachers and parents.

4.7 Assessment

Although MSBP was first described in the literature more than 30 years ago, it is a
difficult syndrome to identify. A major barrier to detection is the failure of the health
professional to consider that a parent may be abusing her child through such means
(Siegel & Fischer, 2001). Historically, there was strong professional and societal
resistance to early accounts of child physical and sexual abuse, and the deliberate

Table 4.1 Assessment of MSBP: Warning signs

1. The child's illness is unexplained, prolonged, or extraordinary, with no clear explanation
   (a) The child is presented frequently for medical care
   (b) Symptoms are incongruous and only observed when the perpetrator is present
   (c) Attempted treatments have proven ineffective
   (d) There are differences between what the parent and child report regarding symptoms
2. The perpetrator, usually the mother, is constantly with her child, not even leaving the hospital for brief outings
   (a) The mother has formed unusually close relationships with medical staff
   (b) The mother does not appear to be as concerned about her child's illness as doctors and nurses
   (c) The mother welcomes invasive testing and procedures for her child
   (d) The mother displays unusual medical knowledge and may even become involved in the care of other hospital patients
3. There appears to be tampering with the child and/or his medical situation, including specimens and test results
4. A sudden, unexplained infant death has occurred in the family
5. No external motivation for the illness, such as economic gain, is present

induction or fabrication of illness in a child may be even more difficult to consider for many people. Some physicians may suspect MSBP, but may be hesitant to make a diagnosis because of the legal ramifications that could result from misidentification. Indeed, legal action has been taken against doctors who have incorrectly labeled MSBP in parents (Rosenberg, 2003). In addition to the legal battles that can ensue, a misdiagnosis of MSBP can have detrimental psychological effects on the mother. One study suggested that as many as 60% of mothers who were falsely accused had attempted suicide (Bütz et al., 2009). Furthermore, most doctors are trained to rely on information from parents, particularly mothers, and many do not doubt the information relayed to them. The mother is, essentially, at the same time abusing her child and seeking medical assistance for him, which is discrepant behavior. Most of the mothers who engage in the behaviors associated with MSBP do not fit the stereotype of the abusive mother and, in many cases, the parent–child relationship appears to be mutually close (Siegel & Fischer). This paradox could cause a doctor to miss warning signs of illness fabrication. Finally, there is no standard psychological profile or diagnostic tool that can be used in assessment of MSBP. Rather, diagnosis is made by excluding other plausible hypotheses (Shaw et al., 2008). These factors can make the disorder a difficult one to detect and diagnose, but given the oft times deleterious outcomes of MSBP, it is important for health care providers to be alert to warning signs.

Table 4.1 summarizes the work of various researchers (i.e., APA, 2000; Ayoub & Alexander, 1998; Kahan & Yorker, 1991; Meadow, 1985; Rosenberg, 2003; Siegel & Fischer, 2001) who have suggested a list of common signs to look for in assessment of MSBP.

Kahan and Yorker (1991) warn that no one indicator in isolation proves the existence of MSBP. However, the presence of any one sign should raise suspicion.

When MSBP is suspected, measures should be undertaken to heighten surveillance of the parent and child and to protect the child from further injury. Increased surveillance may involve seeking information from the father, review of the mother's own medical history for factitious illness, and detailed charting to allow the physician to detect patterns in the child's symptoms (e.g., symptoms that abate when the mother is not present). If permitted, it may also help to contact school personnel, friends, or family members who have been reported as witnesses to symptoms, or who have knowledge of the family's personal and social history (Kahan & Yorker).

Child characteristics may also alert the health care provider to the potential presence of MSBP. Initially, when the child is presented for care, he shows few physical signs and those that are found, generally are incidental to the presenting complaint. However, his mother will describe numerous physical symptoms that usually are not conforming to any easily recognized condition. These symptoms will be unusual or serious, but also unverifiable. For example, the mother might describe sudden, sharp pains that her child experiences, but the doctor might never observe such. In addition, the mother may make extensive claims of serious illnesses that have been identified by other doctors and may offer witnesses in support of these claims. Many times these "witnesses" will have status to emphasize reliability, such as a friend who is a nurse (Eminson & Postlethwaite, 1992).

As Eminson and Postlethwaite (1992) noted, confirmation of MSBP is a long, painstaking process. These authors suggested that diagnosis occurs in three stages. In the first stage, the doctor should take a very detailed history of the child's present and past illnesses, including agreement between the parents as to what has occurred. It is also important to gather as much information about the family as possible in the first stage. For example, the doctor should ask questions about the health of the patient's siblings and parents and about the family's current social circumstances, stresses, and supports. During this initial stage, the child should be thoroughly examined, preferably through the least invasive means, to rule out true physical explanations for symptoms. Finally, the doctor should seek consent to seek records from other agencies at this time (Eminson & Postlethwaite).

In the second stage of confirmation, the doctor will want to provide care to the child as he would any other child with puzzling symptoms. Although the physician may suspect MSBP, it is essential that he see the child when symptoms are present (Eminson & Postlethwaite, 1992). During this time, the doctor will want to observe the mother's behavior. If she believes that the doctor is suspicious of her behavior, she may begin to seek help elsewhere, such as employing another general practitioner or taking her child to a different hospital. The mother may also present her child to the doctor with new symptoms, explaining that the original presenting problem is no longer troublesome. During this second stage, if the mother does not appear reassured by the explanation that her child shows no ill health, or that he does not require further tests and treatments, the doctor should investigate further for possible MSBP (Eminson & Postlethwaite).

In the third stage of confirmation of MSBP, the doctor has the duty to investigate his suspicions (Eminson & Postlethwaite, 1992). The doctor should carefully consider the mother's health-seeking behavior and decide whether she is able to distinguish her own needs from her child's To aid in this process, the doctor may want to seek consultation with a child psychiatric colleague. In addition, the doctor might think about referring the mother for psychiatric or psychological help (Eminson & Postlethwaite).

4.7.1 Burden of Proof: Video Surveillance

It is very difficult to prove that a parent is engaging in the behaviors associated with MSBP because, generally, evidence is circumstantial (Hall, Eubanks, Meyyazhagan, Kenney, & Johnson, 2000). In cases where actual proof is obtained, it is usually serendipitous, such as when a medical professional catches a mother smothering her child or when an offending agent introduced by the mother is detected in a blood test. However, without definitive and timely diagnosis, the child who is a victim of MSBP is at great risk. Undetected cases can lead to permanent damage to a child's organ systems, or even death. Given the deleterious outcomes often associated with the disorder, it has been proposed that covert video surveillance (CVS) be used in suspected cases of MSBP (Greiner et al., 2007; Hall et al., 2000).

In a study completed in a tertiary care children's hospital in the southern United States, facilities and protocols for CVS were developed. Hidden video cameras and audio equipment were used to determine how valuable covert monitoring was in identifying cases of MSBP in 41 families (Hall et al., 2000). Before CVS was used, a multidisciplinary team considered the pros and cons of its use within each of the cases. CVS was only used when the team believed that MSBP was the most likely cause of a child's presenting symptoms. Consent for closed circuit monitoring was obtained from all families upon the child's admission to the hospital and was permitted everywhere, but the bathroom (Hall et al.).

Results of the study indicated that of the 41 original cases, 23 were classified as certain cases of MSBP. Of the 23 identified, CVS was required for definitive diagnosis in 13 (56.1%), used as supporting documentation in 5 (21.7%), and was not needed in 5 (21.7%). In those five cases wherein CVS was not needed to confirm diagnosis, MSBP was definitively diagnosed through laboratory testing in two cases, through direct observation by a staff member in two cases, and through confession by the mother in one case. When video tapes were reviewed in these five cases, no evidence of illness fabrication or inducement was observed. CVS was used with these patients because laboratory tests had not yet been completed, or to provide support for the observations of medical personnel. Of the 23 cases included in the certain MSBP category, 10 parents were classified as fabricators, 2 as inducers, and 11 as both. CVS was required for definitive diagnosis in 80% of the cases where illness was created exclusively by fabrication (Hall et al., 2000).

CVS tapes revealed not only direct actions by mothers to induce illness in their offspring, but also another notable behavior. In many instances, mothers were observed on hospital phones making calls to friends and relatives in which they greatly exaggerated their children's symptoms (Hall et al., 2000). For example, one woman told a listener that doctors wanted to operate on her child, but that she would not consent, when in fact doctors were trying to convince the family that the child was healthy. In another case, a mother told family members over the phone that her child was having constant seizures, when no seizure activity had been observed (Hall et al.).

Although there may be a tendency to want to identify MSBP on certain warning signals, Hall et al. (2000) caution that these patterns may not be sensitive enough to warrant diagnosis. For instance, they found that only 12 of the 23 mothers in their study appeared to be unusually knowledgeable about medical symptoms and procedures and that only 9 of 17 suggested tests to the attending physician. Further, only 8 of 17 mothers suggested a diagnosis for her child and only 9 of 20 appeared to have an unusually close relationship with staff (Hall et al.). In this study, the researchers used CVS to validate the existence of MSBP and such was needed to make a definitive diagnosis in more than half of the cases (Hall et al.). Given the individual differences across families, CVS may be a valuable diagnostic tool. For ethical reasons, medical personnel should warn parents upon admittance to the hospital that they and their child may be taped and the benefits of such a procedure clearly explained.

Foreman and Farsides (1993) contend that CVS is ethical only when it provides information to doctors and authorities that would not otherwise be available in identifying a case of MSBP. If a doctor is sufficiently certain that the parent is harming the child through other evidence, such as improvement in the child when he is separated from the mother or the discovery of foreign agents in blood or urine samples, CVS is not necessary. In fact, CVS infringes upon the rights of the family to privacy, honesty, and autonomy. The lack of trust between parent and doctor could even cause the family to withdraw necessary medical tests and treatments for the child. Foreman and Farsides suggest that CVS should be restricted in its use to those cases in which it is necessary for identification of harmful parental behaviors and should not be used routinely.

4.7.2   MSBP: To Label the Perpetrator or Not

Although there are many case studies to suggest that MSBP can have deleterious effects on children and families, Fisher and Mitchell (1995) suggested that it should not be diagnosed by physicians at all. These authors posited that the wide variations in presentation and perpetrator psychopathology do not satisfy criteria for acceptance as a discrete medical syndrome. Rather than making a diagnosis of MSBP, Fisher and Mitchell recommended that the physician diagnose specific fabricated or induced illness in the child and leave the perpetrator's behavior to the psychiatrist or psychologist to define. In addition, they believe that MSBP should only be diagnosed when the parent has Munchausen's syndrome herself *and* manifests her psychopathology via her child (Fisher & Mitchell).

Along these same lines, Meadow (1995) suggested that it may be more prudent to label the behaviors, rather than the perpetrator of the type of abuse associated with MSBP. A danger in applying the term to the mother is that there is an implication that MSBP has a single cause and, therefore, a single remedy. Studies of the disorder have revealed that there are many different types of perpetrator characteristics. Also, identifying people, rather than behaviors, may lead those in authority to erroneously believe that MSBP abuse could be diagnosed solely by psychiatrists, when differentiating between natural and fictitious illness in a child can be an exceptionally difficult task (Meadow).

4.8 Treatment and Intervention

When MSBP has been identified within a family, the chance for successful rehabilitation is poor, if the child remains in the parent's care. In one study involving 119 cases, 40% of the children who had been poisoned and 50% of the children who had been suffocated experienced further abuse (Klepper et al., 2008).There is also high risk of abuse for siblings of the child victim. Follow-up in cases of MSBP is essential to ensure the child's and his siblings' safety, especially when the children remain in the home with the abusive parent (Klepper et al.).

4.8.1 Confrontation of the Caregiver

In a paper on the management of Munchausen syndrome by proxy, Meadow (1985) discussed confronting the mother with her behavior. As he states, this is a difficult task to undertake, especially when one may have doubt. Meadow suggested that the best approach is to confine conversation to fact and to approach the offending parent alone. Although it is customary to speak to parents together about their child's health, in the case of suspected MSBP, doing so could cause the father to become angry and engage in denial. The purpose of confronting the mother is not to prove her wrong, but to understand the meaning of the symptoms in her child in order to help. The doctor should explain to the parent that her actions are harming her child and could have long-term consequences for his health and well-being. During this time, the doctor should also explain what information will be shared with the child's father. The meeting should not be hostile or condemnatory in nature, but supportive. A goal should be to determine other sources of satisfaction in the mother's life that could replace the personal gains she has received from harming her child and to motivate her to seek treatment and help (Meadow).

4.8.2 Placement in Protective Custody

When MSBP is suspected, most of the time the child victim will be placed under protective care in the hospital (Meadow, 1985). The decision as to what to do next involves a number of factors, including: (a) whether the abuse has involved suffocation or poisoning, which can cause death; (b) the age of the child; (c) unexplained deaths of other children in the family; (d) a mother who fabricates or induces illness in herself; (e) parental drug or alcohol abuse; and (f) persistence of the fabrication, even after confrontation. These factors have been deemed as the most dangerous to the child and presence of any one may result in the child becoming a ward of the court, which results in the child being placed in protective custody, such as foster care. Whatever the arrangement, it is imperative that the doctor continue to see the child for a long time to monitor his health (Meadow).

4.8.3   Therapeutic Intervention

4.8.3.1   Therapy with the Mother

In addition to ensuring the safety of the child, it is also important to provide therapeutic services for the mother and family. Leeder (1990) suggested a three stage process for treatment that includes engagement, development, and termination. Within this framework, therapy is first conducted with the mother alone, then with her partner, if he is still present within the family. Next, the couple enters the therapeutic relationship together. Finally, the child victim, if he is old enough, enters the process. The first stage in therapy, engagement, involves building rapport and gaining the trust of the client. During this stage, the therapist takes considerable time to get to know the mother and the dynamics of her relationships with other family members, including her spouse. Within the second stage, development, the therapist and the client work together to uncover themes in her life that may be motivating and maintaining behaviors. Finally, the final stage in the process, termination, involves ending or fading the therapeutic relationship, depending on the client's needs (Leeder).

An initial task in providing therapy to the mother involves gaining her trust (Leeder, 1990). The therapist may need to spend considerable time listening to details of the child's symptoms and hospitalizations. Once trust has been established, the therapist can begin to explore the mother's background, including her medical history. During this stage, it is also useful to ascertain information about the woman's relationship with her own parents and with her husband. Once this work has been accomplished, the therapist can begin to help the woman identify and explore themes in her life. As the mother gains insight, she should begin to move toward resolution. At this time, the woman may realize that she is dissatisfied with the confines of the mothering role and, thus, treatment should include teaching her to identify her needs and to explore options for meeting them. The therapist should also help the woman to understand that her needs were unmet in childhood and that her behaviors in inducing or fabricating illness in her child were a method for meeting such. When the mother is able to identify other means for meeting her own needs, the next stage of therapy can be entered. If possible, this is the point in the process where work with the woman's husband should begin (Leeder).

4.8.3.2   Therapy with the Husband and as a Couple

Before engaging in therapy with the couple, the practitioner may want to see the husband alone for a few sessions. Generally, his wife should consent, so that she does not feel colluded against. When working with the husband, the therapist should attempt to ascertain his understanding of the situation and his role in it (Leeder, 1990). Once the husband understands his wife's needs, couple therapy can begin. Joint counseling allows for exploration of the relationship dynamics between the partners. The woman can begin to discuss her needs with her husband and he can begin to discuss his feelings regarding the situation. Leeder suggests encouraging the couple to tell the entire story of their relationship because it can have the healing effect of rekindling old positive feelings for one another. The therapist can help the couple identify themes in their relationship that may be problematic and to determine how individual needs can be met. If the woman does not have a partner, treatment can be very difficult because she will have no one to turn to for assistance in parenting or in obtaining support in developing a healthy concept of self. In this case, another family member or trusted friend can be enlisted to work with the woman in the process (Leeder).

Leeder (1990) stated that it is difficult to know when therapy with a family affected by MSBP can be successfully terminated. She suggested assessing how well the couple is communicating and how well each is attempting to recognize and fulfill his/her own needs before ending the relationship. If the decision to terminate is made, it may be wise to schedule periodic follow-up appointments with the mother. Maintaining contact may bring comfort to the woman because she will have someone in authority to contact, in the event that problems resurface (Leeder).

4.8.3.3   Therapy with the Child

If he is old enough, the therapist may also want to work with the child victim, as well as his parents. Although she admitted to having limited experience with this population, Leeder (1990) suggested that play therapy might be a viable option. The therapist's goal should be to help the child escape from an "invalid mentality" and regain a healthy self-image. Much more work is needed in the area of treatment for the child victim of MSBP. It is unknown to what extent the effects of such abuse will impact future behaviors in health seeking and self-care.

4.8.3.4   Narrative Family Therapy

Sanders (1996) proposed utilizing a narrative approach to therapy with the family who has been affected by MSBP. Essentially, the theory behind this approach posits that each human being has a narrative through which we describe ourselves and others, and which influences our behaviors and interactions. Treatment invites the individual to challenge problem stories and to discover the existence of alternatives. When applied to the family in which MSBP behaviors exist, the suggestion is that the family has created an "illness story." The aim of therapy is to assist the family in creating a "health story," through which they will abandon falsification, exaggeration, and induction of illness. This approach includes the development of a treatment contract and parental, family, and child therapies (Sanders).

The treatment contract should include a statement about the limitations of confidentiality within the therapy process and a detailed plan of action. The plan should state what the process will look like, including who will attend therapy sessions and when. There should also be a statement regarding reunification requirements when the child has been removed from the home (Sanders, 1996). Typically, the contract will state that the therapist will work with the parents first, prior to involving children in the process. Individual sessions with the mother may prove beneficial, if it appears that she will be more forthcoming in sessions when her spouse does not attend (Sanders).

Initial work with the mother involves reviewing her past to gather information about her dominant life story. Past experiences such as illness and abandonment in childhood are explored and the therapist helps the woman to determine how these childhood events have contributed to her present behaviors (Sanders, 1996). During the process, the mother is also encouraged to explore obstacles that may be preventing her from accepting responsibility for her MSBP behaviors, such as fear of rejection by her spouse. The therapist and the woman explore the positive and negative effects of her behavior and begin to explore alternative stories. When appropriate, the spouse and children can be brought into the therapeutic process and engaged in the reunification plan. Therapy for children is similar to that used with other abused youngsters, e.g., talk or play therapies (Sanders).

4.8.3.5 Treatment for Educational MSBP

When it comes to providing services for the child who has been affected by EMSBP, Jennens (2009) suggested that the school be alert to discrepancies between the mother and the educational professionals as to what evaluations or programs a child needs. School personnel should be careful to avoid reinforcing maternal factitious behaviors. Direct communication between all professionals involved with the child will help to limit the opportunities the mother has to convey inaccurate information. In addition, when medical professionals are involved with the child (e.g., a neurologist or psychiatrist), the school should appoint a liaison who can translate the terminologies of each profession to minimize misinformation between the systems. A coordinated effort among service providers can help to protect the child from the potentially serious consequences of fabricated or exaggerated learning problems (Jennens). However, because there is no direct physical harm to the child with EMSBP, it may be difficult to protect the child fully or to force the mother to seek treatment.

4.8.3.6   Therapeutic Case Study

Nicol and Eccles (1985) presented a case study in which psychotherapy was used as treatment for a woman who had induced illness in two of her children. Because the mother had confessed to the abuse, it was decided that she was ready for the therapeutic process; she had admitted that there was a problem with her behaviors. A care order was put into place that stated that her children could remain in her care under strict supervision, as long as she participated in the psychotherapy treatment (Nicol & Eccles). At the start of treatment, the mother appeared to be an intelligent woman who had a strong desire to understand her actions. Thus, an active, deep form of interpretive therapy was undertaken. Therapeutic sessions were conducted on a weekly basis for 6 months, then biweekly for another 6 months. At termination, family supervision by a social worker and health care provider continued. All therapy sessions were conducted by a child psychiatrist (Nicol & Eccles).

Early in the therapeutic process, the mother admitted that she enjoyed the sympathy shown her when her child was ill. In fact, the mother stated that she needed her daughter to be ill, so that she felt important. The mother also shared that she had taken pleasure in outsmarting her child's doctors (Nicol & Eccles, 1985). As therapy progressed, the woman expressed two noteworthy affective states – remorse and depression. Remorse surfaced in early sessions and resurfaced throughout the therapy relationship. The woman's report of depression was not clinically diagnosed, but was often a topic of sessions. The depression appeared to consist of an infantile rage coupled with low self-esteem. It was concluded in therapy that the woman's motivation for the behaviors associated with MSBP arose from the patterns of dominance and submission that were established early in her life within her family of origin. As a result of the work done in therapy, several changes were apparent in the woman's life: (a) no further abuse to her children had occurred over a 15-month follow-up period; (b) there was a cessation in her own abnormal illness behavior; (c) she became more assertive in her relationship with her father; (d) she became a "warmer" person in her interpersonal relationships; and (e) she expressed relief at having been discovered harming her children because she had been able to get help for her problems (Nicol & Eccles).

4.8.3.7   Conclusions Regarding Treatment for MSBP

The aforementioned therapies suggest intensive work with the mother who perpetrates harm to her child. However, it may be valuable to focus treatment on the relationship between mother and child because the mother's maladaptive behaviors are vividly expressed through this relationship (Lyons-Ruth, Kaufman, Masters, & Wu, 1991). Generally, the mother somatizes and projects her emotional needs onto the child. This suggests that she may have difficulty in recognizing and verbalizing her emotional experiences within a traditional psychotherapy model (Lyons-Ruth et al., 1991). Much more research in this area is needed before a prescriptive course can be suggested and it may be discovered that no one approach will work, given that MSBP involves a complicated relationship between mother and child.

4.9   Outcome and Prognostic Factors

Often times, MSBP goes undetected because the parent gives the illusion of being attentive and caring. She demonstrates concern and personal sacrifice as she endures her child's prolonged medical tests and treatment regimens (Kannai, 2009). Thus, actual prevalence is difficult to document (Schreier & Libow, 1993). However, in cases where MSBP has been detected, the outcomes are grim. The mortality rate for youngsters affected is approximately 10%. In many of these cases, a sibling has already died under mysterious circumstances (Kahan & Yorker, 1991). If the child remains in the home after discovery, the likelihood of rehabilitation is poor and the risk for further abuse is high (Klepper et al., 2008). Also, the child victim may suffer enduring psychological and physical effects of the abuse. The psychological effects include depression, dependency, shame, immaturity, separation anxiety, phobias, and passivity in tolerating invasive medical procedures (Gross, 2008; Shaw et al., 2008). The physical problems the child may suffer include multiple scars, organ damage or loss, chronic illness, or a compromised immune system (Gross, 2008). The impact that MSBP has on a child's life can be devastating.

Although there is little research to indicate which type of family system has the greatest chance for recovery, it has been suggested that differences across families (e.g., evidence of induced illness or extreme denial of MSBP behaviors) may warrant different treatment approaches (Sanders, 1996). Treatment might be composed of psychological therapy for the mother, child, and family, psychoeducational interventions, and an active approach to risk management (Adshead & Bluglass, 2005). Fisher and Mitchell (1995) suggested that the key to treatment is to understand the motivation of the perpetrator in causing harm to her child. This understanding will help the professionals involved with the case to formulate a policy for safe parenting and to prevent future harm to the child (Fisher & Mitchell). However, there will still be cases wherein the abuse persists and the child is placed at high risk for permanent disability or even death. In these cases, further treatment is not warranted and the only option is to terminate parental rights (Sanders, 1996). Much more research is needed to determine why some mothers and families respond to treatment and others do not.

4.10   Future Directions

Along with a discussion of future research directions should occur a discussion of research avenues that should *not* be pursued because they will not ultimately lead to increased understanding or improved treatments for MSBP. Eminson and Jureidini (2003) demonstrated this point clearly. First, these authors suggested that the study of individuals who engage in MSBP behaviors is unlikely to promote understanding of the phenomenon because there is no single or specific cause. MSBP is variable in its manifestation across cases and rather than examining psychopathology in the parent, it may prove more beneficial to approach research from a sociological perspective. Eminson and Jureidini make an analogy between MSBP and crime that illustrates this approach well. The rates of bicycle theft will depend on the prevalence of bicycles, their utility as a mode of transportation, and their monetary value. The bicycle thief may lack morals, or just be desperate for transportation. He may be a thrill seeker, or an impulsive risk taker who seizes an opportunity to steal. The prevention of bicycle theft may not lie so much as with understanding thieves' motivations, as it does with prevention – strong locks and secure bicycle sheds. Furthermore, improving socioeconomic conditions so that everyone can afford a bicycle might reduce the rate of the crime. Along this line of thinking, it may be more productive to examine existing medical practices in the prevention of MSBP (analogous to securing bicycles or making them available to all), than it may be to study the psychopathology of maternal perpetrators (Eminson & Jureidini).

The metaphor described above will also aid in our understanding of how to determine the risks of repeat MSBP behaviors, once abuse has been detected. Again, rather than looking at psychopathology within the mother, it is important to approach research from an etiological perspective. There are systemic factors, including the parent's history, family relationships, social circumstances, treatment resources, and health care setting that will affect recidivism (Eminson & Jureidini, 2003). Future exploration should focus on finding the factor, or combination, that best predicts recurrence. This knowledge would enable prevention strategies to be formulated that would either stop further abuse from occurring or that would prevent initial factitious behaviors from escalating.

Eminson and Jureidini (2003) also suggested that more research into somatization is needed. Potential risk factors for MSBP that might be investigated include: (a) parents with a past or current history of somatization; (b) mothers with high levels of unexplained symptoms during pregnancy; (c) a history of frequent visits to medical facilities with a child; and (d) a clinician's report that a parent may have distorted beliefs about her child's health. Examination of these variables may lead to prevention strategies. Again, the focus should not be on identifying psychopathology within the mother, but on these behaviors within the sociological and cultural contexts. What combination of factors causes one mother with symptoms of somatization to engage in behaviors associated with MSBP, while another does not?

Finally, given the deleterious effects that MSBP can have on its child victim, longitudinal research needs to be conducted to examine outcomes for these children. It has been suggested that as a child matures, he may begin to participate in his parent's deceit (Meadow, 1985). Future studies should examine the personality traits of these children in an attempt to determine which are at risk for developing factitious behaviors themselves. Also, it is unknown to what extent victims grow up to abuse their own children in the same manner. Research into this area could help to break the cycle and ensure that MSBP does not rob a future child of a happy and healthy childhood.

References

Adshead, G., & Bluglass, K. (2005). Attachment representations in mothers with abnormal illness behaviour by proxy. *The British Journal of Psychiatry, 187*, 328–333.

American Psychiatric Association. (2000). *Diagnostic and statistical manual of mental disorders* (4th ed., rev.). Washington, DC: Author.

Ayoub, C. C., & Alexander, R. (1998). Definitional issues in Munchausen by proxy. *The APSAC Advisor, 11*, 7–10.

Ayoub, C., Schreier, H., & Keller, C. (2002). Munchausen by proxy: Presentations in special education. *Child Maltreatment, 7*, 149–159.

Bande, C. S., & García-Alba, C. (2008). Munchausen syndrome by proxy: A dilemma for diagnosis. *Rorschachiana, 29*, 183–200.

Bools, C., Neale, B., & Meadow, R. (1994). Munchausen syndrome by proxy: A study of psychopathology. *Child Abuse & Neglect, 18*, 773–788.

Bütz, M. R., Evans, F. B., & Webber-Dereszynski, R. L. (2009). A practitioner's complaint and proposed direction: Munchausen syndrome by proxy, factitious disorder by proxy, and fabricated and/or induced illness in children. *Professional Psychology: Research and Practice, 40*, 31–38.

Eminson, M., & Jureidini, J. (2003). Concerns about research and prevention strategies in Munchausen syndrome by proxy (MSBP) abuse. *Child Abuse & Neglect, 27*, 413–420.

Eminson, D. M., & Postlethwaite, R. J. (1992). Factitious illness: Recognition and management. *Archives of Disease in Childhood, 67*, 1510–1516.

Fisher, G. C., & Mitchell, I. (1995). Is Munchausen syndrome by proxy really a syndrome? *Archives of Disease in Childhood, 72*, 530–534.

Foreman, D. M., & Farsides, C. (1993). Ethical use of covert videoing techniques in detecting Munchausen syndrome by proxy. *British Medical Journal, 307*, 611–612.

Grenier, D., Elliott, E. J., Zurynski, Y., Rodrigues Pereira, R., Preece, M., Lynn, R., et al. (2007). Beyond counting cases: Public health impacts of national paediatric surveillance units. *Archives of Disease in Childhood, 92*, 527–533.

Gross, B. (2008, Summer). Caretaker cruelty: Munchausen's and beyond. *The Forensic Examiner*, 54–57.

Hall, D. E., Eubanks, L., Meyyazhagan, S., Kenney, R. D., & Johnson, S. C. (2000). Evaluation of covert video surveillance in the diagnosis of Munchausen syndrome by proxy: Lessons from 41 cases. *Pediatrics, 105*, 1305–1312.

Heubrock, D. (2001). Münchhausen by proxy syndrome in clinical child neuropsychology: A case presenting with neuropsychological symptoms. *Child Neuropsychology, 4*, 273–285.

Horwath, J., & Tidbury, W. (2009). Training the workforce following a serious case review: Lessons learnt from a death by fabricated and induced illness. *Child Abuse Review, 18*, 181–194.

Howe, G. L., Jordan, H. W., & Lockert, E. W. (1983). Munchausen's syndrome or chronic factitious illness: A review and case presentation. *Journal of the National Medical Association, 75*, 175–181.

Jennens, R. (2009). Munchausen syndrome by proxy: Implications for professional practice in relation to children's education. *Child Care in Practice, 15*, 299–311.

Kahan, B., & Yorker, B. C. (1991). Munchausen syndrome by proxy: Clinical review and legal issues. *Behavioral Sciences & the Law, 9*, 73–83.

Kannai, R. (2009). Medical family therapy casebook: Munchausen by mommy. *Families, Systems, & Health, 27*, 105–112.

Klepper, J., Heringhaus, A., Wurthmann, C., & Voit, T. (2008). Expect the unexpected: Favourable outcome in Munchausen by proxy syndrome. *European Journal of Pediatrics, 167*, 1085–1088.

Leeder, E. (1990). Supermom or child abuser? Treatment of the Munchausen mother. *Women and Therapy, 9*, 69–88.

Libow, J. A., & Schreier, H. A. (1986). Three forms of fictitious illness in children: When is it Munchausen syndrome by proxy? *The American Journal of Orthopsychiatry, 56*, 602–611.

Lyons-Ruth, K., Kaufman, M., Masters, N., & Wu, J. (1991). Issues in the identification and long-term management of Munchausen by proxy syndrome within a clinical infant service. *Infant Mental Health Journal, 12,* 309–320.

Mart, E. G. (2004). Factitious disorder by proxy: A call for the abandonment of an outmoded diagnosis. *The Journal of Psychiatry & Law, 32,* 297–314.

Meadow, R. (1977). Munchausen syndrome by proxy: The hinterland of child abuse. *Lancet, 2,* 343–345.

Meadow, R. (1985). Management of Munchausen syndrome by proxy. *Archives of Disease in Childhood, 60,* 385–393.

Meadow, R. (1995). What is, and what is not, 'Munchausen syndrome by proxy'? *Archives of Disease in Childhood, 72,* 534–538.

Nicol, A. R., & Eccles, M. (1985). Psychotherapy for Munchausen syndrome by proxy. *Archives of Disease in Childhood, 60,* 344–348.

Patterson, R. (1988). The Münchhausen syndrome: Baron von Münchhausen has taken a bum rap. *Canadian Medical Association Journal, 139,* 566–569.

Plassmann, R. (1994). Münchhausen syndromes and factitious diseases. *Psychotherapy and Psychosomatics, 62,* 7–26.

Rosenberg, D. A. (1987). Web of deceit: A literature review of Munchausen syndrome by proxy. *Child Abuse & Neglect, 11,* 547–563.

Rosenberg, D. A. (2003). Munchausen syndrome by proxy: Medical diagnostic criteria. *Child Abuse & Neglect, 27,* 421–430.

Sanders, M. J. (1996). Narrative family treatment of Munchausen by proxy: A successful case. *Families, Systems & Health, 14,* 315–329.

Schreier, H. A., & Libow, J. A. (1993). Munchausen syndrome by proxy: Diagnosis and prevalence. *The American Journal of Orthopsychiatry, 63,* 318–321.

Shaw, R. J., Dayal, S., Hartman, J. K., & DeMaso, D. R. (2008). Factitious disorder by proxy: Pediatric condition falsification. *Harvard Review of Psychiatry, 16,* 215–224.

Sheridan, M. S. (2003). The deceit continues: An updated literature review of Munchausen syndrome by proxy. *Child Abuse & Neglect, 27,* 431–451.

Siegel, P. T., & Fischer, H. (2001). Munchausen by proxy syndrome: Barriers to detection, confirmation, and intervention. *Children's Services: Social Policy, Research, and Practice, 4,* 31–50.

Wilde, J. (2004). The educational manifestation of Munchausen by proxy. Retrieved October 30, 2010, from http://www.edfac.unimelb.edu.au/research/resources/student_res/postscriptfiles/vol5/vol5_1_wilde_1.pdf.

Chapter 5
Feral Children

with
Fred W. Greer III

> ...he concluded from hence that he was an Animal,
> endu'd with a Spirit of an equal Temperature, as all the
> Heavenly Bodies are,
> and that he was a distinct Species from the rest of the Animals,
> and that he was created for another end,
> and design'd for something greater than what they were
> capable of.
>
> – Abu Bakr Ibn Turalil (1929)
> *The History of Hayy Ibn Yaqzan*

5.1   Overview

Feral children are familiar figures in popular lore and literature. The story of children growing up alone or raised by wild animals, untouched by human society, has a global and persistent appeal. Contemporary fiction's Mowgli from *The Jungle Book* (1894) and *Tarzan of the Apes* (1914) – both translated into every major language – have enjoyed popularity across world cultures, have remained in print since initial publication, and have been adapted into numerous television and film productions. Such tales are not an invention of modern times, however. Feral children feature in Arabic and Turkic literature to at least the seventh century B.C.E. (Findley, 2005; Ibn Tufail, 1929) and the wolf-suckling twins Romulus and Remus are known from Roman mythology (Malson, 1972).

The idea of feral children may draw its appeal from their unusual position of occupying the gap between animal and human, an extension of the conceptual continuum running from civilization to savagery. Just as the legend of Romulus and Remus offers an explanation for the foundation of Rome, other feral child lore promises insight into the origin and nature of all humans. Before we can learn from feral children, we must learn about them, which leads to the question: Do feral children exist?

S.C. Dombrowski et al., *Assessing and Treating Low Incidence/High Severity Psychological Disorders of Childhood*, DOI 10.1007/978-1-4419-9970-2_5,
© Springer Science+Business Media, LLC 2011

By definition, feral children live outside of human contact, and therefore documentation of wild animals feeding and nurturing them does not exist (Dennis, 1941). Reports of feral children have stated that they were discovered in the proximity of animals, but no credible accounts relate witnessing animals caring for children. In the strictest sense, then, there is no direct evidence for the reality of the feral child as customarily described in literature and folklore. Even in those cases in which a child recovered from the wild is supposed to have lived on its own, without the aid of wildlife, no documentation exists to verify a period of feral existence. The absence of such data does not refute the existence of *wild* children. Trustworthy eyewitness accounts and records of the circumstances in which children have been recovered are sufficient in many cases to indicate reasonable probability that children have lived in the wild, even among animals. Without these data, however, one must avoid credulity in reading reports of feral children, whose history invites speculation.

Even so, in considering the aforementioned continuum that extends from being reared by wild animals to being raised by responsive, skilled, and affectionate parents amid a resource-rich environment, we quickly encounter authenticated cases of real children, and many of them, who share many of the deleterious circumstances of the archetypal feral child. These are the isolated or abandoned children.

Isolated children are those who have been raised separately from others. Such children include those who have been raised in environments of neglect and privation with limited human contact.

More common than isolated children are the abandoned children. These individuals are so frequently encountered in some urban areas that they have been referred to as a group by the term *children of the street* (World Health Organization, 2000). Although they are sometimes referred to as *feral* (Moura, 2002), they are not subject to the same conditions of deprivation and isolation considered in this chapter. Nevertheless, *children of the street*, have been deserted, entirely or largely, to their own caretaking or that of other children and sustain some of the physical and affective needs deficits borne by feral children. They may, therefore, be at risk for some of the same developmental delays and dysfunctions as feral children, albeit under less pervasive environmental stressors.

5.2   Historical Context

The concept of the feral child has long existed in lore, but entered the realm of academic attention by the eighteenth century. The 1724 discovery of a feral 12-year-old, who came to be known as Wild Peter, in Germany caught the attention of scholars. The mute boy "behaved like a wild animal, eating raw birds and vegetables, and when threatened, he sat on his haunches or on all fours looking for opportunities to escape" (Loffstadt, Nichol, & de Klerk, 2006, p. 233). This first famous case of a feral child initiated discussion of the implications for humankind when isolated from the influence of society and culture (Candland, 1993, p. 16). The cases of the wild girl of Songi (1731), Victor of Aveyron (1797), and other reports emerge in the same century (Zingg, 1940a), along with a classification for *homo ferus* in 1758, by the Swedish taxonomist Linneaus (Candland). By the time Kaspar Hauser was found in 1828 in Germany (Singh & Zingg, 1942), the topic of feral children crossed from its home in lore toward the domain of scientific subject.

Interest in feral children has always exceeded actual information, a situation of opportunity for authors gifted in imagination and skilled in fakery, and a pitfall for enthusiastic, but insufficiently critical, journalists and scholars. Hoaxes such as the Wild Boy of Burundi (Lane & Pillard, 1978) – alleged to have been raised by monkeys – have exploited developmentally delayed orphans, while others have been fabricated in their entirety, such as the Syrian Gazelle Boy (Syria: Triumph of Civilization, 1948). Ogburn (1959) relates his investigation into the case of the wolf boy of Agra. News reports told of a 1-year-old suddenly missing from the household and his mother seeing a wolf running away from the home. The arrival of a waif of the appropriate age and appearance over 4 years later was declared the return of a wolf-reared boy. Ogburn's examination of what proved to be a false story, however, revealed how miscommunication, misattribution, and wishful thinking had swiftly adapted to the feral child myth, duping both the parents and the popular press. Note that the academic press has been immune to similar missteps. A psychologist at George Washington University rushed to report "the first case of a human child adopted and reared by infrahuman primates," Lucas, the baboon boy who was alleged to have been found amid a troop of baboons in 1903 South Africa (Foley, 1940, p. 129). The American Journal of Psychology article was retracted by its author after researcher, Robert Zingg, proved the case to have been a hoax (Zingg, 1940b).

It was Zingg, himself, who credibly presented the case of wolf children of Midnapore, India to the world. The two girls, Amala, aged 2, and Kamala, aged 8, were allegedly recovered in proximity of a wolf and her cubs by Reverend Singh and a group from an area village (Singh & Zingg, 1942). The missionary's extensive account of the childrens' discovery, behavior, and subsequent therapeutic progress is regarded as an honest record, even among the more skeptical literature on feral children. Their case became the first of the twentieth century to receive extensive attention from the more rigorous scientific standards of modern times.

Amala and Kamala were subject to intensive study by the scientific community of their day. However, the story of their origin remained suspect to many. It has been suggested that locals arranged for Singh to "discover" the girls nearby the wolves in order that he might relieve the "native community from the burden of caring for two mentally retarded children" (Favazza, 1977, p. 107). Bettelheim (1959) also challenged the notion that the children's behaviors were the result of having been raised by animals. He attributed all of their functional impairments to autism, except for Amala and Kamala's quadruped locomotion.

One of the more famous and well-documented cases of feral children in the later twentieth century was that of Genie, a 13-year-old girl discovered in Los Angeles in 1970. It was found that she had been physically restrained for over a decade and subjected to beatings for any vocalizations. Genie bore many similarities to earlier feral children. She could not stand erect, could barely walk, incontinent, and only whimpered. Susan Curtiss, a member of Genie's hospital intervention team, described her as "unsocialised, primitive, hardly human" (Curtiss, 1977, p. 9). Genie's case is also notable for the controversy – and attending legal action – regarding her being used as an experiment in reputedly poorly managed, unproductive research (Secret of the Wild Child, 1997, para. 152–180).

An 8-year-old feral child, Oxana Malaya, was found in Ukraine in 1991. According to an article in the British newspaper Daily Telegraph (Grice, 2006), she reportedly lived for 5 years among wild dogs in a kennel by her family's house. Little additional information is available as to her developmental history prior to being consigned to life among animals by her alcoholic parents, though she is said to have had some language prior to her isolation. At the time of her rescue, she was described as essentially nonverbal, barking, and moving on all fours. Oxana's case is one of the handful wherein animal-like behavior related to a particular species is distinctive and documented.

Cases of children found kept in isolation continue to arise. In Austria, Natascha Kampusch was abused and kept bound in a cellar for over 8 years from age 10, her sole contact being with her captor before her escape in 2006 (Kampusch, 2010). Two years later in the same country, Elisabeth Fritzl was found after being confine to the basement by her father for 24 years. Three of the seven children she bore by her father had also been imprisoned with her all their lives, two 5-year-olds and one aged 18. While details of the children's functioning in this relatively recent case are few, psychiatrist Berthold Kepplinger described the communication of the youngest two children as "anything but normal" (BBC News, 2008).

5.3 Description and Diagnosis

No single definition for feral child has been established. Linnaeus attempted a taxonomy of *Homo ferus* characteristics *mutus*, *tetrapus*, and *hirsutus* – mute, four-footed, and abnormally heavy hair covering (Candland, 1993). According to Favazza (1977), the taxonomist selected these traits based upon approximately ten feral child reports, including the Irish sheep-boy and the Hessian wolf boys, but he drew particularly from the cases of Wild Peter and the Sogny girl from Champagne. Linnaeus' definition, however, is overly restrictive for the inclusion of the majority of reported feral children, who do not possess each of these characteristics. The eighteenth and nineteenth century Europeans developed a more general concept of feral children that Candland relates as that of "children presumably raised outside culture and civilization – who were presumably raised by animals" (p. 3).

McNeil, Polloway, and Smith (1984) note that Linneaus' characteristic of *tetrapus*, quadruped locomotion, has been present in the majority of feral child reports. Most feral children have been successful in returning to bipedal locomotion. They found only three cases of *hirsutis*, however, among the 31 cases reported by Zingg (1940a). This characteristic, hypertrichosis, may be related to be the phenomenon of lanugo hair sometimes produced by malnutrition (Castellani, 1947). McNeil et al.

(1984) point out that the characteristic of *mutus* established by Linnaeus was consistent with 36 of 46 cases of feral children reports available for their review. Also, of these 36 children, who were reportedly mute or unintelligible, they found that 23 were claimed or suggested to have never learned to speak subsequent to recovery into society.

In their review of literature on feral children, McNeil et al. (1984) distinguish four subgroups of these *atypically reared children*: "those reared by animals; those reared in the wilderness; those reared in confinement; and those reared in confinement with limited human contact" (p. 70). The first of these groups is similar to that described by Candland (1993), and the researchers note that it is the most fitting of the term *feral*. Nonetheless, the remaining subgroups share several characteristics associated with the original concept of feral children.

5.3.1 Animal-Reared Children

Feral children of this type are believed to have been fed and nurtured by animals. When recovered into the care of humans, these children are ordinarily said to exhibit many of the characteristics of their animal "parents" that are not typical among children reared in human society (McNeil et al., 1984).

The two girls recovered from a wolf den in India in 1920 are likely the most famous of the feral children thought to have been raised by animals. They both walked on all fours at the time they were found in the company of a female wolf and her cubs. The girls were described to share other animal-like behaviors as well: for example, eating like dogs, "lowering their mouths to the plate," and lapping at liquids; bearing their teeth at perceived threats; and raising their noses to sniff at the air (Singh & Zingg, 1942, p. 27). The Ukrainian girl, Oxana Malaya (Grice, 2006), too, may be considered to have a combination of the animal-reared and confined-with-limited-human-contact subgroups.

5.3.2 Children Reared in Wilderness Isolation

Unlike the previous subgroup, these children were not fed and nurtured by animals. McNeil et al. (1984) define these feral children as having been initially "reared by humans at least through infancy… later lost to their families, and survived alone in the woods through their on resourcefulness" (p. 73). While feral children from this subgroup are also fearful of humans at the time of their recovery, they do not share the animal traits of the first subgroup.

The Wild Boy of Aveyron provides an example of this feral child subgroup. Victor sought to evade capture and when discovered and was mute – and remained so (Itard, 1962).

5.3.3   Children Reared Isolated in Confinement

These children have been housed and fed by humans – the minimum requirements for sustaining life – but have been starved of nurturing physical, social, and emotional human contact. Reports of feral children from this subgroup often feature the child's begin kept locked in a room or container, sometimes shackled, to maintain their isolation.

Kasper Hauser is the exemplar of this subgroup. Information provided by Kasper following his appearance yielded the speculation that he had been kept in a wooden box from age 3 to 17. During this period, he never saw anyone. A soporific drug was believed to have been used to induce the deep sleep during which he was bathed and clothed throughout his captivity (McNeill et al., 1984, p. 75). A similar example, in 1938 in Pennsylvania, an emaciated 6-year-old, Anna, was discovered bound in a small room, where she had kept from five-and-a-half months of age (Davis, 1940, p. 556). Her only human contact was with her mother, who seldom spent time with Anna except to feed her milk (McNeill et al., p. 75).

5.3.4   Children Confined with Limited Human Contact

The circumstances of this subgroup of feral children are nearly identical to those of the previous group. The difference is that they have exposure to some human contact. In some reported cases, the feral child has contact with an adult who keeps the child in confinement, At other times, the human contact is with another feral child in confinement.

A 1938 case in the USA provides an example of this subgroup. A 6-year-old girl was discovered to have been kept secluded in a dark room with her deaf-mute mother all the child's life (Davis, 1947, p. 436). When she was found she could only croak and behaved similarly to an infant.

LaPointe (2005) relates another case of this subgroup, a 33-year-old male who "was found chained to a post in a chicken yard when he was 8 years old, having lived primitively with chickens for most of his developmental years, supposedly shunned by the family for reasons not clearly discoverable" (p. vii) According to an audiology and speech scholar, the man had neither meaningful verbal nor nonverbal communication, though he emitted "primitive screeching sounds." Though he may be considered to have been in the confined with limited human contact subgroup, like the Ukrainian girl Oxana, he was described to act similarly to the animals around him: "He squats and uses his hands in a prehensile pecking manner, consistent with the behavior of chickens hopping around" (p. vii)

5.4   DSM-IV TR

There is no disorder designation specific to feral children. Among the documented cases of feral children, however, behavioral descriptions often report symptoms associated with mental retardation, communication disorders, pervasive developmental disorders, and reactive attachment disorder. It is unknown what portion of such deficits is related to the children's social isolation and other environmental factors, or, in some cases, if these disorders may have contributed to caretakers' decision to abandon or neglect the children.

5.5 Prevalence and Incidence

The literature regarding feral children is consistent in viewing them as exceedingly rare. In his 1942 review of the subject, Zingg states that no more than 40 cases were known to have ever been reported. The difficulty in establishing an estimate of incidence is found in two of the same problems that limited Zingg in the last century: definition and authentication.

Explicit delineation of the circumstances that identify an individual as within the concepts feral or isolated child is difficult to set. Even if a standard is established, substantiation of facts remains as challenging as ever. A search of a world newspaper database yields dozens of reports of feral children in this century, all purportedly recovered from the wild or raised by animals. How many fit within the feral concepts outlined by McNeill et al. (1984)? Of these, how many would be determined to be false as Ogburn (1959) revealed the wolf boy of Agra to be?

While verifiable instances of children found raised in extreme isolation continue to surface, the rarity of cases makes it difficult to establish their prevalence as well. Constructing a reliable body of information on contemporary isolated children is further hindered by legal considerations and the personally sensitive nature of cases. Children found in circumstances are usually the victims of abuse, and criminal proceedings against their abusers offer one possible avenue for researchers to gather data on isolated child cases – but complete information ordinarily is not disclosed until all matters, criminal and civil, are resolved after a period of years. Efforts to protect isolated children following their discovery and intake into social services also limit the availability of confidential physical and mental health data for research.

5.6 Assessment

Multidisciplinary assessment is indicated for any child subjected to chronic situations of neglect or deprivation. Malnutrition, developmental delay, and physical trauma are frequent factors in feral and isolated children. In addition, visual, aural, tactile, gustatory, and olfactory impairment or dysfunction has been reported in several cases (Itard, 1962; Zingg, 1940a), suggesting a need for sensory assessment by medical professionals.

Speech delays have been associated with nearly all cases of feral and isolated children. In addition to hearing assessment and evaluation by a speech-language pathologist, a physical examination is indicated to rule out congenital or trauma-related

88 5 Feral Children

impairments to speech production. Such a physical limitation, in fact, may explain Victor of Aveyron's failure to attain functional oral communication (Lane, 1976).

Motor skills must also be assessed. Impairments of gross motor skills have been reported for many feral and isolated children (Singh & Zingg, 1942). The classification criterion for *homo ferus* of quadruped locomotion originally set by Linneaus (Candland, 1993) has been noted frequently in cases, from the wolf girls of Agra to the 2004 discovery of an isolated family in South Africa (Loffstadt et al., 2006). While deficits in fine motor skill development have been inconsistently reported among cases of feral and isolated children, the deprivation of sensory experience and unfamiliarity with the materials and tools of society place them at risk for fine motor skill delays and indicate the need for assessment.

A comprehensive psychological evaluation is essential for any individual taken from the conditions of neglect and deprivational abuse that define feral and isolated persons. Intelligence should be assessed to determine any areas of cognitive delay. Social–emotional evaluation will be required to diagnose any mental disorders, regardless of their etiology. Educational assessment, too, will be necessary for any child that has been subjected to neglect and isolation. Appropriate evaluation techniques will likely include the use of nonverbal instruments and behavioral observation systems.

5.7 Etiological Hypotheses and Theoretical Frameworks

While the origin of feral childrens' entry to the wild is as individual as it is unknown, isolated children are the victims of active neglect or what Golden, Samuels, and Southall (2003) refer to as "deprivational abuse" (p. 105). They include "forced isolation, food deprivation, or the withholding of love…used deliberately, as punishment, sadistically, or to induce illness" (p. 105) within their definition, though the specifics of motivation are second to the element of active abuse.

In addition to intrapersonal factors contributing to vulnerability and resiliency, the timing of deprivation can determine the degree of neuropsychological insult. As Loffstadt et al. (2006) explain:

> The nervous system of young children is malleable and depends on experience to shape the behavior and skills needed for life. If abandoned while very young, they may never make up for the experience. This is known as the critical period of brain plasticity. The idea of critical periods teaches us that for some aspects of brain development, timing of environmental input is crucial, and that important abilities will be lost or diminished if stimulation does not occur at the right time (p. 233).

Cognitive, language, and motor development delays as well as sensory and affective dysregulation are common features among reports feral and isolated children. Loffstadt et al. (2003) state that "the specific dysfunction will depend upon the timing of the insult…, the nature of the insult (e.g., a lack of sensory stimulation due to neglect), and the pattern of the insult (e.g., a chronic experience)" (p. 234).

5.8   Treatment and Intervention

The greatest step in intervention for feral or isolated children is also the first, removing them from their state of deprivation or abuse. Planning subsequent treatment efforts is surely made more difficult by the complexity of comorbidities that exist in every reported case.

The salient feature of feral and isolated children is their disconnection from human contact. Therefore, socialization will always be necessary. As Smith (1997) points out:

> Children reared by animals are not animals but neither are they fully human in a social or cultural sense. Whether reared by animals or growing up with only limited contact with other people, such children are in critical need of human socialization once they are found and placed in a cultural context (p. 32).

Socialization was a central objective in the case of the Indian girl, Kamala. Singh and Zingg (1942) reported that regular massage contributed to her therapy. He wrote, "The human touch in the massage had an especially soothing influence on her to give up her ferocious animal nature, an developed in her in its place a sort of crude affection towards [Mrs. Singh]" (p. 115). This treatment modality is detailed in several places in Singh's record of the wolf girls, and he credits its therapeutic benefit more than once. The merit of the intervention's obvious lack of language component is highlighted when one considers its utility in working with nonverbal feral children such as Kamala.

Terr (2003) describes a girl, Cammie, with severe posttraumatic stress disorder subsequent to suffering physical violence, sexual abuse, and likely witnessing the slaughter of animals and murder of her sister. As a toddler, the child growled and hissed, shuddered at the approach of people, sniffed adults' sexual organs, and bit people. Her psychiatrist noted that she "strongly resembled the 'feral children' described in classic psychiatric and psychological literature" (p. 1402).

Successful intervention for Cammie was implemented over 12-year course of monthly psychotherapy sessions based on three principles. Terr (2003) states that these are "abreaction (full emotional expression of the experience), context (understanding and gaining experience on the experience), and correction (finding ways personally or through society to prevent or repair such experiences)" (p. 1403). Developmentally appropriate psychotherapy was designed for Cammie based on these principles, including the modalities of play therapy and cognitive-behavioral interventions, beginning at 29 months. In combination with family counseling, medical, educational, and speech interventions, this course of psychotherapy yielded unpredicted improvements in Cammie, whom Terr described as developing into socially and emotionally high-functioning adolescent, participating in gifted education, and continuing to benefit from psychotherapeutic support.

Kenneally, Bruck, Frank, and Nalty (1998) relate the case of an adult female, Rose, following 30 years of social isolation and neglect. Developmental delays had begun at 9 months of age following an illness accompanied by seizures. Rose was cared for in a playpen until age 5. From age 6, she was confined in a small room

with a mattress and blanket, reportedly living on a diet of "four items: coffee, cook-
ies, carnation milk, and candy" (p. 17). Unclothed, incontinent, and without sanita-
tion, Rose remained in this situation until age 36. During this time she "received
only limited contact" with her custodian grandmother, except for occasional visits
to a physician to obtain prescriptions for an antipsychotic. Rose was rescued from
her confinement and neglect following her grandmother's death. At this time she
had pica, was aggressive, acting out self-injurious behaviors, and nonverbal. Rose's
communication deficits were such that she was initially thought to be blind and
deaf, even though this was not the case.

Therapists set three communications objectives for Rose: association of meaning
with picture symbol cards, comprehension and executing one-step directives, and
use of hand gestures. Although progress was achieved toward each of the objectives,
after 2 years of language intervention, Rose was only able to meet the success criterion for following simple directives.

5.8.1   Pharmacological

Pharmacological interventions, of course, are not indicated for the status of feral,
isolated, or *of the street* children. The physical health problems consequent to the
risks posed by neglect, deprivation, and abuse, however, may require medical treatment. Psychotropic drugs have been applied as an adjunct to psychological interventions for specific disorders of children from situations associated with feral and
isolated children. Terr (2003), for example, reports that methylphenidate was incorporated into the treatment of Cammie's ADHD-related symptoms, as well as a
selective serotonin reuptake inhibitor, over the years of her psychotherapy.

5.9   Outcome and Prognostic Factors

Outcomes depend, in part, on the degree to which environmental cues neurological
development are limited by the privations suffered by feral and isolated children.
Loffstadt et al. note that "disruption of the pattern, timing, or intensity of these cues
can lead to abnormal neurodevelopment and severe dysfunction, since the developmental experiences determine the organizational and functional status of the mature
brain" (p. 234).

The prospects for feral and isolated children are quite individual and strikingly
unpredictable. Temperament, neuropsychological function, physical and mental
health as well as variable treatment support influence childrens' progress from a
broad variety of circumstances and unique, scarcely known, histories.

Victor of Aveyron developed communication, self-care, and communication
skills (Itard, 1962), and Kasper Hauser acquired these to an even greater degree,
learning some facility in Latin and working as a clerk (McNeill et al., 1984, p. 75).

The Midnapore girls, found in a state of more severe delay and deprivation, could not reach such outcomes. Amala made progress but died 1 year after their discovery. Kamala grew away from many of her animal-like behaviors, used three-word sentences from her vocabulary of 45 words, and socialized with others in the orphanage. As McNeill et al. emphasize, her "advances have to be viewed in terms of a continuum of change…. Kamala did not just attain a developmental age of three, she changed from a 'wolf-child' to a 'human-child'" (p. 73).

Some isolated children have made remarkable recoveries, despite the severe abuse they have suffered. Natascha Kampusch escaped a cellar in which she had been held by a man for more than 8 years. In addition to Natascha's isolation, the she was assaulted daily, had her head shaved, kept seminaked, and starved. Natascha attempted suicide several times before her escape. Since then she has hosted a television program and written a book on her ordeal (Kampusch, 2010).

It must be remembered, though, Natascha was a normally developed 10-year-old at the time of her abduction into isolation. In general, the earlier in life children are exposed to environmental deprivation and abuse, the more severe, extensive, and enduring are their deficits and dysfunction. Exceptions occur, however. Koluchová reported the case of identical twin males, raised "isolated and cruelly treated" from the age of 18 months to 7 years, who could not speak or walk and were cognitively in the "range of severe subnormality" ("Koluchova's Twins," 1976, p. 897). Following their rescue and placement in a nurturing foster family, the twins steadily improved in every area of development and functioning. Wechsler IQ standard scores increased from 40 at the boys' first assessment to 80 and 72 the next year. By age 18, the twins' Wechsler Adult Intelligence Scale IQ scores were both above average, about 113. They developed proficient motor skills, "harmoniously formed personalities" (Koluchová, 1992, p. 50), and many intellectual interests over the years. As adults, the brothers were described as socially emotionally normal, each professionally established and enjoying good marriages with children (Koluchová).

Prognosis for feral and isolated children also relies on effective and sustained intervention. Until at least age 23, the Ukrainian Oxana lived in the care of an Odessa clinic, where she has acquired substantial social, speech, and adaptive skills, according to reports. She has been diagnosed with cognitive delays and continues to have affective and speech limitations (Grice, 2006).

5.10   Future Directions

The twenty-first century world's increasingly dense population and great availability of travel and communications have combined so that true isolation seems rare. In these times, it seems improbable that new cases of documentable feral children will come to light. Isolated children will surely continue to surface, however, in exceptional, atypical situations perhaps even under the rubric of Munchausen by proxy.

Encountering feral and isolated children will always provoke intense intellectual curiosity, a desire for inquiry that must be approached with regard to the individual. In a public broadcasting documentary on Genie's psychologist, Harlan Lane, acknowledged the tension between the need to learn more about the effect of extreme neglect and isolation and aiding its victims, saying, "Look, there's an ethical dilemma in this kind of research. If you want to do rigorous science, then Genie's interests are going to come second some of the time. If you only care about helping Genie, then you wouldn't do a lot of the scientific research" (Secret of the Wild Child, 1997, para. 190). In the case of feral children, the question remains. Are they able to be rehabilitated to become productive citizens? The evidence suggests that this is improbable, but not impossible. Although the vast majority of feral children will remain in a nexus between an animal and human state, there are others who can be sufficiently rehabilitated so that they may at the very least be integrated to some degree into society. Still, the scars of abandonment and lack of human contact remain with these children throughout the remainder of their lives.

References

BBC News. (2008, April 30). *Austria seeks to 'rescue image'*. Retrieved from http://news.bbc.co.uk/2/hi/europe/7374965.stm.

Bettelheim, B. (1959). Feral children and autistic children. *The American Journal of Sociology, 64*(5), 455–467.

Candland, D. K. (1993). *Feral children and clever animals: Reflections on human nature*. New York: Oxford University Press.

Castellani, A. (1947). Hypertrichosis of the lanugo hair in malnutrition. *British Medical Journal, 2*(4517), 188.

Curtiss, S. (1977). *Genie: A psycholinguistic study of a modern-day "wild child"*. New York: Academic.

Davis, K. (1940). Extreme social isolation of a child. *The American Journal of Sociology, 45*(4), 554–565.

Davis, K. (1947). Final note on a case of extreme social isolation of a child. *The American Journal of Sociology, 52*(5), 432–437.

Dennis, W. (1941). The significance of feral man. *The American Journal of Psychology, 54*(3), 425–432.

Favazza, A. (1977). Feral and isolated children. *The British Journal of Medical Psychology, 50*(1), 105–111.

Findley, C. V. (2005). *The Turks in world history*. New York: Oxford University Press.

Foley, J. P. (1940). The 'baboon boy' of South Africa. *The American Journal of Psychology, 53*(1), 128–133.

Golden, M. H., Samuels, M. P., & Southall, D. P. (2003). How to distinguish between neglect and deprivational abuse. *Archives of Disease in Childhood, 88*, 105–107.

Grice, E. (2006, July 17). Cry of an enfant sauvage. *The Telegraph*. Retrieved from http://www.telegraph.co.uk.

Ibn Tufail, A. B. (1929). *The history of Hayy Ibn Yaqzan*. New York: Frederick A. Stokes Publishers.

Itard, J.-M.-G. (1962). *The wild boy of Aveyron*. New York: Appleton-Century-Crofts.

Kampusch, N. (2010). *3,096 Days*. New York: Viking.

Kenneally, S. M., Bruck, G. E., Frank, E. M., & Nalty, L. (1998). Language intervention after thirty years of isolation: A case study of a feral child. *Education and Training in Mental Retardation and Developmental Disabilities, 33*(1), 13–23.

Koluchovà, J. (1992). Deprivation and its reparation in children of Czechoslovakia. *Child Abuse Review, 1*, 49–51.

Koluchova's Twins. (1976). *British Medical Journal, 2*(6041), 897–898. Retrieved from http://www.jstor.org/stable/20411792.

Lane, H. (1976). *The wild boy of Aveyron.* Cambridge, MA: Harvard University Press.

Lane, H., & Pillard, R. (1978). The wild boy of Burundi: A study of an outcast child. New York, Random House.

LaPointe, L. L. (2005). Children aren't dogs; adults aren't gods. *Journal of Medical Speech-Language Pathology, 13*(1), vii–ix.

Loffstadt, H., Nichol, R. J., & de Klerk, B. (2006). *African Psychiatry Review, 9*(4), 231–234.

Malson, L. (1972). *Wolf children and the problem of human nature.* New York: Monthly Review Press.

McNeil, M. C., Polloway, E. A., & Smith, J. D. (1984). Feral and isolated children: Historical review and analysis. *Education and Training of the Mentally Retarded, 19*(1), 70–79.

Moura, S. L. (2002). The social construction of street children: configuration and implications. *British Journal of Social Work, 32*, 353–367.

Ogburn, W. F. (1959). The wolf boy of Agra. *The American Journal of Sociology, 64*(5), 454–459.

Secret of the Wild Child. (1997, March 4). *NOVA [Television Program].* Retrieved from http://www.pbs.org/wgbh/nova/transcripts/2112gchild.html.

Singh, J. A. L., & Zingg, R. M. (1942). *Wolf-children and feral man.* New York: Harper & Row.

Smith, J. D. (1997). Liddy, a child found and lost: A voice across time. *Journal of Developmental and Physical Disabilities, 9*(1), 31–38.

Syria: Triumph of Civilization. (1948, September 9). *Time.* Retrieved from http://www.time.com/time/magazine/article/0,9171,855406,00.html.

Terr, L. C. (2003). "Wild child": How three principles of healing organized 12 years of psychotherapy. *Journal of the American Academy of Child and Adolescent Psychiatry, 42*(12), 1401–1409.

World Health Organization. (2000). *Working with street children.* Retrieved from http://www.unodc.org/pdf/youthnet/who_street_children_introduction.pdf.

Zingg, R. M. (1940a). Feral man and extreme cases of isolation. *The American Journal of Psychology, 53*(4), 487–517.

Zingg, R. M. (1940b). More about the 'baboon boy' of South Africa. *The American Journal of Psychology, 53*(3), 455–462.

Chapter 6
The Youth Gang Member

All I'm trying to do is survive and make good out of the dirty,
nasty, unbelievable lifestyle that they gave me.

–Tupac Shakur (1971–1996)

6.1 Overview

Few social issues are more troubling than that of youth gangs and their impact on society. Early views of gangs and gang members depicted these individuals as outcasts of society who banded together to cause trouble. The perception of youth gang members was aptly depicted in Charles Dicken's *Oliver Twist* whose characters were a group of orphans living on the street, stealing food, and snatching wallets and purses in order to survive. In the present day, when people think about a gang, they typically picture notorious groups like the Crips, the Bloods and perhaps even the Hell's Angels. Yet scholars and researchers believe that most people identify gangs and their members with an exaggerated, sensationalized image (Tobin, 2008). The modern image of a street gang has, in some form, been influenced by the media which has not adequately reflected the character of the problem (Spergel, 1995). Life as a gang banger has often been glamorized by the entertainment industry with some characters becoming popular cultural icons (e.g., Tupac Shakur). Movies and songs about gang life, like *Gangsta's Paradise*, have popularized the notion of gangs within our culture. Hard-core rap artists often rap about revolutions and killing. This music has integrated itself with the hip-hop scene and is in great demand from mainstream adolescents. But in spite of this more romanticized view of gangs, the reality is that gangs have an extremely damaging impact on the individual and society as a whole. Members often become involved with a gang at an early age and the course of their lives is dangerously directly and indirectly controlled by their affiliation with a gang. In many cases, the eventual outcome for the individuals is tragic.

S.C. Dombrowski et al., *Assessing and Treating Low Incidence/High Severity Psychological Disorders of Childhood*, DOI 10.1007/978-1-4419-9970-2_6, © Springer Science+Business Media, LLC 2011

People have formed groups throughout human history to fulfill the important psychological need of belonging. By joining a group, an individual becomes part of a whole (Delaney, 2006). Within a group, an individual acquires both an individual and collective identity, both of which are essential for human development. Abram Maslow's (1943) hierarchy of human needs identifies that a sense of belonging and establishing affiliations with others is essential to one's psychological development. Almost everyone has been a part of a group, be it a sports club, a member of a religious group, or having a collective group of friends. Involvement in a gang, therefore, fulfills an essential human need to band together with others for a common purpose and such belonging needs explains why youth gangs can become so powerful.

In more recent times, the role of youth gangs in our society has become more prominent, with their presence often reflecting the significant sociological problems in society such as poverty and discrimination. At present, gangs have pervaded our entire social structure, with notorious gangs attaining significant financial, political, and social power to the point of becoming a major threat to national and international security.

Gangs are a global entity, identified throughout the world, with each continent having its own unique history. Current gang research indicates that gangs are expanding throughout the world (Covey, 2010). This is likely a function of improved technology, primarily through the World Wide Web which has facilitated the increased globalization and communication around the world. Communication across continents is now almost instantaneous with virtually anyone having access to this information super highway. The growth of gangs throughout the world is a topic unto itself (Covey), and for the current chapter, a historical overview will primarily focus on youth gangs in the USA and Canada.

It is important to note that there are multiple perspectives, theories, and explanations of youth gangs and youth gang membership stemming from the contributions of sociology, psychology, criminology, and justice. The topic is so expansive that there are many levels and disciplines that attempt to provide grounded theories and descriptions of youth gangs. Because of the role of youth gangs in crime, the majority of theories and descriptions of gang activity come from a legal and justice perspective. This chapter reviews major theoretical perspectives from various disciplines but will highlight the psychological aspects of the youth gang member.

6.2   Historical Context

> Gang violence in America is not a sudden problem. It has been a part of urban life for years, offering an aggressive definition and identity to those seeking a place to belong in the chaos of large metropolitan areas.
>
> –Dave Reichart, US Congressman

Gangs can be traced back as far back as recorded history. The fact that gangs have such a deep and prolonged history is an interesting phenomenon, suggesting that there are conditions in society and culture that facilitate the emergence and sustainability of gangs. In more recent times, scholars have sought to delineate what may best explain and even predict the emergence of gangs. Many authors now suggest that the evolution of gangs, especially in North American Society, is inextricably linked with two momentous sociological forces: economic disadvantage and racism (Pyrooz, Fox, & Decker, 2010a). Pratt and Cullen (2005) conducted a meta-analysis of predictors of aggregate crimes rates and found economic disadvantage to be one of the strongest macrolevel predictors of youth crime. Other factors suggest that youth gangs are often concentrated in disadvantaged neighborhoods characterized by economic deprivation, high residential mobility, and racial and ethnic heterogeneity (Pyrooz et al., 2010). Christopher Adamson (2000) captures this sentiment in his statement that, "indeed, the effects of racial and class structures on the behavior of American youth gangs have been so profound that scholars who sought to develop race-invariant theories of gangs and delinquency have been stymied" (p. 272). More detailed descriptions of theories and etiological hypotheses will be outlined in subsequent sections of this chapter. With this context in mind, we set the stage for the brief overview of the past.

Early records of what might be described as "gang activity" are loosely defined, given the breadth of behavior that could be defined as belonging to gangs. For instance, early historical writings provide many accounts of bands of individuals who pillaged, burned, and ransacked towns, cities, to inflict damage on victims for personal gain (Delaney, 2006). The Old Testament provides accounts of warring cultural factions at odds with the people of Israel who, during times of war, raided peaceful tribes. Savelli (2001) states the word *thug* originated in India in the 1200s (A.D. 2000) and referred to a gang of criminals that roamed the country pillaging towns along their path. These bands of thugs were known to have their own symbols, hand signs, rituals, and slang (Delaney).

During the Roman age, suburban criminal gangs were reported to disrupt life with riots and mayhem. These gangs were believed to begin such practices at kidnapping for ransom and aligning with barbarians to aid in their antisocial activity. Pearson (1983) described fourteenth- and fifteenth-century London as a place where citizens were terrorized by gangs such as the Mims, Hectors, Bugles, and Dead boys. Perhaps the most famous and fabled gang was Robin Hood and his Merry Men. Folklore depicted Robin Hood's gang of thieves to be uniquely prosocial, helping the poor victimized common folk of England to fight against the corrupt political and social powers that oppressed them.

Christopher Adamson (2000) compared the emergence of European American and African American youth gangs in American history and found that in spite of similarities between the two groups, the two gangs were profoundly different historical creations. Black gangs were not recognized as a social problem until the early 1910s during the great migration that took place during that time. While black gangs in the 1800s existed, they were not distinct identifies (i.e., they had no names) and, important for that historical periods, these gangs did not make claims about specific territories within cities. Thus, they were seen as an extension of the community in which they lived.

White gangs, in contrast, appeared as the American Revolution ended and their activities became increasingly visible during the formation of neighborhoods in big cities like Boston, Philadelphia, Chicago, and New York. Many believe that the rapid changing economics of big cities, especially New York, gave rise to a number of immigrants from distinct ethnicities. As more immigrants gathered to form their own communities, the result was increased tension among these groups as they sought to establish their identities. This was fueled by environmental and economic factors in which the cities grew too fast to allow for proper housing, jobs, and access to resources leading to gross over population, limited access to jobs and education.

Adamson argues that white youth gangs enjoyed a measure of support from the adult population which fostered their growth. These gangs were often supported by politically powerful adults who rewarded them for defending local neighborhoods. Thus, these gangs were reinforced for serving a protective function. As a result, gangs allied themselves with social and political clubs and often took direction from political bosses (Adamson, 2000).

By the early 1900s, the populations in big cities exploded. The economics of the time created the need for a blue-collar work force. In the context of increasing urbanization, a transient inner city population, and few social/community supports, children were increasingly left alone. Furthermore, with increased competition for resources, gangs became more territorial. It is interesting that during this period, gangs were more concerned about the territory they protected than the ethnicity of their group members. While politically powerful adults frowned upon the activities of these gangs (such as breaking windows, defacing streets, disturbing the peace), there continued to be an approval of the role gangs played in maintaining quality of community life (like keeping others away from their neighborhoods). However, over time, clashes between ethnic minorities, especially whites and blacks became more frequent. This was thought to arise from the eroding of the political positions held by whites (Adamson, 2000). In addition, the rapidly growing urban African American community led to an increased number of African American gangs. These groups increased their presence and by nature of the very tense political relationships that emerged between blacks and whites, racial segregation, and limited economic options, the incidence of warfare between these gangs increased. This was most evident in cities like Los Angeles and Chicago.

Delaney (2006) proposes that the philosophy of youth gangs changed past the middle part of the twentieth century. The early history of youth gangs suggested that they formed protective-type groups to increase their survival and to protect their own "turf." This changed as gangs expanded into the black market of trading goods and increased involvement in drug trafficking, all of which increased their access to resources. Delaney suggests that today's youth gangs are for more offensive in that they "seek larger territories, they have become more mobile, and conduct such behaviors as drive-by shootings, and have seemingly taken claim to the economically profitable illegal drug industry" (p. 60). Others (Moore, 1991) agree, pointing to the increased lethal violence pervasive through many large urban centers throughout North American. There has been a significant increase in the number of youth gangs since the early 1980s. Some of these gangs have become involved in international terrorism (Covey, 2010). In addition, there has been a spread of gangs to smaller urban cities and Native-American reservations likely a result of deindustrialization. Furthermore, the continued influx of immigrants to North American has resulted in the formation of other ethic gangs. For instance, recent violent crime across cities in North America has been attributed to Somalian gangs (Associated Press, 2009). Below is a brief history of several notorious gangs in North America now follows.

6.2.1 Prominent Gangs in North America

6.2.1.1 The Crips

One of the most well-known gangs of Los Angeles, the Crips was reportedly founded by Raymond Washington in 1968. At the time many black youths were ostracized from organizations like Boy Scouts because of race, and began to form their own gangs. Washington originally started a gang known as the "Baby Avenues" but after a fight with a fellow gang member, split off to form his own gang. Apparently, a friend of Washington's had a limp and was referred to as a cripple by his peers. The distinct walk was emulated by the growing members of the gang, and soon others referred to them as "crips." The name held. Stanley "Tookie" Williams joined with Washington a few years later. The gang became popular among disillusioned black youth, and many young and vulnerable youths became targets for recruitment. Members adopted a similar dress style of jeans, a blue shirt, and dark blue suspenders. The shooting death of one of its early members who wore a blue banana further entrenched this color as part of its identity. As gang membership grew, members formed groups within their own neighborhoods taking on names that reflected their locale (e.g., The Avalon Garden Crips). Folklore suggested these gangs evolved as a protest to the treatment of Black Panther members in the USA and sought political justice. However, scholars dispel this myth, pointing out that the primary activity of these gangs was to socialize its members and engage in violence with warring gang members. The increasing clashes between gangs led to large-scale violence in major urban centers. Currently, it is estimated that there are over 800 sets of Crips gangs that have spread to many parts of the USA, most notably in big urban centers. It is noted that some gangs in various cities take on the name of the Crips, even without any affiliation, to try to enhance their status (Covey, 2010).

6.2.1.2 The Bloods

This gang evolved primarily in response to the Crips. There are various folklores about the events that actually gave the impetus to the formation of the bloods, but a more common belief was that some youths from Centennial High in Los Angeles fought and defeated some members of the Crips (Morales, 2010). This group originally known as the Piru street gang began to ally with other smaller gangs to assert their influence and compete with the Crips, who, in the early 1970s in Los Angeles, outnumbered other gangs 3–1 (Wolf, 2010). To assert their power and influence, members of the Bloods became increasingly violent, especially when warring against members of the Crips. To this day they are considered one of the more violent gangs, with their trademark being the use of knives and razors often for initiation purposes, hence the referral to the name Bloods. The United Blood Nation, or simply, "The Bloods" expanded into prisons in the 1990s to rival The Latin Kings (Morales). However there are varying opinions regarding how the prison gangs actually began. Like many other gangs, recruitment focuses on youth living in impoverished neighborhoods. The gangs offer a sense of protection, a sense of belonging, and the promise of power and riches. The Bloods have their unique dress style which almost always involves the color red. A prominent sign among the Bloods is a crossed out C which serves as a form of disrespect toward the Crips.

6.2.1.3   The Almighty Latin King and Queen Nation (ALKQA)

The Latin Kings originally emerged out of Chicago in the 1940s where small groups of Puerto Rican and Mexican male youths organized in order to protect their neighborhoods. The impetus behind the Latin Kings was to fight against the oppression and discrimination felt by Latino minorities. The name refers to a uniting of all individuals of Latino heritage. Like other gangs, a common bond was a fight against racism and oppression that faced so many of these youths. Over time, the ALKQA followed a path toward crime and violence with its members being associated in drug trafficking, turf wars with other gangs, and participating in riots. The ALKQA is believed to be Chicago's largest gang with over 25,000 members in that city alone. Chapters of the ALKQA are spread throughout most large urban settings in the USA and Canada. A unique identifying aspect of the ALKQA is the emphasis on establishing community among Latino's with some chapters having formed their self-proclaimed religion of "Kingism." In addition, this gang is known for its strong organization, structure, and harsh discipline of its members. The gang stresses basic principles of respect, honesty, unity, knowledge, and love among members, with these principles forming the five points to the crown that symbolizes their gang.

6.2.1.4   MS-13

Salvadoran migrants who had escaped El Salvador's civil fighting established the Mara Salvatrucha (MS-13) gang in Los Angeles during the 1980s (Ribando, 2007). These migrants found difficult work and social conditions in Los Angeles, particularly with the city's established gangs including African Americans in the Crips or Bloods, and Mexican-Americans or illegal Mexican immigrants in the EME, also known as the Mexican Mafia (Bruneau, 2005). Some of the migrants joined the Mexican founded M-18 gang, which had started to encompass multiple nationalities including Hispanics (Bruneau). In response to this viewed betrayal and the other established gangs, a portion of the remaining Salvadorans created the Mara Salvatrucha (Bruneau). Also known as MS-13, for the 13th street in Los Angeles, the gang's territory now spans a transnational region, including Central America, the USA, and even Canada (Bruneau). This widespread range is largely attributed to the mass deportation of imprisoned Salvadoran gang members from the USA, which led to the San Salvadoran establishment of the Mara Salvatrucha (Bruneau). As membership is dynamic, and census taking is rudimentary, numbers are roughly estimated to be 7,000 in El Salvador, 20,000 in the USA, and 4,000 in Canada (Bruneau). The gang identifies itself through written and hang signaled language, as well as tattoos (Bruneau). However, it most distinguishes itself through its use of violence, a theme intimately wrapped within its discipline and hierarchy, from membership initiation to leadership ascension (Bruneau). For instance, part of the ascension process includes "Sangre Afuera, Sangre Adentro" (blood outside and blood inside), which is killing a person without reason, other than displaying the ability to do so (Bruneau).

There are many other notable gangs throughout the USA and Canada that are not presented here. Some of these gangs, like the Wah Ching gang from southern California, have become well known for their violence and criminal behavior. In sum, the roots of most known gangs indicate they are established to retaliate against the violence from other gangs and become involved in drug trafficking and criminal activity.

6.3 Description and Diagnostic Classification

6.3.1 Definitions

Defining a gang is not easy, given the broad range of descriptions and perspectives of a gang. Researchers, theorists, and policy makers focus on different attributes of youth gang activity given their unique perspectives. In fact, many contemporary gang researchers indicate that in spite of the multiple efforts at addressing youth gangs in society, there continues to be an absence of a definitional consensus (Esbensen, 2000). Charlie Brown and his friends from the Peanuts gang could, loosely speaking, fit the definition of a gang. However, widely used benchmarks for defining whether a social group is a youth gang depends on their youth status (generally ages 10 to early 20s) and the engagement by group members in law-violating behavior, or at minimum, imprudent behavior (Esbensen, 2000). Of interest, traditional researchers like Thrasher (1927/1963) and Klein (1971) who have spent time living among gangs argued pervasively for the self-definition of gang members, that is, they let the individual make the designation of whether they are a member of a gang or not. In fact, Esbensen (2000) argues that from a research perspective, self-nomination was a particularly robust measure of gang membership capable of distinguishing gang from nongang youth.

An important attempt at consensus came when the Office of Juvenile Justice and Delinquency Prevention (OJJDP) conducted its first National Youth Gang Survey (National Gang Crime Research Center, 1996) of the nearly 55,000 law enforcement agencies. The NYGS defined a gang as "a group of youths or young adults in your jurisdiction that you or other responsible persons in your agency or community are willing to identify or classify as a gang" (Sheldon, Randall, Sharon, & Brown, 2001). In 2000, the OJJDP set criterion for youth gang membership to have:

- More than two members.
- Fall within a limited age range (generally between 12 and 24 years of age).
- Have a sense of shared identify (including a name and/or associated symbols to claim gang affiliation).
- Show some degree of permanence, generally lasting over 1 year.
- Involvement in criminal activity.

The latter point is an important one for distinguishing youth gangs from non-criminal youth groups. Tobin (2008) cautions that gangs are easily misunderstood and that there is variation in the gang world that is not presented in the movies, on TV, or in the newspaper. In addition, some critics cite the NYGS's early definition was not restricted enough, leading to an overestimate of youth gangs in the USA by 35% (Esbensen, Winfree, He, & Taylor, 2001) leading to an over estimate of the number of youth gang members. However, at present, this remains the most widely used definition. Thus, the term "youth gang" will use the definition provided by the OJJDP, but also relates to other group activities involved in crime as well. Finally, the term "gang banger" is often used in the media to refer to gang members. The term was originally used to describe someone who participates in group sex, but has become a descriptor for gang members who engage in violence and crime.

6.3.2   Descriptions and Diagnosis

What does a youth gang member look like? How would they best be described? What do they wear and what do they do? Most people have an image of a gang member influenced by what they have witnessed in the media. Often depictions of a gang member rely on the many stereotypes regarding gangs and gang behavior (Delaney, 2006). As a result, most people believe the typical gang member "is male, lives in the inner city, and is a member of a racial or ethnic minority" (Esbensen, 2000).

Gang membership is not a criterion for psychopathology in the Diagnostic and Statistical Manual of Mental Disorders, fourth Edition (DSM-IV; 2000) or the International Classification of Diseases, tenth Edition (ICD-10, WHO, 2010). However, severely trouble youth, particularly those with conduct disorder (DSM-IV: 302.8 or ICD-10: F91), have a high incidence of involvement in gang activity due to the antisocial features of this disorder. Descriptors of predictive variables of gang membership are outlined in greater detail below.

6.3.3 Prevalence/Incidence

According to statistics from 2008 National Youth Gang Survey, there were approximately 27,900 gangs and 774,000 gang members (Egley, Howell, & Moore, 2009). Like most official data sources, questions of validity are prevalent, and this result represents an underestimate of active members. According to the OJJDP (2010), all cities with a population above 250,000 reported gang activity and 87% of cities with more than 100,000 also reported gang activity. Cities like Los Angeles, New York, and Chicago are best known for their historic gang problems. Results estimate that over 2,300 cities in American have active gangs. Los Angeles, which has the dubious distinction of being the street gang capital, is reported to have over 100,000 gang members and one half of all homicides are reported to be gang-related (Delaney, 2006). In Canada, Criminal Intelligence Service Canada (CISC, 2006) reported 344 Street gangs with 11, 900 active members in rural, urban, and aboriginal reserve areas across Canada. Most researchers agree there has been a dramatic increase in gang activity in the last 30 years, and now every state reports youth gang activity (Miller, 2001). Given the increased prevalence of national task forces and increased support of policing of gang activity, statistics suggest that since 1996, the number of gang and gang members has declined slightly, but the opposite trend is true of larger cities (Egley, 2002).

There are different ways to measure the incidence of gang involvement among youth, but these statistics can be challenging to understand. For instance, most statistics come from the Department of Justice that tabulates the incidence of crime among youth. However, this does not necessary reflect gang involvement. The average age of a youth gang member is approximately 17-year-old, but gang members can be much younger than that (Egley, 2002). Nationwide, 23% of students report the presence of gangs at their schools (Dinkes, Kemp, & Baum, 2009), and approximately 35% of law enforcement agencies indicate gang problems (such as gang-related crime) in their jurisdictions (Egley & O'Donnell, 2009). Self-reported youth surveys show varying estimates of gang membership, from single digits among a national sample of students to about 30% among high-risk youth in large cities (Howell & Egley, 2005). Recently, the National Council on Crime and Delinquency (2009) indicated that 5% of all youth reported gang involvement. Perhaps the most interesting measure of youth gang involvement comes from youth themselves. When urban youth are asked to report affiliation with a gang, the bulk of studies suggest approximately 15% of youth indicate they have belonged to a gang (Delaney, 2006; Esbensen, 2001; OJJDP, 2004; Tobin, 2008). This number, of course, relies on the person's perspective of a "gang" and therefore, these numbers may be skewed. However, it represents a significant number of adolescents within North American culture.

6.3.4 Ethnicity

There are many types of youth gangs and they are most often categorized according to ethnicity (e.g., Asian gangs and African American gangs) or by association [e.g., a bike gang like Hell's Angels or a prison gang like the Black Guerilla Family. Gangs are, in principle, but not exclusively minority in ethnicity or race (Klein)]. The NYGC estimates that 36% of all gangs were reportedly mixed race. Those that are defined by their ethnicity are prominently Hispanic (46%), followed by African American (34%), Caucasian (12%), Asian (6%), and other (2%). Of interest, Caucasian gangs represented 30% of gangs found in small cities and 27% of gangs present in rural counties (National Youth Gang Center, 2000). There has been an alarming increase in the number of Native-American gangs, and it is estimated that there are approximately 800–1,000 gangs in the Prairie Provinces of Canada (Totten, 2009).

6.3.5 Gender

Historically, youth gangs have been principally male, with virtually all research showing a much higher percentage of male gang members than female members. In history, there have been several notorious female gangsters like Belle Starr who lived in the early 1800s was known to carry guns, rob stage coaches, and associate with other devious men. Thrasher's (1927/1963) famous early research of gangs identified females as "auxiliaries" and most female gang members were described in terms of their sexual role. Sadly, female gang members are often victimized and subjected to manipulation and objects of sexism within a gang. There continues to be the notion that many females are regarded as possessions of their male counter-parts, and subjugated to increased violence, and control (Totten, 2001). However, Delaney cautions that the treatment of female members by a gang is very individual, and in some gangs females are treated as equals.

Statistics from law enforcement agencies report that only 6% of gang members are female (National Council on Crime and Delinquency, 2010). It is also estimated that 39% of gangs have some female members (Esbensen & Osgood, 1997). Other statistics from the NYGC (1996) reported 8% of gang members were female. One 11-city survey of eighth grades found that 38% of gang members were female (Esbensen & Osgood), and the discrepancy is likely a function of how the gang member is defined. More recent statistics suggest that 32% of youth gang members are female (Glenman, Krisberg, & Marchionna, 2009). Initial estimates suggested that all female gangs represented under 10% of all gangs (Egley, Howell, & Major, 2006), but recent evidence suggests this is on the rise (Moriconi, 2006). According to the Bureau of Justice Statistics, the number of female juvenile offenders increased at a much higher rate than males from 1995 to 2004 (Moriconi). The discrepancy among the statistics provided reflects the different perspectives of how youth gangs are defined and also whether loosely affiliated youth are included or excluded in these statistics. As noted above, in many instances, female youth are loosely tied to gang activity.

Statistics also suggest that females are much less likely to be involved in crim-inal behaviors than males, but can often be accomplices to criminal activities

(Moore & Hagerdorn, 2001). However, females are still likely to be involved in gang fights, and a majority report carrying a weapon for protection (Deschenes & Esbensen, 1999). Females may also become more enmeshed in the gang lifestyle because of economic pressure (Anderson, Brooks, Langsam, & Dyson, 2002). Finally, other data suggest that female involvement in serious crime remains minimal and stable over time (Egley, 2002).

6.3.6 Leaving the Gang

It is believed that leaving a gang can have disastrous consequences for the individual (and potentially family members) and in most cases the results is inevitable death. However, this is regarded as a myth by many gang researchers (Curry & Decker, 2003; Delaney, 2006) who assert that this belief is propagated by the media and even by gang members themselves. Decker and Van Winkle (1996) conducted many interview with gang members about leaving the gangs reported the high stakes of leaving a gang, insisting that their departure would lead to likely death. Yet, data from national and local surveys does not support this belief. Research indicates that the typical gang member is active for less than a year (Esbensen et al., 2001; Thornberry, Huizinga, & Loeber, 2004), and that up to 60% of males and 70% of females will leave after 1 year (these survey involved over 5,000 youths). These researchers believe that threats of violence and death are instituted to maintain gang solidarity and enforce the importance of their collective bond. This is not so say there are not situations where individuals have suffered severe consequences for leaving a gang. For instance, gang members who have considerable knowledge of gang activities or who was a troublemaker while in the gang are often targeted for exit beatings (Delaney). The term "blood out" refers beating an individual for leaving a gang. "Aging out" refers to an individual who leaves again as they mature and seek other direction in life.

While the act of leaving a gang does not seem to consistently result in consistent dire consequences, leaving their *environment of the gang* does. Many youths who leave gangs live in impoverished environments where little positive opportunities exist. They face the arduous task of dealing with rejection from their peers, the lack of social companionship, change patterns of delinquent behavior, deal with drug and alcohol issues, and finding legitimate means that lead to positive outcomes. Moreover, former gang members may continue to be targeted by rival gangs (Tobin, 2008). The Rochester Youth survey (of over 1,000 youth) suggested that by the age of 30, former gang members were much more likely to report being unemployed, receiving welfare, committing a crime, or carrying a gun than peers who had never joined a gang (Thornberry, 2005; Thornberry & Krohn, 2003). Other studies suggest Gang membership remained a significant predictor of ever having been incarcerated and acquiring income from illegal sources (Levitt & Venkatesh, 2001). For males, stable gang membership remained significant for all the problematic transitions except for early nest leaving. For females, gang membership was significantly related to early pregnancy, teenage parenthood, and unstable employment even after controlling for the other eight variables (Thornberry, Krohn, Lizotte, Smith, & Tobin, 2003). Finally, it is important to note that research suggests the shorter time that a youth spends with the gang results in a decreased likelihood to commit a crime (Krohn & Thornberry, 2008).

6.4 Assessment Approaches

Because gang membership is not classified as mental health disorder, there are no specific assessment approaches from a mental health perspective. That is, there is no specific diagnosis of a "youth gang member." However, many youth gang members have disturbed psychological functioning. For instance, some studies suggest approximately 50% of youth gang members have diagnoses including conduct disorder and oppositional defiant disorder (Hirschfield, Maschi, White, & Traub, 2006). One study found that between 20 and 50% of youth gang members were diagnosed with substance abuse (Vermeiren, 2003). Finally, mood disorders have also been found at a much higher rate among delinquent youth involved in gangs (Hirschfield et al., 2006).

As noted above, children with more severe forms of psychopathology involving problems of conduct are often implicated in delinquent behavior. Thus, screening for a child's history of significant disturbances of conduct is an important component of assessing a child's risk for youth gang involvement. Conduct disorder is a psychological diagnosis that is the most common among youth gang members given the definition that youth gang members are involved in crime and likely to violate the law. Both the DSM-IV TR (APA, 2000) and ICD-10 provide diagnostic descriptors of conduct disorder (F91). The ICD-10 provides describes subtypes of conduct disorder. The essential features of conduct disorder, according to the ICD-10 are as follows:

- Conduct disorders are characterized by a repetitive and persistent pattern of dissocial, aggressive, or defiant conduct. Such behavior, when at its most extreme for the individual, should amount to major violations of age-appropriate social expectations, and is therefore more severe than ordinary childish mischief or adolescent rebelliousness. Isolated dissocial or criminal acts are not in themselves grounds for the diagnosis, which implies an enduring pattern of behavior.
- Features of conduct disorder can also be symptomatic of other psychiatric conditions, in which case the underlying diagnosis should be coded.
- Disorders of conduct may in some cases proceed to dissocial personality disorder (F60.2). Conduct disorder is frequently associated with adverse psychosocial environments, including unsatisfactory family relationships and failure at school, and is more commonly noted in boys. Its distinction from emotional disorder is well validated; its separation from hyperactivity is less clear and there is often overlap.

Socialized conduct disorder (F91.2) is a subtype of conduct disorder characterized by persistent dissocial or aggressive behavior (meeting the overall criteria for F91 and not merely comprising oppositional, defiant, disruptive behavior) occurring in

individuals who are generally well integrated into their peer group. Often the disturbance of conduct occurs outside the family and includes, "offenses committed in
the context of gang membership." However, gang membership that occurs outside
the context of a psychiatric disorder is one of the exclusionary criteria, meaning that
an individual may be part of a gang without having conduct disorder.

Overall, the bulk of psychological assessment approaches to determine risk
factors for youth gang membership involve individual assessment of a child's
psychopathology. Screening a troubled adolescent will include assessment of mood
disorders, history of delinquent behavior, patterns of substance abuse, and other
measures of psychological stress. There have been some attempts to develop instruments that may determine the risk of a youth for gang involvement. One of the earliest
measures was the *Gang Membership Inventory* (Pillen & Howeing-Robertson,
1992) that was developed to screen high-risk youth in urban centers. It was normed
with 650 adolescents and psychometric properties suggested that it was a promising
tool, but it subsequently fell out of use. More recently, Malcolm Klein, a retired
professor from the University of Southern California, developed a screening tool to
identify youth at risk for gang membership (Casey, 2009). This tool asks a range of
questions on issues ranging from past relationships, drug use, and attitudes toward
violence. The test is being piloted in Los Angeles and results are not yet known.
Critics are concerned that the test would be too narrow and potentially miss children
who would benefit from gang-prevention programs (Casey).

6.5   Etiological Hypotheses and Theoretical Frameworks

> Anyone who has studied gangs over a period of time will admit that the more one studies
> them, the more complex they are. At best, we can come to understand a bit about certain
> features of gangs at given points of time. Gangs are dynamic, flexible and ever-changing.
>
> –William B. Sanders (1994)

Theories and etiologies of youth gang membership are extremely complex, with
each disciplines having its own theoretical formulations. There are both macrolevel
explanations (e.g., economic deprivation, high residential mobility, and racial and
ethnic heterogeneity) and microlevel explanations (psychological, family, and peer
factors; Tobin, 2008). Recently, researchers from the National Gang Center (OJJDP,
2010) organized the risk factors for serious and violent delinquency according to
five developmental domains: individual, family, school, peer group, and community.
Research has shown that risk and protective factors in these five domains function
as predictors of juvenile delinquency, violence, and gang membership at different
stages in social development (Howell & Egley, 2005; Thornberry, 2005; Thornberry
et al., 2003). This research also indicates that these risk factors have a cumulative
impact in that the greater number of risk factors experienced by the youth, the
increased likelihood of gang involvement. These risk factors come into play long
before youths reach the typical age for joining a gang, and can occur as early as ages
3–4. Table 6.1 taken from the OJJDP provides an extensive list of the risk factors for

Table 6.1 Risk factors for juvenile delinquency and gang involvement (ages 12–17)

Individual

Antisocial/delinquent beliefs[a]

Drug dealing

Early dating/sexual activity/fatherhood[a]

Few social ties (involved in social activities, popularity)

General delinquency involvement[a]

High alcohol/drug use[a]

High drug dealing

Illegal gun ownership/carrying

Life stressors[a]

Makes excuses for delinquent behavior (neutralization)[a]

Mental health problems[a]

Physical violence/aggression[a]

Violent victimization[a]

Family

Antisocial parents

Broken home/changes in caretaker[a]

Delinquent/gang-involved siblings[a]

Family history of problem behavior/criminal involvement

Family poverty/low family socioeconomic status[a]

Family violence (child maltreatment, partner violence, conflict)

Having a teenage mother

High parental stress/maternal depression

Lack of orderly and structured activities within the family

Living in a small house

Low attachment to child/adolescent[a]

Low parent education[a]

Parental use of physical punishment/harsh and/or erratic discipline practices

Poor parental supervision (control, monitoring, and child management)[a]

Poor parent–child relations or communication

School

Bullying

Frequent school transitions

Low academic aspirations[a]

Low math achievement test scores (males)[a]

Low parent college expectations for child[a]

Low school attachment/bonding/motivation/commitment to school[a]

Poor school attitude/performance; academic failure[a]

Poorly organized and functioning schools/inadequate school climate/negative Labeling by teachers[a]

Community

Availability and use of drugs in the neighborhood[a]

Availability of firearms[a]

Community disorganization[a]

Economic deprivation/poverty/residence in a disadvantaged neighborhood[a]

Exposure to violence and racial prejudice

Feeling unsafe in the neighborhood[a]

High-crime neighborhood[a]

(continued)

Table 6.1 (continued)

Low neighborhood attachment[a]
Neighborhood physical disorder
Neighborhood youth in trouble[a]

Peer
Association with antisocial/aggressive/delinquent peers; high peer delinquency[a]
Association with gang-involved peers/relatives[a]
Gang membership

[a]Risk factors for gang membership

teenage youth. The potential etiologies to gang membership are extremely expansive and the various perspectives cannot be effectively synthesized in a single chapter. For the purposes of this chapter, a brief overview of the macrolevel and microlevel perspectives will be provided.

6.5.1 Sociological Theories

Social Disorganization Theory: Frederic Thrasher (1927/1963) was one of the first individuals to conduct studies of gangs and relied on patterns of urbanization in explaining gang formation in slum areas. His research was furthered by Park and Burgess (1925/1984). Essentially, this theory postulates that rapid growth and change within an urban center leads to increased economic disadvantage, residential instability, and racial heterogeneity. As a result, the surrounding community cannot impose its social control. Institutions like churches, schools, and community organizations cannot instill common values, resulting in disorganization among specific subgroups. Thrasher felt that natural adolescent development requires peer group interaction, but in disorganized areas, these peer groups are largely left unsupervised and are at high risk for engaging in delinquent behavior.

Strain Theory: Robert Merton, a prominent Sociologist (1938), popularized this theory. Merton argued that crime and organized crime is a product of the discrepancy between the emphasis on economic success and access to legitimate means to attain this success. The strain is seen most clearly in limited or blocked opportunities to achieve economic vitality. Those in economically deprived areas either give up altogether or find ways to achieve this success.

Other Theories: Social disorganization theory and strain theory are the most prominent sociological explanations although others have followed. For instance, Cohen's 1960 book, "Delinquent Boys" was the precursor to what came to be known as status frustration theory in which delinquency arises because of the desire to attain status, but not necessarily financial status. Lower class youth typically have difficulties in achieving success and are associated with others who face similar strain.

The collective force ultimately sets the foundation for the formation of gangs with attaining status in a different form can be idealized. Other sociological theories include Cloward and Ohlin's delinquency and opportunity theory (1960).

6.5.2 Biological Theories

Biological theories of gangs and gang membership have sought to determine a potential genetic basis. The belief that an individual's character could be read from their physical appearance dates back to the ancient Greeks and Romans. This study, known as "physiogamy," postulated that physical features such as the size of one's skull, faces, and other physical features could, in fact, reveal a person's natural disposition. There were such outlandish beliefs in medieval times that if two people were suspected of having committed the same crime, the uglier one should be regarded as more likely the guilty party (Curran & Renzetti, 1994)! In psychology, Franz Gall, known as the father of phrenology, continued this thinking with the belief that one's personality and developed mental and moral faculties could be determined by evaluated the shape of the skull. While phrenology and physiogamy have been discredited as plausible theories, the debate that one's biological make-up could be a predetermined factor for criminal activity and gang membership continues. The overriding belief is that one's genetic make-up coupled with specific environmental conditions may lead to the propensity of specific antisocial behavior including joining a gang.

Genetics: New research indicates that genetics may be linked with personality and behavioral traits that are common among gang members (Hill, Howell, Hawkins, & Battin-Pearson, 1999). The particular gene, low-activity mononoamine oxidase A (low MAOA), has previously been connected to criminal behavior, cognitive dysfunction, maladaptive behavior, and a range of psychopathologies and is now linked with both gang membership and use of a weapon in gang fights (Beaver, DeLisi, Vaughn, & Barnes, 2010). Found on the X chromosome, MAOA is a polymorphic gene with two forms – a low MAOA activity group and a high MAOA activity group (Haberstick et al., 2005; Levy et al., 1989). In order to exhibit multiple phenotypes, MAOA is thought to affect the regulation of emotion and cognition through the limbic system (Meyer-Lindenberg et al., 2006). For example, increased amygdala arousal and decreased reactivity of the regulatory prefrontal cortex is seen in male carriers of low-activity MAOA (Meyer-Lindenberg et al.).

It is low MAOA's location on the X chromosome that determines its differential role between genders (Beaver et al., 2010). With females, the presence of the gene does not show significant predictability for gang membership or using a weapon as a gang member (Beaver et al.). Where low MAOA's strong predictability of criminogenic effects lies with males. Male carriers of the gene are found to have an increased risk of gang membership, as well as using a weapon in gang fights (Beaver et al.). Therefore, not only is low MAOA demonstrating a link to predicting whether males join gangs, the preliminary research also indicates it can differentiate the type of violence exhibited as a gang member.

Although this relatively new research finding will require further studies to understand how it applies to the general public, it holds important implications for assessing and treating gang members. Gang formation and activity can now be considered not only a sociological and psychological phenomenon, but also a product of gene–environment interplay (Beaver et al., 2010). How this genotype–environment interaction works and how intervention can be applied will be critical areas of future research.

6.5.3 Psychological Theories

There are many psychological factors that are associated with youth gang involvement (see Table 6.1). There are a myriad of factors underscore the complexity of involvement in youth gangs. Psychological theories provide a framework that explains how psychological variables influence human behavior toward deviant behavior and specifically to gang involvement.

6.5.3.1 Social Learning Theory

Social learning theory is an expansion of the ideas rooted in the work of Sutherland's differential association theory (1947). Essentially, Sutherland believed that deviant behavior is learned from primary social groups, with those that we interact with most often, and with those who are important to us. Akers (1985) furthered this theory by applying the principles of learning to deviant behavior. Specifically, he proposed that behavior is a result of instrumental conditioning or differential reinforcement. Behavior that is reinforced is likely to continue but behavior that is punished is likely to be reduced. Criminality (and gang membership) occurs when social reinforcement (as in the form of gang acceptance) is more reinforcing than the punishment.

6.5.3.2 Goldsteins's Hyperadolescence Theory

Goldsteins's hyperadolescence theory (1991) builds upon Erik Erikson's theory to identity development, and emphasizes that adolescence is an essential time period for developing one's identity. Adolescents who are gang affiliated are "hyperadolescents" in that they exhibit similar needs and behaviors of most adolescents *but* to a much greater degree. Thus, the gang member is much more prone to the effects of peer pressure and peer identification. Personality traits like neuroticism, oppositional behaviors, adventure-seeking, and experimentation behaviors are more pronounced, leading to a more likely affiliation with deviant groups.

6.5.3.3   Personality Theory

This theory is much aligned with biological/genetic theories of gang membership in that personality traits are believed to be innate and therefore, predispose an individual to certain types of behavior. As noted above, there is considerable research suggesting genetic markers to conduct disorder which may predispose a person to gang membership. Other research proposes that gang members show other traits that set them apart from juveniles not affiliated with gangs or with normal youth. For instance, a study by Alleyne and Wood (2010) identified that gang members were more antiauthority than nongang youth, and both gang and peripheral youth valued social status more than nongang youth. Gang members were also more likely to blame their victims for their actions and use euphemisms to sanitize their behavior than nongang youth, whereas peripheral youth were more likely than nongang youth to displace responsibility onto their superiors. Low self-esteem has a significant relationship with delinquency, antisocial behavior, and aggression, elements characteristic of gang membership (Donnellan, Trzesniewski, Robins, Moffitt, & Caspi, 2005). Some research supports the premise that youth with less confidence and self-esteem, and weak bonds with a prosocial environment and network (i.e., schools and family) are more likely to look toward gangs than youth who are more confident (Dukes, Martinez, & Stein, 1997).

6.5.3.4   Causal Model

A more recent theoretical approach to gang membership is a causal model postulated by Thornberry et al. (2003). Based on the interactional theory of delinquency, they suggest that a collection of structural and developmental shortages increase the chances of joining a gang. They argue that many conventional gang theories explain why gangs emerge, but do not account for why particular adolescents join gangs and others do not (Thornberry et al.). They further state that traditional sociopsychological causal theories of juvenile delinquency are not developed enough in gang theory (Thornberry et al., 2003).

   Thornberry et al.'s (2003) causal model is based on interactional theory which holds three premises; behaviors manifest through development rather than being set in childhood, factors have bidirectional causality on each other, and finally, that social structural influences affect the growth of misdemeanors (Thornberry & Krohn, 2001). Thornberry et al. (2003) applied this theory to gangs and systematically derived which factors worked together to increase risk of membership. In their application of interactional theory, they note that factors such as structural variables do not directly lead to gang membership, but rather through a series of indirect paths, causing youth to develop a higher propensity for gang membership (Thornberry et al., 2003). For example, structural disadvantages can increase antisocial influences directly or indirectly through the mediation of social bonds like academic performance (Thornberry et al., 2003). Overall, their study suggests youth who experience structural adversity, poor performance in school, involvement in antisocial networks and behaviors, and higher than average life stresses have an increased chance of joining a gang (Thornberry et al., 2003).

6.5.4 Summary

For an overall perspective, Davis (1993) reviewed sociological and psychological literature on gang formation etiology and found little agreement as to which approach was best (Davis, 1993). He noted that psychological and sociological factors can be used interchangeably in gang research and it was unclear how either variable differentially affected gang formation (Davis, 1993). Studies either argued that psychological approaches were less essential or even nonessential for gang conduct or were significant and required more credit as explanatory factors. This was also found with sociological factors. Davis (1993) stressed that a synthesis of both approaches was likely required for effective application because both have shown significant effects on juvenile gang formation and perseverance. Furthermore, he also postulated a biological basis be synthesized with the two theoretical approaches, a notion that is more important now with recent research suggesting a genetic basis for gang formation exists in the low MAOA gene (Beaver et al., 2010; Davis, 1993).

   In conclusion, not only are there a great number of theories that explain the etiology of gang formation, there is also disagreement in determining which models are best in use (Davis, 1993). In particular, with the advent of the newly discovered genetic basis for gang formation, a further synthesis of ideas will be necessary to continue the shaping of a working model for the future. Overall, it is evident that theories on youth gang etiologies are multifaceted and require an understanding from multiple perspectives.

6.6 Treatment/Intervention

Authorities agree that there is a serious youth gang problem in North America. As discussed, there are many reasons why youth choose to become involved with gangs and therefore solutions must be multifaceted. Covey (2010) states that "numerous antigang approaches have been attempted in North American including approaches that involve suppression, social intervention, recreation, cultural competence, outreach workers, information sharing, community mobilization, job services, extended incarceration medication, specialized gang units, antigang laws, gang sweeps, and others" (p. 70). Single-focused approaches to gang intervention have not proven successful (Covey). Thus, a combination of the efforts is essential. As Delaney (2006) writes:

> The techniques implemented by various policy makers are determined by their ultimate goal. Prevention efforts are those methods designed to stop youths from joining gangs in the first place. Suppression efforts are attempts by law enforcement and judicial bodies to punish existing gang members. Treatment programs are designed to rehabilitate gang members so they can become positive members of society (p. 251).

OJJDP's Comprehensive Gang Model: The OJJDP recently published the second edition of its Best Practices to address community gang problems in October, 2010 (OJJDP, 2010). It is the only national assessment of organized agency and community response groups to gang problems in the USA. The multimillion dollar initiative began in 2003 and was designed to "reduce gang crime in targeted neighborhoods by incorporating research-based interventions to address individual, family, and community factors that contribute to juvenile delinquency and gang activity. The program leveraged local, state, and federal resources in support of community partnerships that implement progressive practices in prevention, intervention, suppression, and re-entry" (OJJDP). The model essential components of this initiative included five strategies:

1. *Community Mobilization*: Involvement of local citizens, including former gang-involved youth, community groups, agencies, and coordination of programs and staff functions within and across agencies.
2. *Opportunities Provision*: Development of a variety of specific education, training, and employment programs targeting gang-involved youth.
3. *Social Intervention*: Involvement of youth-serving agencies, schools, grass roots groups, faith-based organizations, police, and other juvenile/criminal justice organizations in "reaching out" to gang-involved youth and their families.
4. *Suppression*: Formal and information social control procedures, including close supervision and monitoring of gang-involved youth by agencies of the juvenile/ criminal justice system and also by community-based agencies, schools, and grass roots groups.
5. *Organizational Change and Development*: Development and implementation of policies and procedures that result in the most effective use of available and potential resources, within and across agencies, to better address the gang problem.

These components were the product of considerable research among multiple agencies. The project is ongoing and will continue to implement its objectives in key cities throughout the USA.

6.6.1   Community Prevention Programs

Because of the global impact of gangs in society, many interventions for gang membership have come at the community level. Some researchers suggest that massive changes in society would need to be made in order for community prevention programs to be effective. As Esbensen (2009) writes, "the traditional image of American youth gangs is characterized by social disorganization and economic marginalization"; the housing projects or barrios of Chicago, Los Angeles, and New York are viewed as the stereotypical homes of youth gang members. Thus, to positively impact the youth gang problem, significant social changes would need to occur. Regardless, the origin of gang problems primarily resides within local communities. Therefore, communities are viewed as the focal point for preventing youths from joining gangs.

The Office of Juvenile Justice and Delinquency Prevention (OJJDP) acknowledged that community programs must be flexible, since programs that are effective in one area may not be in other areas. However, a primary facet of effective intervention is mobilization of community efforts. Because theories of social disorganization suggest that gang problems are a result of ineffective communities, measures to improve community strength are targeted. The Chicago Area Project (CAP) and Philadelphia Youth Violence Reduction Partnership (YVRP) are examples of programs designed to bring communities together. Irving Spergel (2007) developed a multi-faceted, community-based model, entitled "Little Village Gang Project" which incorporated multiple institutions and agencies, including gangs, in addressing the gang problem. The outcome of this project was promising, with evidence of decelerated gang violence and reduction of gang drug arrests. However, results also suggested an acceleration of gang drug problems. Moreover, surveys of residents within this locale of Chicago reported reduction of gang crime and gang violence in spite of increased gang drug problems (Spergel).

6.6.2   Social Interventions

These interventions are grounded in theories that address individual-level risks for gang membership. Many of these interventions include educational programs designed to teach youth prosocial values. One nationally promoted program is Gang Resistance Education and Training (G.R.E.A.T) which is a school-based program often taught by law enforcement officers who talk about the consequences of joining a gang. Evaluations of G.R.E.A.T are modest suggesting that students completing the G.R.E.A.T program have lower rates of gang affiliation and self-reported delinquency than do students in the control group (Esbensen & Osgood, 1999). In addition, the G.R.E.A.T students report a number of more prosocial attitudes, including more positive attitudes to the police, than do the control students. Other programs, such as the Boys and Girls Club of America's Gang Prevention through Targeted Outreach (GPTTO), provide programs with multiple prosocial activities. Results showed more positive outcomes for high-risk than low-risk youths. GPTTO had stronger effects on school engagement and achievement, as well as positive use of leisure time, than on delinquency. GPTTO did not appear to impact gang membership, however (Esbensen & Osgood, 1999).

6.6.3 Cognitive-Behavioral Intervention

Cognitive-behavioral interventions are designed to address cognitive deficits in order to reduce maladaptive or dysfunctional behavior. The goal of cognitive behavior therapy (CBT) is to help individuals solve problems concerning dysfunctional emotions, behaviors, and cognitions through a systematic process of challenging underlying thoughts that influence behavior. Research has generally shown that CBT is one of the more efficacious psychotherapeutic treatments and has been used for to treat a wide range of psychological disorders including oppositional defiant disorder and other behavioral difficulties (Lambert, Bergin, & Garfield, 2004). Several meta-analyses have found that cognitive-behavioral programs are effective in reducing recidivism of juvenile and adult offenders (Landenberger, & Lipsey, 2005; Lipsey, Chapman, & Landenberger, 2001; Pearson, Lipton, Cleland, & Yee, 2002; Wilson, Bouffard, & MacKenzie, 2005). One of the most comprehensive reviews was recently conducted by Fisher, Gardner, and Montgomery (2008) who completed a meta-analysis of randomized controlled and quasi randomized controlled studies of cognitive-behavioral interventions for gang prevention. Overall, results were weak and the study did not find evidence of significant main effects. The authors conclude that results suggest an urgent need for additional primary evaluations of cognitive-behavioral interventions for gang prevention and higher standards of research conducted to provide meaningful findings.

6.6.4 Other Approaches

More generic counseling approaches to intervening with youth gangs seems logical, given that the majority of these individuals are troubled individuals with considerable stressors in their lives. Thus, provision of supportive counseling service makes sense. Earlier research by Sherman et al. (1997) conducted a meta-analysis of over 24 studies using counseling as an intervention for youth involved in gangs. Overall, the effect size was essentially zero, indicated that there was no evidence of significant findings. However, the authors are quick to point out that this did *not* mean counseling should never be used for youth. Rather they suggested that counseling should be used in the context of other activities. This again points to the complex nature of youth gangs and that single interventions are likely to be ineffective. The most common criticism is that the effectiveness of counseling does not generalize outside the counseling setting (Greenwood, 2006). Thus, it is difficult for the individual to apply what they have learned in their home or community setting where outside pressures are enormous.

While the bulk of studies evaluating counseling have not demonstrated positive results, most experts agree that counseling and therapy is an important *component* of a gang reduction strategy (Covey, 2010). Of note, one series of studies demonstrated that crisis intervention was helpful in reducing youth gang involvement. The Crisis Intervention Services Project which took place in Chicago included both patrols and counseling for youth gangs and their family. This treatment demonstrated significant reductions in youth gang involvement (OJJDP, 2010).

6.6.5 Pharmacological Treatment

It should be noted that treatment with medication is unlikely to be efficacious with most youth gang members, especially the "hard-core" members. Treatments are likely to be unsuccessful given issues with compliance, the need for follow-up with a physician, interest in using drugs for criminal purposes, etc. Thus, pharmacological treatment should only be provided in a context of a structured outpatient program where significant monitoring and control could be implemented.

As with the treatment of most mental health disorders, pharmacological treatments are used to improve symptoms. Pharmacological treatments not considered to be helpful in isolation, but should be incorporated in a multifaceted program. Given that gang membership is not considered a specific mental health disorder, there are no consistent pharmacological treatments for youth gang members. Rather, the treatment requires appropriate treatment of potential underlying psychological disorders including conduct disorder, ADHD, and other related mood and substance disorders. The first step in providing pharmacological treatment for a youth gang member would be the identification and diagnosis of a specific mental health condition.

Because of the multifaceted nature of conduct problems, particularly related to comorbidities (such as ADHD, ODD, and substance abuse disorders), treatment usually includes a combination of treatments including medication, teaching parenting skills, family therapy, and consultation with the school. No medications have been consistently effective in treating persons with CD. Substance abuse occurs in a high number of children with CD whether or they have been treated with stimulant medication (used to treat ADHD). From a treatment perspective, a great deal of caution needs to be taken when prescribing stimulants because they can be sold illegally.

Evidence suggests that antipsychotics, antidepressants, mood stabilizers, antiepileptic drugs, stimulants, and adrenergic drugs can be well tolerated and effective therapeutic options for individuals with conduct disorder and comorbid psychiatric conditions. However, the most successful therapeutic outcomes are likely to be achieved by combining the current advances in psychopharmacology with behavioral and psychosocial interventions, aimed at modifying the excessive patterns of maladaptive behaviors observed in conduct disorder (Tcheremissine & Lieving, 2006).

6.7 Future Directions

The role of youth gangs in society has a long and storied history. Perhaps more than any other arcane disorder of youth, involvement in gangs is the most complex given the many etiologies and facets that are involved. As noted by the OJJDP (2010), there are multiple-risk factors that may predispose youth to joining gangs. It is clear that these factors are extremely variable and have differential impact on each youth. For some, growing up in poverty, family dysfunction, and too much time alone are key factors related to joining a gang. For others, personality traits and even one's genetics may be the most significant factors that predict youth gang membership.

In spite of the complex etiologies of youth gang membership, what is clear is that there has been little improvement with prevalence rates remaining significantly elevated in recent years. Recent statistics from the OJJDP (2010) indicate a decrease in gang activity in smaller cities and rural settings. However, there have been increases in both gangs and gang membership observed in larger cities, especially those with more than 250,000. This suggests that sociological and economic factors are closely tied to youth gang activity. This is very consistent with the findings of Pratt and Cullen (2005) who indicated that economic disadvantage was the most significant factor for predicting youth crime and likely gang membership.

Current research provides convincing evidence that single-faceted approaches for treating the youth gang problem are not successful. While these approaches may be helpful for specific individuals (like counseling/psychotherapy and education), they do not provide a global solution. The most promising approaches are those that involve targeting the communities where gang membership is believed to be most prominent. Specifically, multilevel approaches that involve education, available of alternative activities for youth within those communities, family support, positive peer modeling, and involvement of gang members themselves have been most effective in slowing the gang problem. It is evident that the impact of drugs and drug trafficking has become intertwined with violence and gang activity among youth and augments the underlying sociological and psychological issues of youth. More recent research has provided evidence that genetics may play a role in the behavior of youth, especially male youth. In sum, gang activity remains a widespread problem in North America and requires a multifaceted, multidisciplinary collaborative effort from many aspects of society.

References

Adamson, C. (2000). Defensive localism in white and black: A comparative history of European-American and African-American youth gangs. *Ethnic and Racial Studies, 23*(2), 272–298.

Akers, R. L. (1985). *Deviant behavior: A social learning approach* (3rd ed.). Belmont, CA: Wadsworth.

Alleyne, E., & Wood, J. L. (2010). Gang involvement: psychosocial and behavioral characteristics of gang members, peripheral youth, and nongang youth. *Aggressive Behavior, 36*(6), 423–436.

American Psychiatric Association. (2000). *Diagnostic and statistical manual of mental disorders – Text revision* (4th ed. rev). Washington, DC: Author.

Anderson, J. F., Brooks, W., Jr., Langsam, A., & Dyson, L. (2002). The new female gang member: Anomaly or evolution. *Journal of Gang Research, 10*, 47–65.

Associated Press. (2009). *Minneapolis struggles with Somali gangs*. Retrieved November 15, 2010 from http://www.msnbc.msn.com/id/32010471/ns/us_news-crime_and_courts.

Beaver, K. M., DeLisi, M., Vaughn, M. G., & Barnes, J. C. (2010). Monoamine Oxidase A genotype is associated with gang membership and weapon use. *Comprehensive Psychiatry, 51*, 130–134.

Bruneau, T. C. (2005). The Maras and National Security in Central America. *Strategic Insights, 4*, 1–12.

Casey, N. (2009). *A new approach to gang violence includes a multiple-choice test.* Retrieved November 22, 2010 from http://online.wsj.com/article/SF124276162416235869.html.

Cloward, R. A., & Ohlin, L. E. (1960). *Delinquency and opportunity: A theory of delinquent gangs.* New York: Free Press.

Cohen, A. K. (1960). Delinquent Boys: *The Culture of the Gang.* Glencoe, IL: The Free Press.

Covey, H. C. (2010). *Street gangs throughout the world* (2nd ed.). Springfield: Charles C. Thomas Publisher.

Criminal Intelligence Service Canada (CISC). (2006). *Project spectrum: 2006 situational overview of street gangs in Canada.* Ottawa: Author.

Curran, D., & Renzetti, D. (1994). *Theories of crime.* Boston, MA: Allyn and Bacon.

Curry, G. D., & Decker, S. H. (2003). *Confronting gangs: Crime and community* (2nd ed.). Los Angeles: Roxbury.

Davis, J. (1993). Psychological versus sociological explanations for delinquent conduct and gang formation. *Journal of Contemporary Criminal Justice, 9*, 81–93.

Decker, S. H., & Van Winkle, B. (1996). *Life in the Gang: Family, Friends, and Violence.* New York, NY: Cambridge University Press.

Delaney, T. (2006). *American street gangs.* New Jersey: Pearson Prentice Hall.

Deschenes, E. P., & Esbensen, F.-A. (1999). Violence in gangs: Gender differences in perceptions of behaviour. *Journal of Quantitative Criminology, 15*, 63–96.

Dinkes, R., Kemp, J., & Baum, K. (2009). *Indicators of school crime and safety: 2008.* Washington, DC: National Center for Education Statistics, Institute of Education Sciences, US Department of Education, and Bureau of Justice Statistics, Office of Justice Programs, US Department of Justice.

Donnellan, M. B., Trzesniewski, K. H., Robins, R. W., Moffitt, T. E., & Caspi, A. (2005). Low self-esteem is related to aggression, antisocial behavior, and delinquency. *Psychological Science, 16*, 328–355.

Dukes, R. L., Martinez, R. O., & Stein, J. A. (1997). Precursors and consequences of membership in youth gangs. *Youth & Society, 29*, 139–165.

Egley, A. (2002). *Highlights of the national youth gang survey trends from 1996 to 2000. OJJDP Fact Sheet.* Washington, DC: U.S. Department of Justice, Office of the Juvenile Justice and Delinquency Prevention.

Egley, A., Jr., Howell, J. C., & Major, A. K. (2006). *National Youth Gang Survey 1999–2001.* Washington, DC: U.S. Department of Justice, Office of the Juvenile Justice and Delinquency Prevention.

Egley, A., Jr., Howell, J. C., & Moore, J. P. (2009). *Highlights of the 2008 National Youth Gang Survey.* Washington, DC: U.S. Department of Justice, Office of the Juvenile Justice and Delinquency Prevention.

Egley, A., Jr., & O'Donnell, C. E. (2009). *Highlights of 2007 National Youth Gang Survey. OJJDP Fact Sheet.* Washington, DC: U.S. Department of Justice, Office of the Juvenile Justice and Delinquency Prevention.

Esbensen, F.-A. (2000). *Preventing adolescent gang involvement.* Washington, DC: U.S. Department of Justice, Office of the Juvenile Justice and Delinquency Prevention.

Esbensen, F.-A., & Osgood, D. W. (1997). *National evaluation of G.R.E.A.T. research in brief.* Washington, DC: U.S. Department of Justice Office of the Juvenile Justice and Delinquency Prevention.

Esbensen, F. A., & Osgood, D. W. (1999). Gang resistance education and training (GREAT): Results from the national evaluation. *Journal of Research in Crime and Delinquency, 36*, 194–225.

Esbensen, F.-A., Winfree, F. M., Jr., He, N., & Taylor, T. J. (2001). Youth gangs and definitional issues: When is a gang a gang, and why does it matter? *Crime and Delinquency, 47*, 105–130.

Fisher, H., Gardner, F., & Montgomery, P. (2008). Cognitive-behavioural interventions for preventing youth gang involvement for children and young people (7–16). *Cochrane Database of Systematic Reviews 2008*, Issue 2. Art. No.: CD007008. DOI: 10.1002/14651858.CD007008. pub2.

Glenman, C., Krisberg, B., & Marchionna, S. (2009). *Youth in gangs: Who is at risk?* Oakland, CA: National Council on Crime and Delinquency.

Goldstein, A. P. (1991). *Delinquent gangs: A psychosocial perspective*. Champaign, IL: Research Press.

Greenwood, P. (2006). *Changing lives: Delinquency prevention as crime-control policy*. Chicago, IL: University of Chicago Press.

Haberstick, B. C., Lessem, J. M., Hopfer, C. J., Smolen, A., Ehringer, M. A., Timberlake, D., et al. (2005). Monoamine oxidase A (MAOA) and antisocial behaviors in the presence of childhood and adolescent maltreatment. *American Journal of Medical Genetics, 135B*(1), 59–64.

Hill, K. G., Howell, J. C., Hawkins, J. D., & Battin-Pearson, S. R. (1999). Risk factors for adolescent gang membership: results from the Seattle social development project. *Journal of Research in Crime and Delinquency, 36*, 300–322.

Hirschfield, P., Maschi, T., White, H. R., & Traub, L. G. (2006). Mental health and juvenile arrests: Criminality, crimininalization, or compassion? *Criminology, 44*(3), 593–630.

Howell, J. C., & Egley, A., Jr. (2005). Moving risk factors into developmental theories of gang membership. *Youth Violence and Juvenile Justice, 3*(4), 334–354.

International Classification of Diseases (ICD-10). *World Health Organization*. Retrieved November 15, 2010 from http://www.who.int/classifications/icd/en/.

Klein, M. W. (1971). *Street gangs and street workers*. Englewood Cliffs, NJ: Prentice-Hall.

Krohn, M. D., & Thornberry, T. P. (2008). Longitudinal perspectives on adolescent street gangs. In A. M. Liberman (Ed.), *The long view of crime: A synthesis of longitudinal research* (pp. 128–160). Washington, DC: National Institute of Justice.

Lambert, M. J., Bergin, A. E., & Garfield, S. L. (2004). Introduction and historical overview. In M. J. Lambert (Ed.), *Bergin and Garfield's handbook of psychotherapy and behavior change* (5th ed., pp. 3–15). New York: Wiley.

Landenberger, N., & Lipsey, M. (2005). The positive effects of cognitive behavioral programs for offenders: A meta analysis of factors associated with effective treatment. *Journal of Experimental Criminology, 1*, 451–476.

Levitt, S. D., & Venkatesh, S. A. (2001). *An analysis of the long-run consequences of gang involvement*. Paper presented at the 2001 Harvard Inequality Summer Institute, Harvard University.

Levy, E. R., Powell, J. F., Buckle, V. J., Hsu, Y. P., Breakefield, X. O., & Craig, I. W. (1989). Localization of human monoamine oxidase-A gene to Xp11.23-11.4 by in situ hybridization: implications for Norrie disease. *Genomics, 5*, 368–370.

Lipsey, M. W., Chapman, G. L., & Landenberger, N. A. (2001). Cognitive behavioral programs for offenders. *The Annals of the American Academy of Political Science, 578*, 144–157.

Maslow, A. H. (1943). A theory of human motivation. *Psychological Review, 50*(4), 370–396.

Merton, R. K. (1938). Social structure and anomie. *American Sociological Review, 3*, 672–682.

Meyer-Lindenberg, A., Buckholtz, J. W., Kolachana, B., Hariri, A. R., Pezawas, L., Blasi, G., et al. (2006). Neural mechanisms of genetic risk for impulsivity and violence in humans. *Proceedings of the National Academic of Sciences, 103*, 6269–6274.

Miller, W. B. (2001). *The growth of youth gang problems in the United States, 1970–1998*. Washington, DC: U.S. Department of Justice, Office of Juvenile Justice and Delinquency Protection.

Moore, J. W. (1991). *Going down in the barrio: Homeboys and homegirls in change*. Philadelphia: Temple University Press.

Moore, J., & Hagerdorn, J. (2001). *Female gangs: A focus on research*. Washington, DC: U.S. Department of Justice, Office of the Juvenile Justice and Delinquency Prevention.

Morales, G. C. (2010). *The bloods*. Retrieved November 18, 2010 from http://www.gangpreventionservices.org/bloods.asp.

Moriconi, L. H. (2006). *Girl gangs on the rise, involved in violence in the major cities in the USA*. Retrieved November 17, 2010 from http://www.communidadesegura.org/?q=en/node/155.

National Council on Crime and Delinquency. (2010). *Children exposed to violence*. Retrieved November 25, 2010 from http://www.nccd-crc.org/nccd/dnld/Home/focus0809.pdf.

National Gang Crime Research Center. (1996). Preliminary results of the 1995 Adult Corrections Survey: A special report of the National Gang Crime Research Center. *Journal of Gang Research, 3*, 27–63.

National Youth Gang Center. (2000). *1998 National Youth Gang Survey*. Washington, DC: U.S. Department of Justice, Office of Juvenile Justice and Delinquency Prevention.

Office of Juvenile Justice and Delinquency Prevention (OJJDP). (2004). *OJJDP fact sheet*. Washington, DC: U.S. Department of Justice.

OJJDP Model Programs Guide. (2010). *The office of Juvenile Justice and Delinquency Prevention model programs guide*. Retrieved November 5, 2010 from http://www.dsgonline.com/mpg2.5/mpg_index.htm.

Park, R. E., & Burgess, E. W. (1925/1984). *The city*. Chicago, IL: University of Chicago Press.

Pearson, G. (1983). *Hooligan: A history of reportable fears*. New York: Shocken Books.

Pearson, F. S., Lipton, D. S., Cleland, C. M., & Yee, D. S. (2002). The effects of behaviour/cognitive-behavioural programs on recidivism. *Crime and Delinquency, 48*(3), 476–495.

Pillen, M. B., & Howeing-Robertson, R. C. (1992). *Determining youth gang membership: development of a self-report instrument*. Bloomington, IL: Chestnut Health Systems.

Pratt, T., & Cullen, F. (2005). Assessing macro-level predictors and theories of crime: A meta-analysis. In M. Tonry (Ed.), *Crime and justice: A review of research*. Chicago, IL: University of Chicago Press.

Pyrooz, D. C., Fox, A. M., & Decker, S. H. (2010a). *Gang violence worldwide: Context, culture, and country*. Cambridge: Cambridge University Press.

Pyrooz, D. C., Fox, A. M., & Decker, S. H. (2010b). Racial and ethnic heterogeneity, economic disadvantage, and gangs: A macro-level study of gang membership in urban America. *Justice Quarterly, 27*, 867–891.

Ribando, C. M. (2007). *Gangs in Central America*. Washington, DC: Congressional Research Service.

Sanders, W. B. (1994). *Gangbangs and drive-bys: grounded culture and juvenile gang violence*. New York: Aldine de Gruyter.

Savelli, L. (2001). *Gangs across America and their symbols*. New York: Looseleaf Law Publications.

Sheldon, W., Randall, G., Sharon, S. K., & Brown, W. B. (2001). *Youth gangs in American society*. Belmont, CA: Wadsworth.

Sherman, L. W., Gottfredson, D., MacKenzie, D., Eck, J., Reuter, P., & Bushway, S. (1997). *Preventing crime: What works, what doesn't, what's promising (Report to the United States Congress)*. Baltimore, MA: University of Maryland, Department of Criminology and Criminal Justice, Office of Justice Programs.

Spergel, I. A. (1995). *The youth gang problem: A community approach*. New York: Oxford University Press.

Spergel, I. A. (2007). *Reducing youth gang violence: The little village gang project in Chicago*. Lanham, MD: AltaMira.

Sutherland, E. H. (1947). *Principles of criminology*. Philadelphia: L.B. Lippincott.

Tcheremissine, O. V., & Lieving, L. M. (2006). Pharmacological aspects of treatment of conduct disorder in children and adolescents. *Central Nervous System Drugs, 20*, 549–565.

Thornberry, T. P. (2005). Explaining multiple patterns of offending across the life course and across generations. *The Annals of the American Academy of Political and Social Science, 602*, 156–195.

Thornberry, T. P., Huizinga, D., & Loeber, R. (2004). The causes and correlates studies: Findings and policy implications. *Juvenile Justice, 9*, 3–19.

Thornberry, T. P., & Krohn, M. D. (2001). The development of delinquency: An interactional perspective. In S. O. White (Ed.), *Handbook of youth and justice* (pp. 289–305). New York: Plenum.

Thornberry, T. P., & Krohn, M. D. (2003). *Taking stock of delinquency: An overview of findings from contemporary longitudinal studies*. New York: Kluwer/Plenum.

Thornberry, T. P., Krohn, M. D., Lizotte, A. J., Smith, C. A., & Tobin, K. (2003). *Gangs and delinquency in developmental perspective*. New York: Cambridge University Press.

Thrasher, F. M. (1927/1963). *The gang: A study of 1,313 gangs in Chicago*. Chicago, IL: University of Chicago Press.

Tobin, K. (2008). *Gangs, an individual and group perspective*. New Jersey: Pearson Education Inc.

Totten, M. D. (2001). *Guys, gangs, & girlfriend abuse*. Orchard Park, NH: Broadview.

Totten, M. (2009). *Preventing Aboriginal youth gang involvement in Canada: A gendered approach*. Retrieved November 7, 2010 from http://www.turtleisland.org/resources/gangsnwac09.pdf.

Vermeiren, R. (2003). Psychopathology and delinquency in adolescents: A descriptive and developmental perspective. *Clinical Psychology Review, 23*, 277–318.

Wilson, D. B., Bouffard, L. A., & MacKenzie, D. L. (2005). A quantitative review of structured, group-oriented, cognitive-behavioral programs for offenders. *Criminal Justice and Behaviour, 32*(2), 172–203.

Wolf, R. (2010). *The bloods: A look at the notoriously dangerous gang from Los Angeles*. Retrieved November 1, 2010 from http://www.associatedcontent.com/article/2926702/the_bloods_a_look_at_the_notoriously_pg2.html?cat=7.

Chapter 7
Impulse Control Disorders

with
Jennifer Gordon

> *I am, indeed, a king,*
> *because I know how to rule myself.*
>
> –Pietro Aretino (1492–1556)
> *Italian Author, Poet & Playwright*

7.1 Overview

Extreme patterns of impulsivity can be problematic, harmful, and may require formal assessment and intervention. A number of complex and maladaptive behaviors have been classified in the DSM-IV TR, under "impulse control disorders-not elsewhere classified (ICDs-NEC)." These behaviors have been categorized together because they do not meet criteria for specific impulse disorders and are distinguishable from other DSM-IV TR disorders that share symptoms of impaired impulse control (e.g., ADHD and conduct disorder; American Psychiatric Association (APA), 2000; Hollander, Baker, Kahn, & Stein, 2006).

The following chapter provides a brief historical context and description of impulse control disorders, then moves to a discussion of three ICDs that are of particular relevance and interest in childhood and adolescence: (1) trichotillomania, (2) kleptomania, and (3) intermittent explosive disorder (IED). In so doing, this chapter aims to increase familiarity and understanding of ICDs in order to facilitate more comprehensive assessment, diagnosis, and intervention plans for children and adolescents suffering with this group of disorders. It is important to note that current knowledge in this area is limited, and accordingly, much of the information presented should not be seen as conclusive. Gaps in current knowledge and future directions in ICD research are underscored in a final section of this chapter.

S.C. Dombrowski et al., *Assessing and Treating Low Incidence/High Severity Psychological Disorders of Childhood*, DOI 10.1007/978-1-4419-9970-2_7,
© Springer Science+Business Media, LLC 2011

7.2   Historical Context

Whether the behavior is impulsive hair-pulling, stealing, explosive anger, or pathological gambling, individuals with ICDs are essentially unable to control or stop
engaging in behaviors which are experienced as anxiety reducing and gratifying
(APA, 2000). ICD-NEC became an Axis 1 diagnostic category in the DSM-III R in
1987. The DSM-III R sought to categorize a diverse set of behaviors that had a common key feature of impulsivity, not better accounted for by other psychiatric or
medical conditions, under a common nomenclature (APA, 2000, 2010; First &
Tasman, 2004). Aside from establishing impulsivity as the essential component of
ICDs, diagnostic criteria for specific ICDs has changed over time to fit improved
research in this field. Furthermore, there has been much historical debate regarding
whether ICDs would be better conceptualized as part of other clinical spectrums,
such as obsessive-compulsive, behavioral additions, and affective spectrum disorders,
due to similar clinical features and high rates of co-morbidity between ICD and
these other disorders (e.g., depression, eating disorders, anxiety, obsessive compulsive disorder (OCD), substance abuse; Dannon, 2002; Dell'Osso, Altamura,
Allen, Marazziti, & Hollander, 2006; Grant, 2008; Grant, Mancebo, Eisen, &
Rasmussen, 2010; Grant & Potenza, 2008; McElroy, Hudson, Pope, Keck, & Aizley,
1992; Potenza, Koran, & Pallanti, 2009). This continued debate as to whether
ICDs warrants distinct diagnostic categorization is far from resolved at present,
and will likely depend on continued research and improved understanding of this
group of disorders in the future.

7.3   Definition and Description

Currently, ICD-NEC is broadly defined by DSM-IV TR diagnostic criteria as
having the following essential elements:

- An inability or failure to resist an impulsive act or behavior that may be harmful
  to self or others.
- An increasing sense of arousal or tension prior to engaging in the behavior.
- An experience of either pleasure, release of anxiety or tension, or temporary
  reduction of the urge when committing the act or behavior.

Children and adolescents with ICDs are unable to stop the temptation to engage
in certain behaviors which are brought about by an increasing sense of tension or
anxiety that is temporarily relieved by engaging in the act (APA, 2000). These
defining components are common to all ICDs, regardless of the behavioral presentation of the disorder. Individuals with ICDs generally understand that their behaviors
are out of control and harmful, yet repeatedly engage in them despite negative
personal consequences (Dell'Osso et al., 2006; Grant, 2008). Their failure to stop
their behaviors ultimately creates significant distress and impairment in day-to-day

functioning (e.g., social and academic), and may additionally create much distress and frustration for those involved in the management of their care (Grant).

7.4 Trichotillomania

April began pulling out hair from her eyebrows, eyelashes and scalp when she was 13 years old. Now, at age 19, she frequently spends a half hour each day pulling, and has noticeable bald patches where the pulling has occurred. April expresses embarrassment and distress for this behavior, and is often teased at school. Nonetheless she cannot stop herself from engaging in this behavior. Her pulling seems to increase during times of stress, or when she is bored studying, reading and lying in bed falling asleep; at times she doesn't even realize she is doing so.

7.4.1 Historical Context

Trichotillomania has been reported to first emerge in the literature in 1889 by a French dermatologist, Dr. Francois Hallopeau, who published case reports of a man who had pulled out all of his body hair (Chamberlain, Menzies, Sahakian, & Fineberg, 2007; Christenson & Mansueto, 1999; Walther, Tucker, & Woods, 2010). Trichotillomania was not included in psychiatric nomenclature until the DSM-III R edition in 1987 (APA, 1987 as cited in Walther et al., 2010). During the subsequent edition of the DSM (i.e., DSM-IV), trichotillomania was considered for inclusion as an anxiety disorder, due to the perceived commonalities to OCD, as well as considered a disorder of childhood and adolescence due to fact that it frequently occurs prior to adulthood (Christenson & Mansueto). Like the DSM-III R, however, the DSM-IV, and its text revision (DSM-IV TR) have kept Trichotillomania in the general category of impulse control disorders: NEC.

7.4.2 Description and Diagnosis

The DSM-IV TR defines trichotillomania (TTM) as having the follow elements: (a) Recurrent pulling of one's hair, resulting in noticeable hair loss; (b) An increasing sense of tension immediately before pulling out the hair or when attempting to resist the behavior; (c) Pleasure, gratification, or relief when pulling out the hair. Furthermore, (d) hair-pulling is not better accounted for by another mental disorder and is not caused by a general medical condition (e.g., a dermatological condition); and (e) the disturbance causes clinically significant distress or impairment in social, occupational, or other important areas of functioning (APA, 2000).

Age of onset typically occurs between 9 and 13 years (Bloch, 2009; Christenson & Mansueto, 1999; Grant, 2008; O'Sullivan, Keuthen, et al., 1997; Yong-Kwang,

Levy, & Metry, 2004). However, a subgroup of children experience early onset (2–6 years; Christenson & Mansueto; Walther et al., 2010). Hair-pulling is usually chronic in nature, although it has been reported to be more transitory in young children (Christenson, Mackenzie, & Mitchell, 1991; Mansueto, Ninan, Rothbaum, & Reeve, 2010; O'Sullivan, Keuthen, et al.). In particular, in early childhood onset, chronic hair-pulling may be a benign habit, as it associated with less severe symptoms and a more limited course, and may remit without intervention (Chamberlain et al., 2008; Duke, Keeley, Geffken, & Storch, 2009; First & Tasman, 2004; Miller & McMichael, 2010). Alternatively, later onset of TTM (i.e., older children and adolescence) is associated with more severe pulling behaviors, more resistance to treatment intervention, and more co-morbid psychopathologies (Duke et al., 2009; Mancini, Van Ameringen, Patterson, Simpson, & Truong, 2009).

The precise prevalence of TTM is unclear due to low rates of referral, disclosure, and diagnosis. Some research report that approximately 1–3% of the total population (Bloch, 2009; Grant, 2008; Walther et al., 2010) and 1–2% of children and adolescents meet current TTM criteria (APA, 2000; Christensen, Pyle, & Mitchell, 1991; Mancini et al., 2009). The prevalence for young children remains unknown. Furthermore, it has been consistently noted that among preadolescents to young adults, TTM affects more females than males (2:1 ratio; Dell'Osso et al., 2006; O'Sullivan, Keuthen, et al., 1997). This estimate may be confounded, however, due to the noted tendency of females to seek professional help more often than males (Woods et al., 2006). Among young children, hair-pulling may be as common in boys as it is in girls (APA; Christenson & Mansueto, 1999; Cohen et al., 1995; Reeve, 1999; Woods et al., 2006).

Hair-pulling can occur from any part of the body, but in youth ages 10–17, pulling most frequently occurs from the scalp region, followed by eyelashes and eyebrows (Cohen et al., 1995; Franklin et al., 2008). Some children with TTM have also been noted to impulsively pull hair from pets, dolls, and fibrous materials (APA, 2000; First & Tasman, 2004). Children and adolescents may not understand why they engage in repetitive hair-pulling (Duke et al., 2009), but research has reported that episodes are often triggered and exacerbated with environmental stress and negative emotional states (Diefenbach, Mouton-Odum, & Stanley, 2002; Diefenbach, Tolin, Meunier, & Worhunsky, 2008) as well as during sedentary activities (e.g., reading, homework, watching television, and when falling asleep; Adamec, 2008; Christenson & Mansueto, 1999; Hanna, 1997; O'Sullivan, Keuthen, et al., 1997).

Adolescents diagnosed with TTM may pull for an hour or more each day (Grant, 2008; Yong-Kwang et al., 2004). Pulling may occur in frequent and short episodes throughout the day or during less frequent and longer periods of pulling (APA, 2000; First & Tasman, 2004). Moreover, individuals may have set behaviors associated with pulling, such as touching or stroking the hair prior to pulling, and playing with and eating the hair afterwards (Christenson et al., 1991; First & Tasman; Franklin & Tolin, 2007; Yong-Kwang et al., 2004). Repeatedly pulling hairs is thought to temporality alleviate anxiety, tension, "itch-like" somatic sensations, and other negative emotional states, and create emotional relaxation and gratification (Duke et al., 2009; First, Frances, & Pincus, 2004; First & Tasman; Meunier, Tolin, & Franklin, 2009;

Ninan, Rothbaum, Marsteller, Knight, & Eccard, 2000). However, aversive emotions after pulling episodes (e.g., guilt, distress) may supersede any temporary relief experienced during the pulling, which in turn may lead to greater anxiety and tension that perpetuates future episodes (Diefenbach et al., 2002; Dell'Osso et al., 2006; Shusterman, Feld, Baer, & Keuthen, 2009; Woods et al., 2006). Undoubtedly, significant functional and interpersonal impairment is associated with this disorder.

The tension-relief requirement for a TTM diagnosis remains controversial because some individuals who meet DSM-IV TR criteria may not actually experience this cycle (APA, 2010; Christenson et al., 1991; Franklin & Tolin, 2007; Hanna, 1997). For instance, Hanna found in a small sample of children and adolescents, in which only half experienced tension-relief cycles. This, however, may reflect limitations in younger children's ability to describe their psychological states prior to and after pulling (Franklin & Tolin; Hanna; Meunier et al., 2009). Other individuals with TTM may have features of both compulsive and impulsive behavior; compulsively driven behaviors to decrease feelings of anxiousness, and impulsive behavior to achieve feelings of relaxation and gratification (Hanna; Hollander et al., 2006). Consequently, there has been recent consideration for potential change in the DSM-V (APA), which involves re-categorizing TTM as an obsessive-compulsive spectrum disorder. Although impulsive and compulsive behaviors both imply underlying problems with inhibitory control, it has been further noted that they stem from different motivating factors that perpetuate the behavior (e.g., engaging in the behavior without forethought vs. in response to an obsession; APA, 1994, 2000; Chamberlain et al., 2008). This potential re-categorization is consistent with research which has found shared clinical characteristics (e.g., urges to repeatedly engage in unwanted acts), and a high co-prevalence between TTM and OCD (Christenson, 1995; Meunier et al.; O'sullivan, Keuthen, et al., 1997; Potenza et al., 2009). Re-classification presents as a contentious issue, however, as TTM and OCD has also been found to differ with regard to age of onset, gender prevalence, cognitive mechanisms (e.g., need for control over thoughts), co-morbidity, and response to treatment (Chamberlain et al.; Grant, 2008; Swedo & Leonard, 1992). With improved research and understanding of the neurobiology and etiology of TTM, re-classification may or may not provide more meaningful and relevant classification in the future.

Hair-Pulling Subtypes. Some researchers posit that TTM is a heterogeneous disorder that may be more accurately characterized by different subtypes. In particular, two subtypes (i.e., focused and autonomic) have been frequently reported to occur among children and adolescents with TTM (Christenson et al., 1991; Christenson & Mackenzie, 1994; Flessner, Woods, Franklin, Keuthen, & Piacentini, 2008). *Focused pulling* is described as intentional and goal-directed, where conscious attention is focused on the pulling prior to and during the act, in order to decrease negative emotional states (Flessner et al., 2008). *Automatic pulling*, on the other hand, is pulling that occurs in a disengaged or habitual way, with lack of full awareness that one is even engaging in the behavior. This latter type is most associated with sedentary activities (Flessner et al.). Factor analysis research has supported the presence of both these subtypes in children with TTM (Flessner et al., 2007).

Duke and colleagues (2009) and Flessner and colleagues (2008) noted that focused hair-pulling may increase in intensity across adolescence (i.e., ages 13–18), and thus may be associated with stressors associated with puberty. It is important to note, however, that these subtypes are not mutually exclusive; the majority of children and adolescents with TTM have been shown to engage in both types of pulling (Flessner et al., 2008). Moreover, Flessner and colleagues found significant differences in pulling severity, psychiatric co-morbidity, and degree of functional impairment, depending on pulling styles in adolescents with TTM. In particular, after controlling for pulling severity, adolescents who were high in automatic hair-pulling had more depressed symptoms than those low in automatic pulling, and those high in focused pulling had more anxiety and depressive symptoms than those low in focused pulling. These findings exemplify the need for interventions that focus on children and adolescents' specific TTM presentation.

7.4.3   Etiology and Theoretical Frameworks

Currently, there is little consensus on the etiology of TTM, though as with other ICDs, its development is likely due to an interaction of both biological and psychosocial factors (see Duke et al., 2009).

7.4.3.1   Biological Models

Genetics. It is not clear if genetic factors are involved, though some suggest that heritability may be an important contributor in the development of TTM. For instance, limited studies have found significant differences in concordance rates between identical and fraternal twins, with identical pairs being significantly more likely to met DSM criteria for TTM than fraternal pairs (38.1% vs. 0%; Novak, Keuthen, Stewart, & Pauls, 2009). Furthermore, family studies have found increased rates (5–8%) among family members with TTM compared to the general population (Christenson, Mackenzie, & Reeve, 1992 as cited in Duke et al., 2009; Lenane et al., 1992).

Neuroanatomical. Chamberlain and colleagues (2009) noted that abnormalities in cognitive regions responsible for normally inhibiting behaviors (i.e., prefrontal cortex), regulating affect and arousal (i.e., amygdala and hippocampus), and learning habits (e.g., putamen and basal ganglia) are implicated in individuals with TTM. Specifically, MRI studies have found that left putamen brain structure volume to be significantly smaller in individuals with TTM than normal matched controls (O'Sullivan, Rauch, et al., 1997). As well, heightened brain metabolism in the cerebellum, smaller cerebellar volumes, and increased density in the left striatum and left amygdala-hippocampal formation have been reported in individuals with TTM compared to normal controls (Chamberlain et al., 2008; Duke et al., 2009; Keuthen et al., 2007).

7.4.3.2 Environmental Models

Affective Regulation Theory. As mentioned, the development of ICDs has been conceptualized as a maladaptive way of regulating emotions (Grant, 2008; Shusterman et al., 2009). With specific regard to TTM, pulling behaviors may provide regulation by either serving to increase simulation when under-stimulated (e.g., during sedimentary activities) and/or as a calming function when over-stimulated (First & Tasman, 2004). Hair-pulling then may serve to distract or provide temporality relief from negative emotional or physiological states in individuals who lack alternate and more adaptive mechanisms for coping (Meunier et al., 2009; Shusterman et al., 2009). Thus, pulling becomes a maladaptive yet effective tool for emotional regulation.

Reinforcement Theory. Reinforcement theory asserts that pulling behaviors are perpetuated and maintained because they are negatively and positively reinforced through tension reduction and temporary stimulation (Franklin & Tolin, 2007; Woods et al., 2006). It is important to note however that a predominance of TTM research has been conducted with adults, and consequently, it is not entirely clear whether hair-pulling in children and adolescents serves the same functional (e.g., reinforcing) characteristics. Some preliminary research (i.e., Meunier et al., 2009) with children and adolescents has found that hair-pulling is initially associated with both pleasure and pain, and then becomes associated with pleasure only. Therefore, the factors that maintain hair-pulling episodes (i.e., punishment and reinforcement) may actually change over the course of the disorder. Furthermore, parents' reactions (e.g., attention) may serve as reinforcing factor that maintains pulling behavior (Walther et al., 2010).

Cognitive-Behavioral Theory. Cognitive-behavioral models assert that dysfunctional and irrational beliefs (e.g., negative thoughts about self) underlie intense negative emotions (e.g., anxiety and tension), which in turn lead to pulling behaviors. Engaging in pulling episodes then leads to more negative thinking, which continues this dysfunctional cycle (Franklin & Tolin, 2007).

Early Trauma. TTM has been reported to have a high overlap with posttraumatic stress disorder (PTSD; Chamberlain et al., 2008; Gershuny et al., 2006). This suggests that psychological and traumatic stress early in life may play some role in the development of TTM. Christenson and Mansueto (1999) reported on a previous study (Christenson, 1995) that found adults with early onset of TTM (prior to age 7) had significantly higher incidences of physical and sexual abuse. Thus, early traumatic stress may be one of many contributing factors to TTM. Franklin and Tolin (2007) note, however, that more research in this area is warranted prior to making conclusions on this etiological pathway.

7.4.4 Assessment

Clinicians must assess children based on DSM-IV TR criteria, including hair-pulling severity, potential subtypes, and the extent of functional impact (Woods et al.,

2006). Furthermore, research suggests that TTM is highly co-morbid, with 33–70% of children and adolescents diagnosed with TTM meeting criteria for at least one other DSM-IV TR Axis I disorder (King et al., 1995; Lewin et al., 2009; Tolin, Franklin, Dienfenbach, Anderson, & Meunier, 2007). Mood, anxiety, substance use, body dysmorphic, and eating disorders (i.e., bulimia) are most frequently identified in individuals with TTM (Duke et al., 2009; Franklin et al., 2008; Lewin et al.; O'Sullivan, Keuthen, et al., 1997). In children, co-morbid diagnoses such as ADHD (with or without hyperactivity), tic disorders, OCD, and disruptive behavioral disorders have also been frequently reported (Adamec, 2008; Chamberlain et al., 2008; Franklin et al.; King et al.). Thus, routinely assessing for more common co-occurring medical and psychological disorders is important (Franklin & Tolin, 2007). Practitioners conducting assessment should also be aware of cultural factors that may influence hair-pulling. For example, Duke and colleagues (2009) note that pulling hair may be a normal part of grieving during periods of extreme loss in some cultures. Thus, a comprehensive evaluation must assess multiple factors that may alternatively account for hair-pulling behaviors, and rule them out prior to a TTM diagnosis (APA, 2000; Trainor et al., 2007). In addition, shame and embarrassment frequently results in individuals attempting to hide evidence of hair loss. A skin biopsy from the affected area should aid in confirming or ruling out a diagnosis, particularly when children and adolescents deny their pulling behaviors (APA; First & Tasman, 2004).

At present there is no consensus on standards to best assess for TTM. The following are some rating scales that have been utilized in previous research to aid diagnosis in children and adolescent samples, and may warrant consideration in aiding practitioners through the process of assessment and differential diagnosis.

7.4.4.1   TTM Rating Scales

- *The NIMH Trichotillomania Questionnaire* is a semistructured interview that assesses the severity and impairment of TTM, and has been used with children and adolescents (Franklin, Keuthen et al., 2002 as cited in Franklin & Tolin, 2007).
- *Milwaukee Inventory for Subtypes of Trichotillomania-Child Version (MIST-C).* The MIST-C is designed to assess both automatic and focused TTM subtypes in children and adolescents and has been found to have good validity and reliability for this population (Flessner et al., 2007; Woods et al., 2006).
- *The Trichotillomania Scale for Children.* Tolin and colleagues (2008) has found this measure to be useful for aiding TTM diagnosis in child and adolescent samples. This measure assesses symptom severity and associated distress and interference from hair-pulling, and includes both parent and child versions.
- *The Trichotillomania Impact Survey for Children (TISC).* The TISC is designed to gather a broad range of information on TTM in children and adolescents, including descriptive psychopathology, co-morbidity, and functional impact of the behaviors. This survey also includes both parent and child report sections (Franklin et al., 2008).

Functional assessments to obtain information on behavioral, cognitive, and emotional antecedents of pulling behaviors and consequences (postpulling emotions, thoughts, behaviors) are also available (see Franklin & Tolin, 2007 for a trichotillomania functional assessment protocol). This protocol may be helpful in informing appropriate intervention strategies for children and adolescents diagnosed with TTM.

7.4.5   Treatment and Intervention

7.4.5.1   Pharmacological

To date, very limited intervention studies on children and adolescents diagnosed with TTM are available (Mancini et al., 2009; Trainor et al., 2007). Tricyclic antidepressants (e.g., clomipramine) and SSRIs (e.g., fluoxetine) have been approved for use with older children and adolescents to treat disorders with similar neurobiological links to TTM (e.g., OCD; Chamberlain et al., 2008). Their effectiveness in treating TTM specifically, however, has been inconsistent (Duke et al., 2009; Mancini et al.; Woods et al., 2006), and are limited to open trials and single case reports. Some have concluded that SSRIs with adults have little efficacy in reducing chronic hair-pulling (Franklin et al., 2008; Ninan et al., 2000; van Minnen, Hoogduin, Keijsers, Hellenbrand, & Hendriks, 2003), while others have reported initial decrease in hair-pulling, with subsequent relapse during periods of stress (O'Sullivan, Keuthen, et al., 1997).

On the basis of retrospective case series, Mancini and colleagues (2009) found that antipsychotics were somewhat more effective than SSRIs (89% response rate) in a sample of 11 children (mean age of 11 years), who had TTM. Most of this sample also had other co-morbid diagnoses (ADHD, tics, social phobia). It is important to note however that aversive side effects to these medications were experienced by 7 out of 11 children, though this did not lead to treatment discontinuation. Moreover, Palmer, Yates, and Trotter (1999) reported a case study of a 7-year-old female who had success with the SSRI fluoxetine in decreasing TTM symptoms (after 15 weeks), after she was unsuccessfully treated with another SSRI (fluvoxamine).

In addition, because TTM is commonly accompanied by anxiety and exacerbated by stress, attempts to treat TTM with anxiolytic agents have been proposed (First & Tasman, 2004; Grant, 2008). These agents decrease the activity in the sympathetic nervous system and thereby reduce symptoms of anxiety and tension (APA, 2000; Firestone & Marshall, 2003). No studies found to date have examined treatment efficacy in pediatric TTM samples.

Atypical neuroleptics and opioid blockers have also been reported to have moderate success with adults with TTM (Doughterty, Loh, Jenike, & Keuthen, 2006; Palmer et al., 1999; van Minnen et al., 2003). As mentioned, these drugs decrease the positive reinforcement function of the behaviors through inhibiting dopamine in the brain. Based on an open pilot trial, De Sousa (2008) found that 11 out of 14 children (mean age of 9 years) with childhood onset of TTM responded positively to the opoid blocker, Naltrexone, which was administered for a duration of 10 months. Specifically, these children demonstrated a significant decrease in both the frequency of pulling and in the intensity of the urge to pull.

In sum, results are limited and mixed. Accordingly, considerably more research with larger and more controlled trials is needed before any conclusions are made on effectiveness of this modality of treatment with pediatric TTM cases. Currently, medication may be more effective in treating co-morbid disorders (Franklin et al., 2008).

7.4.5.2   Psychosocial Approaches

Given the paucity of pharmacological research with TTM in pediatric populations, nonpharmacological approaches have been consistently reported to be a first-line treatment approach for children and adolescents with TTM (Chamberlain et al., 2007; O'Sullivan, Keuthen, et al., 1997; Trainor et al., 2007; Woods et al., 2006). These approaches generally focus on the antecedents and consequences of pulling behaviors and have reported benefits in decreasing TTM symptoms (Duke et al., 2009; Ninan et al., 2000). Efficacy research on these approaches for children and adolescents with TTM are also very limited.

Cognitive-Behavioral Therapy (CBT). CBT approaches for TTM generally involve challenging and modifying cognitive distortions associated with hair-pulling (e.g., fear of negative evaluation and negative beliefs about appearance; Franklin & Tolin, 2007; Norberg, Wetterneck, Woods, & Conelea, 2007; Walther et al., 2010). With adults, CBT has been found to be successful in some randomized trials (Woods et al., 2006), and has been shown to be even more effective in decreasing hair-pulling episodes than antidepressants alone (Dell'Osso et al., 2006; Ninan et al., 2000). One open trial of CBT for pediatric TTM found that CBT was also effective for children and adolescents (n=46), with a response rates of 77% posttreatment and 65% at a 6-month follow-up (Tolin et al., 2007). Larger and more controlled studies are needed to evaluate the efficacy of CBT for TTM in pediatric samples (Woods et al.).

Habit Reversal Training (HRT). Randomized controlled trials using behavioral approaches have focused on HRT to treat TTM. HRT involves teaching individuals to recognize and redirect their impulse for pulling. Awareness training is one important component of HRT, which involves identifying and increasing awareness to cues and triggers that lead to pulling (Woods et al., 2006). Self-monitoring is the most common strategy to improve awareness, and generally involves recording either the number of pulling episodes or the actual number of hairs pulled each day (Woods et al.; Vitulano, King, Scahill, & Cohen, 1992). Creating colorful self-monitoring graphs that plot progress may encourage children in this process (Franklin & Tolin, 2007). Competing response training (i.e., engaging in an alternate, more adaptive behavior like fist clenching or squeezing a stress ball in response to triggers), relaxation training, and self-rewards are also important components of HRT (Chamberlain et al., 2008; Duke et al., 2009; First & Tasman, 2004; Franklin & Tolin; O'Sullivan, Keuthen, et al., 1997; van Minnen et al., 2003).

Research has demonstrated that HBT has good short-term effectiveness, though predominately with adult samples. Notably, 12-week sessions of HRT in adults has shown modest reductions in hair-pulling severity and impairment, with improvements maintained at a 3-month follow-up (Woods et al., 2006). Moreover, some studies have shown that HRT is more effective than certain SSRI medication trials (e.g., van Minnen et al., 2003), while others have reported that HRT in conjunction with SSRIs are more advantageous than either one alone (Doughterty et al., 2006). In an early study with a sample having 34 patients (including four children), HRT was found to be superior to negative training practices (i.e., involving acting out motions of hair-pulling without actually pulling it) in significantly decreasing hair-pulling episodes by more than 90% after 4 weeks (Azrin, Nunn, & Frantz, 1980 as cited in Chamberlain et al., 2007). Another study found that HRT, which consisted of awareness training, competing response training (e.g., folding arms or sitting on hands during urges), and social support (i.e., reinforcement from parents) was successful in three preadolescents (age 12) diagnosed with TTM (Rapp, Miltenberger, Long, Elliot, & Lumley, 1998). Positive results were maintained from 18 to 27 weeks posttreatment for two out of three adolescents, though 1–3 booster sessions, starting approximately 2-months after initial treatment, were required to prevent relapse in hair-pulling.

Flessner and colleagues (2008) noted that HRT may be particularly effective for children with a high rate of autonomic pulling, to increase awareness of pulling and to reduce habitual responding. Alternatively, interventions such as CBT may be more effective for those who are predominately focused hair pullers (Flessner et al., 2008; Tolin et al., 2007). Longer-term efficacy of both HRT and CBT with children and youth diagnosed with TTM is not clear (Franklin et al., 2008; Lerner, Franklin, Meadows, Hembree, & Foa, 1998; Ninan et al., 2000; van Minnen et al., 2003).

Stimulus Control. Other behavioral therapeutic strategies include stimulus control procedures which aim to interfere with hair-pulling episodes (Franklin & Tolin, 2007; Mansueto et al., 2010). For example, some researchers have suggested techniques such as utilizing physical barriers to hair-pulling (e.g., hats and gloves); keeping hands occupied; getting children to wear "jingly" bracelets or strong perfume on their wrists to improve awareness when their hands are raised to their head; and using visual cues such as posting reminder signs in "high-risk" areas (Franklin, Tolin, & Diefenbach, 2006; Mansueto et al.). Behavioral approaches aimed at removing and avoiding stimuli that trigger hair-pulling episodes have also been included to help treat individuals with this disorder (Duke et al., 2009). The inclusion of a social support component, such as getting a parent to prompt the use of strategies learned in therapy and rewarding for doing so is also important when treating children and adolescents (Walther et al., 2010).

Relaxation Training. Franklin and Tolin (2007) note that some individuals will find that decreasing their levels of physiological tension and anxiety will result in reduced urges to pull. Franklin and Tolin found, however, that individuals with TTM reported relaxation training as being less helpful than "core" treatment approaches (e.g., self-monitoring, competing response training, and stimulus control). Thus, relaxation and stress management approaches may be more beneficial as an adjunct approach in treating individuals with TTM, and may be most helpful for focused pullers who are triggered by anxiety. The efficacy of relaxation and stress management techniques had rarely been reported for pediatric TTM cases. Vitulano and colleagues (1992) reported three cases of children with TTM where progressive muscle relaxation was well accepted and demonstrated benefits when used in conjunction with other behavioral approaches.

Psychoeducation. Educating children and their families about TTM may be helpful. TTM support groups and information can be found through The Trichotillomania Learning Center (http://www.trich.org).

7.4.6 Prognosis

A dominant factor in the prognosis of TTM is whether an individual receives treatment. When left untreated, the consequences of TTM can be severe. Physical consequences of hair-pulling may occur such as alopecia, scalp infections, neck and back pain from repetitive pulling, and the possible development of gastrointestinal obstruction if hair is repeatedly consumed (Christenson & Mansueto, 1999; Diefenbach, Tolin, Hannan, Crocetto, & Worhunsky, 2005; First & Tasman, 2004; Miller & McMichael, 2010; Woods et al., 2006).

Yong-Kwang and colleagues (2004) noted that children who pull for more than 6 months are generally more difficult to treat than those who have been pulling for less than 6 months. The latter case may be due to coping with stressful environmental circumstances (e.g., divorce of parents), and may remit with or without treatment. Moreover, prognosis is thought to be worst in individuals who have a later onset of TTM (e.g., adolescents; APA, 2000). Feelings of psychological distress as a result of pulling may be exacerbated during adolescence, as it is a time when appearance is particularly tied to self-esteem and sense of competence (Franklin & Tolin, 2007; O'Sullivan, Keuthen, et al., 1997). A great deal of shame and embarrassment often results when evidence of their hair-pulling is noticed by peers (Franklin & Tolin). Moderate to severe social and academic impairment has indeed been found in children and adolescents with TTM (Diefenbach et al., 2005; Franklin et al., 2008; Tolin et al., 2007). In particular, difficulties focusing on school, performing school responsibilities (Bloch, 2009; Franklin et al., 2008), and avoidance of social and sport endeavors as an effort to prevent scrutiny from peers are common (Diefenbach et al.; Wood et al., 2006). Lewin et al. (2009) found that 45% of children with TTM endorsed depressive symptoms and 40% endorsed anxiety symptoms. Franklin and colleagues (2008) further reported that severity of anxiety and depressive symptoms were particularly elevated in youth aged 10–17, and thus may contribute to day-to-day impairment in this age group. Like other ICDs, prognosis is thought to be poor for individuals with more severe pulling behaviors (Yong-Kwang et al., 2004), and for those with co-morbid diagnoses, individuals usually require longer treatment duration (Walther et al., 2010).

Relapse rates are common in individuals with TTM, and particularly so in the presence of stress and after treatment is completed (Mansueto et al., 2010). Thus, relapse prevention training becomes essential during treatment, where individuals are taught how to handle the recurrence of pulling by continuing with follow-up sessions when necessary (Franklin & Tolin, 2007; Mansueto et al.).

7.5 Kleptomania

Laura, a 20-year-old female, reported a history of compulsive and uncontrollable stealing. It began 1–2 times a week 4 years ago, and is now almost a daily occurrence. She steals various, unneeded items that have no significance to her, and of which she can afford. She does not understand why she does this, only reporting that she is simply unable to stop herself and feels a sense of relief when doing so. Laura feels much shame and guilt over these behaviors, and ends up throwing out or surreptitiously returning the items soon after stealing them. She has recently lost a friendship after she was caught stealing from her house, which has served as a motivation for seeking treatment.

7.5.1 *Historical Context*

Although stealing has occurred for centuries, *impulsive* stealing was first described in 1816 by the physician Andre Matthey, after witnessing accounts of individuals who stole without any apparent motive or need (Fullerton & Punj, 2004; Grant, 2008; McElroy, Hudson, Pope, & Keck, 1991). The term Kleptomania was subsequently coined by French physicians C.C. Marc and Jean-Etienne Esquirol in 1838 (Aboujaoude, Gamel, & Koran, 2004; Adamec, 2008; Grant, 2006; Koran, Bodnik, & Dannon, 2010). Historically, Kleptomania has been considered a disorder seen mainly in Caucasian, upper-class women (Kohn & Antonuccio, 2002; McElroy, Hudson, et al., 1991), and was considered alongside female hysteria and pelvic disorders (Grant, 2008; Koran et al., 2010). Kleptomania as a psychiatric disorder began to receive increased clinical and research attention since its inclusion in the third edition of the DSM in 1980. Kleptomania was subsequently categorized as an impulse control disorder-NEC in DSM-III R in 1987 (Grant, 2004; Grant, Kim, & McCabe, 2006). To date, Kleptomania is one of the least researched and poorly understood disorders in the DSM-IV TR (Grant & Kim, 2002a; Hollander, Berlin, & Stein, 2008). Likewise, there is still some controversy as to whether it is a separate disorder or secondary symptom of other disorders (e.g., borderline personality disorder (BPD) or conduct disorder; Aboujaoude et al., 2004; APA, 2000; Grant, 2004). Others contend that Kleptomania is merely theft, and assert that psychological elements are not involved (Bresser, 1979 as cited in Kohn & Antonuccio, 2002). Despite many debatable and uncertain elements of Kleptomania, the substantial financial cost that this ICD creates on economic and legal systems is unquestionable (Grant, Odlaug, Davis, & Kim, 2009; Novak, 2010). Today, many cases of celebrities who have been caught during stealing episodes have increased public awareness of this disorder. True modern day cases of Kleptomania, however, are not common in the general population and warrant comprehensive assessment to determine an accurate diagnosis. Furthermore, within the legal system, Kleptomania is not considered as an insanity defense, rather individuals are held responsible for theft except in cases where there is a complete absence of control of actions and of which can be established accordingly (Koran et al.).

7.5.2 Diagnosis and Description

The DSM-IV TR currently defines Kleptomania (312.32) as having the follow elements: (a) the recurrent failure to resist impulses to steal objects that are not needed for personal use or for their monetary value; (b) Increasing subjective sense of tension immediately before committing the theft; (c) Pleasure, gratification, or relief at the time of committing the theft. Furthermore, stealing is not committed to express anger or vengeance and is not in response to a delusion or a hallucination (d), and is not better accounted for by conduct disorder, a manic episode, or antisocial personality disorder (e).

Individuals with Kleptomania have an inability to stop themselves from stealing although they have the awareness that the act is wrong and senseless, and frequently do not understand why they commit such behaviors (APA, 2000; Dannon, Lowengrub, Iancu, & Kotler, 2004; First & Tasman, 2004; Grant & Kim, 2002a). Unlike shoplifting, those with Kleptomania do not steal for monetary or social gain (e.g., acceptance by deviant peer groups), anger or vengeance, and do not have intentional plans to steal prior to an impulse to do so (APA; Grant, 2008; Grant et al., 2009; Koran et al., 2010). Rather, these individuals are compelled to steal in order to decrease the overwhelming emotional tension that occurs either from attempting to resist the act or due to aversive states such as loneliness, stress, boredom, or anxiety (Aboujaoude et al., 2004; Grant & Kim, 2002a). After the act, items may be kept (e.g., horded), given or thrown away, or surreptitiously returned to others and stores (APA; First & Tasman; Goldman, 1991; Grant, 2006; McElroy, Hudson, et al., 1991). Feelings of shame, guilt, and depression are frequently experienced as a result of the theft (APA; Dannon et al., 2004; Dannon, Aizer, & Lowengrub, 2006; First & Tasman; Grant & Kim, 2002a). Consequently, this disorder causes significant distress and functional impairment for individuals. Most individuals with Kleptomania will attempt to actively hide their impulsive stealing behaviors and items from friends and family to avoid embarrassment, social stigma, and due to fear of apprehension (Grant & Kim, 2002d; Hollander et al., 2008). The intensity of gratification and sense of relief experienced during and immediately after committing the act, however, tend to replace any negative consequences associated with stealing (Grant, 2006; Grant & Kim, 2002a). This makes individuals unable to stop from engaging in subsequent episodes.

Onset of Kleptomania may occur anytime between childhood to adulthood. Some researchers found that onset of Kleptomania peaks by late adolescence (Aboujaoude et al., 2004; Grant & Kim, 2002a; Grant & Potenza, 2008; Grant et al., 2009; McElroy, Pope, Hudson, Keck, & White, 1991) while others suggest a later onset period (e.g., mid-1920s; Dannon et al., 2006; 28–30 years; Bayle, Caci, Millet, Richa, & Olie, 2003). Despite this lack of clarity, Kleptomania has rarely been researched in pediatric and adolescent populations. Diagnosis of Kleptomania has been found to occur up 2–4 times more frequently in females (Bayle et al., 2003; Dannon, 2002; Dannon et al.; Goldman, 1992). Some researchers have further reported an association between Kleptomanic acts and menstruation or premenstrual tension (Dannon; Dannon et al.). Research has also found that females have a later onset than men (20 vs. 14 years of age; Grant & Potenza). There is no consistent evidence, however, to suggest that the clinical presentation of Kleptomania significant varies between genders (Aboujaoude et al.; Grant & Kim, 2002a; Hollander et al., 2008), though Grant and Potenza found that women were more likely to steal household items and hoard items once stolen. For both, onset may be rapid or occur after years of stealing, and results in significant impairment in day-to-day functioning (Bayle et al.; Grant & Potenza; Grant & Kim).

Prevalence rates for Kleptomania are difficult to precisely estimate given the obvious social stigma and legal ramifications that prevents individuals from disclosing this behavior (Bayle et al., 2003). Estimates suggest that less than 1% of the general population, approximately 5% of all shoplifters (APA, 2000; Dannon, 2002; Dannon et al., 2006; First & Tasman, 2004; Grant, 2006; Koran et al., 2010), and up to 8.8% in clinical adolescent populations meet diagnostic criteria (Grant, Williams, & Potenza, 2007). Prevalence rates for Kleptomania in children are unknown. Kleptomania is still most frequently seen in middle to high socioeconomic status (SES) groups, though current definitional criteria (i.e., senselessly stealing unneeded items) may actually exclude individuals in lower SES brackets who may also have the disorder, by presuming that those diagnosed have adequate income to purchase the stolen items (Kohn, 2006; Kohn & Antonuccio, 2002). Kleptomania may occur trans-culturally, as it has been described in both Western and Eastern cultures (APA; First & Tasman).

Individuals with Kleptomania are found to have generally high sensation seeking and risk-taking behaviors, and frequently have co-occurring anxiety disorders (e.g., OCD), mood disorders (e.g., depressive episodes), eating disorders (i.e., bulimia), substance abuse disorders, and other ICDs (Aboujaoude et al., 2004; Bayle et al., 2003; Dannon, 2002; Dannon et al., 2004; Grant, 2006, 2008; Grant & Kim, 2002a; Lejoyeux, Arbaretaz, Mcloughlin, & Ades, 2002; McElroy, Pope, et al., 1991). Interestingly, females diagnosed with Kleptomania have been found to be less likely to have co-occurring ICDs than males (Grant & Potenza, 2008), though this finding requires replication with child and adolescent samples. Some have asserted that Kleptomania is a symptom of antisocial disorder and BPDs, however, co-morbidity rates have been found to be only 3% and 10%, respectively, suggesting distinct psychiatric difficulties (Grant, 2004, 2008).

7.5.3   Etiology and Theoretical Frameworks

7.5.3.1   Biological Models

Genetics. There is a current paucity of genetic and biological research on Kleptomania. The majority of individuals with Kleptomania in a few studies, however, had significant family histories of psychiatric disorders (e.g., mood disorders), substance use disorders, and Kleptomania (Grant & Kim, 2002a; McElroy, Pope, et al., 1991). Family histories of psychiatric illness have further been found be a predictor of developing Kleptomania (Grant & Kim).

Neurobiological. Like other ICDs, frontal lobe dysfunction may be implicated in individuals with Kleptomania (Kozian, 2001). Though studies have found that as a group, individuals with Kleptomania may not demonstrate deficits on executive functioning compared to the normative population; individuals with more severe symptoms of Kleptomania have in fact demonstrated more significant impairment in executive functioning and mental flexibility (Grant et al., 2007). Lower inhibitory mechanisms may also be involved, which results in impulsive and high-risk-taking behaviors (Grant, 2008). Neurochemical abnormalities (i.e., serotonin and dopamine deficiency) may also play a role in Kleptomania, where stealing episodes may be triggered by changes in neurotransmitter levels in the brain (Adamec, 2008; Dannon et al., 2006; Grant). Considerably, more research is needed to confirm these preliminary findings in child and adolescent groups.

7.5.3.2   Environmental Models

Affective Regulation Theory. With specific regard to Kleptomania, the temporary rush or relief associated with stealing may be at maladaptive way to temporarily alleviate and distract themselves from negative states (e.g., anxiety, depression) and life stressors (First & Tasman, 2004). One study in particular found that individuals with Kleptomania reported feelings of relief from depression during and immediately after a stealing episode (Dannon et al., 2004). This is consistent with other findings that have found Kleptomania to be co-existent with unipolar and bipolar mood disorders (41–100% lifetime prevalence; Bayle et al., 2003; Dannon et al.; Grant, 2006, 2008). Like other ICDs, this attempt at symptom relief is misguided and is frequently followed by negative affect (Grant, 2008; Grant & Kim, 2002a).

Early Life Experiences. Some limited studies have empirically examined the role of early experiences of individuals diagnosed with Kleptomania. In particular, Grant and Kim (2002b) found significantly lower levels of maternal and paternal care and more neglectful maternal parenting among those with vs. without Kleptomania. This suggests that low levels of parental care and protection may be a psychosocial antecedent for Kleptomania. Stressors such as major losses may also precipitate impulsive stealing behavior (First & Tasman, 2004).

7.5.4 Assessment

Assessing for Kleptomania can be particularly difficult for practitioners given that those suffering do not generally seek professional help for these issues, or are willingly disclose these behaviors, and generic assessment tools may not adequately detect such covert behaviors (Aboujaoude et al., 2004; Grant, 2006, 2008; Grant & Potenza, 2008). In fact, individuals are typically diagnosed with Kleptomania after they seek psychological help for other difficulties (e.g., depression or anxiety; Dannon et al., 2006; First & Tasman, 2004).

As those with Kleptomania often have many co-morbid difficulties, psychologists need to rule out the possibility that the impulsivity of Kleptomania is not simply the consequence or associated feature of other clinical disorders (First & Tasman, 2004). Furthermore, stealing may be common during childhood and adolescence, and these behaviors need to be differentiated from a clinical behavioral disturbance (APA, 2000). One differentiation is that those with Kleptomania commonly suffer from overwhelming distress and remorse over their behaviors (Aboujaoude et al., 2004; Grant & Kim, 2002a; Grant, 2006). In addition, Kleptomania should only be diagnosed when an individual describes urges to steal that are uncontrollable (APA). Practitioners must ensure that stealing is not motivated by peer pressure, approval, or for monetary gains, or in support of a drug habit (Aboujaoude et al.; APA). Given the infrequency of Kleptomania and the common occurrence of shoplifting, malingering must also be considered as some individuals may mimic symptoms to avoid legal consequences (APA). To this end, practitioners must inquire about symptoms, antecedents, consequences, and functional impact of impulsive stealing behaviors.

The following are scales that have demonstrated utility for assessing Kleptomania, although their utility with children is unknown.

* *The Structured Clinical Interview for Kleptomania* (SCI-K) assesses anticipatory tension and urges, frequency, duration, thoughts, and behaviors, and subjective distress caused by stealing in the previous week (Grant et al., 2006).
* *Improvement Scaling* (IMS; Smith, Cardillo, Smith, & Amezaga, 1998) has been successfully utilized to assess treatment gains (i.e., level of improvement in symptoms) in individuals with Kleptomania (Kohn, 2006; Kohn & Antonuccio, 2002).
* *The Kleptomania Symptom Assessment Scale (K-SAS)* assesses average severity, frequency, duration and level of control over stealing urges and thoughts, emotional states before and after episodes, and degree of functional impairment (Koran et al., 2010).

7.5.5 Treatment and Intervention

Intervention for individuals diagnosed with Kleptomania has generally been centered around improving impulse control and treating co-morbid difficulties such as depression, low self-esteem, and negative self-evaluations (Dannon et al., 2006; Kohn & Antonuccio, 2002).

7.5.5.1 Pharmacological Approaches

Consistent with the role that serotonin and dopamine play in Kleptomania, SSRIs, opiod antagonists, antiepileptics, and mood stabilizers have all been used to treat Kleptomania in adults, with equivocal evidence on their effectiveness (Dannon, 2002; Dannon et al., 2006; Grant & Kim, 2002c; McElroy, Pope, et al., 1991). Antidepressants (i.e., SSRIs) seem to be the most promising and a frequent choice in pharmacological treatment (Dannon; First & Tasman, 2004), although some researchers report studies with low response rates with these agents with adults (Dannon et al.; Grant & Kim, 2002a; McElroy, Pope, et al.). Grant and Kim (2002c) completed one case report of successfully treating an adolescent (13-year-old female) diagnosed with Kleptomania with the opiod blocker, Naltrexone. The lack of trials with pediatric samples severely limits recommendations options to parents with children and adolescents with Kleptomania. Like other ICDs, pharmacological agents may be more promising as an adjunct therapy, and for children and adolescents who demonstrate co-occurring mood and anxiety disorders.

7.5.5.2 Behavioral and Cognitive-Behavioral Approaches

Symptoms of Kleptomania are most frequently treated within a cognitive-behavioral or behavioral framework (Kohn, 2006; Kohn & Antonuccio, 2002). The main goals of CBT and behavioral approaches involve identifying cognitive and behavioral triggers (e.g., wearing loose clothes, shopping at store with minimal security), restructuring irrational beliefs that precede episodes (CBT), generating more adaptive responses to stress, and developing behavioral strategies for relapse prevention (Dannon et al., 2006; Kohn & Antonuccio). Among these:

Cognitive-Behavioral Approaches. Cognitive-behavioral approaches (e.g., rational emotive therapy (RET); Ellis, 1994) are concerned with how individuals interpret events, and how these interpretations influence their behaviors (Firestone & Marshall, 2003). CBT approaches generally involve identifying, evaluating, disputing, and acting against irrational self-defeating beliefs (e.g., "I'm a bad or weak person") that may perpetuate the impulsive stealing episodes (Kohn & Antonuccio, 2002), as well as teach individuals to think systematically about the positive and negative consequences of their stealing behaviors (Glosscock, Rapoff, & Christerpherson, 1988). Although this approach may be promising for Kleptomania, no empirical pediatric trials were found in this review. However, the promotion of more adaptive ways for satisfaction and coping with aversive emotions has been cited to help individual with Kleptomania decrease depressive symptoms, and overcome the need for gratification and tension release presumably gained through stealing (Dannon, 2002).

Covert Sensitization. This approach involves pairing various aversive, imagined consequences (e.g., getting arrested, disappointing loved ones, nausea, and vomiting) with the impulse to steal (Gauthier & Pellerin, 1982 as cited in Kohn & Antonuccio,

2002; Glover, 1985 as cited in Dannon, 2002). Repeated pairings may lead to a decrease in expressed stealing behaviors, though this approach must be accompanied by reinforcement of appropriate behaviors to be beneficial (First & Tasman, 2004). No reports found have examined this approach with children and adolescents with Kleptomania.

Systematic Desensitization. Systematic desensitization is a preventative technique where individuals envision resisting urges while in a relaxed state (Firestone & Marshall, 2003). Specifically, individuals with Kleptomania may describe multiple scenarios where they typically steal or thinking about stealing, which are then ranked according to the degree of difficulty to control the urge. They may be then taught relaxation techniques which are utilized as they imagine these increasingly difficult situations (Grant, 2006). This approach is thought to control impulses to steal through controlling the anxiety and tension that tends to occur prior to the act (Aboujaoude et al., 2004). This approach has been reported to be effective with additive behaviors (e.g., pathological gamblers; Lopez, 1998), and in limited case studies of Kleptomania (e.g., Gudjonsson, 1987 as cited in Grant, 2008). No empirical evidence has been reported on pediatric samples with Kleptomania.

Aversion Therapy. Aversive therapy involves the use of unpleasant stimuli to decrease unwanted behaviors (Firestone & Marshall, 2003). Various aversive therapies have been proposed for Kleptomania treatment, including aversive breath-holding until it becomes mildly painful (Kreutzer, 1972 as cited in Dannon, 2002), or snapping a band around their wrist whenever an urge to steal or an image of it is experienced. In general, few empirical studies have examined the benefits of this approach. Furthermore, aversive therapy has been viewed as controversial, and many doubt that it produces long-lasting changes in behavior (Firestone & Marshall). Thus, this approach may be more valuable as an adjunct to other therapeutic approaches. Research with children and adolescents is greatly warranted.

Behavioral Interruption and Control. Incongruent activities may also be taught and practiced, which aims to block or decrease the plan of stealing during an impulse to do so. For example, individuals may be encouraged to stop to write down a thought, or take out a picture of their loved ones to decrease the urge to steal (Kohn & Antonuccio, 2002). This approach generally aids the implementation of other preventive strategies such as covert sensitization (Kohn & Antonuccio). Behavioral control strategies are additionally employed to prevent individuals with Kleptomania from engaging in impulsive stealing – for example, avoiding stores, shopping only when with someone else, or only shopping in high security stores where there is a high risk of being caught (Adamec, 2008). First and Tasman (2004) noted that a complete abstinence of stores may be the most effective behavioral treatment of all for individuals with this disorder.

It is important to reiterate that although the above therapeutic interventions have been noted to have some success in treating individuals with Kleptomania, there have been almost no controlled treatment studies in the literature to date that have adequately evaluated these approaches with children and adolescents. Accordingly, research is needed in pediatric samples before making any conclusions on the best way to go about treatment planning for children and adolescent who impulsively steal. As with any therapeutic approach, it is crucial to tailor their use to the developmental stages of the child. Young children may not be developmentally ready to introspect and describe their emotional states, cognitions, and behaviors. Accordingly, practitioners will need to adapt many of these techniques to make them applicable for pediatric clients. Planning treatment interventions should also take into account individual's co-morbid conditions (Koran et al., 2010).

7.5.6 Prognosis

The course of Kleptomania may range from brief episodes with long periods of remission to a more chronic course which may persist even after multiple attempts to stop (Grant, 2006; Koran et al., 2010). Despite this variability, the disorder is reported to be most typically chronic, with some increase and decreases in severity over time (Aboujaoude et al., 2004; Grant, 2006, 2008; Grant & Potenza, 2010). Most individuals report stealing episodes for more than 10 years prior to entering treatment (Grant & Kim, 2002d; McElroy, Pope, et al., 1991). Once the disorder is correctly identified and treated, prognosis is improved (Dannon, 2002; Dannon et al., 2006).

Without identification and treatment, the consequences of individuals suffering from Kleptomania may be particularly severe. Undoubtedly, individuals with impulsive and repetitive stealing may face substantial legal consequences. Grant and colleagues (2009) noted that many individuals with Kleptomania (67–87%) become apprehended at some point during the duration of the disorder. In general, these individuals have a high degree of emotional distress, significant functional impairment in social and occupational domains, and a perceived low quality of life (Aboujaoude et al., 2004; Dannon et al., 2006; Grant & Potenza, 2008; Grant & Kim, 2002a; McElroy, Pope, et al., 1991). Interestingly, individuals with Kleptomania have been shown to report significantly more perceived stress (i.e., viewing their life as unpredictable and uncontrollable) than those diagnosed with major depressive disorder (Grant, Kim, & Grosz, 2003). These individuals also have higher rates of psychiatric hospitalization (Grant & Kim) and a substantially higher risk (6–24 times; Grant & Potenza) of suicide when compared to the general population, and significantly more suicide attempts when compared to individuals with depression and other ICDs (Lejoyeux et al., 2002). Individuals who experience global feelings of shame (e.g., stable thoughts that they are a "bad" person) are more likely to have a poorer prognosis that those who experience situation-specific feelings of shame associated with their behavior (e.g., feelings of being an otherwise "good" person; Kohn, 2006; Kohn & Antonuccio, 2002). Lifetime co-morbidity rates have been reported to be approximately 40% for major depressive disorder, anxiety disorders, and other ICDs, and 60% for bulimia nervosa (First & Tasman, 2004). Like other ICDs, individuals with co-morbid diagnoses are likely to have a poor prognosis than those without (Grant & Kim).

7.6   Intermittent Explosive Disorder

Tyler, a 27-year-old male, describes himself as having had a "short fuse" since he was a teenager. In particular, Tyler quickly escalates into a rage when he encounters many minor inconveniences. On many occasions, Tyler has reacted to long lines in the grocery store by throwing items and screaming at the cashier and other customers for their incompetence. In a more serious incident last month, Tyler tailgated another driver for 25 min after he was cut off – honking his horn, screaming, and running the other car off the highway. Tyler expresses much embarrassment and guilt after these explosive episodes, and wishes he could prevent himself from losing control of his behavior.

7.6.1   Historical Context

Intermittent explosive disorder (IED) was first described by French psychiatrist Esquirol, to characterize irrational explosive anger, which was thought to be caused by the possession by spirits and moral weakness (First & Tasman, 2004). IED was not classified as an ICD-NEC by APA until the third edition of the DSM in 1980 (Coccaro & Danehy, 2006; Dell'Osso et al., 2006; Grant, 2008). The concept of impulsive aggression, however, has been part of the DSM since its first edition in 1956; originally defined under "Passive-Aggressive Personality-Aggressive Type," which described individuals with "persistent reactions to frustration with irritability, temper tantrums and destructive behavior" (Coccaro & McCloskey, 2010, p. 221). In the DSM-II, the construct of impulsive aggression was subsequently labeled "Explosive Personality" to describe individuals who exhibited episodic and explosive behavior that varied from their typical behavior (Coccaro & Danehy; Coccaro, Posternak, & Zimmerman, 2005). Narrow criteria in the DSM-II and DSM-III, however, excluded individuals with generalized impulsivity and aggression between explosive episodes from receiving a diagnosis (Coccaro et al., 2005). Consequently, during the DSM-III, prevalence of IED was thought to be less than 2% (Coccaro & Danehy; Coccaro et al.). This exclusionary criterion was deleted in the DSM-IV, allowing for generalized impulsivity and aggression to be present between outbursts. Criteria in the DSM-IV further allowed practitioners to give an additional diagnosis of IED in the presence of another disorder if aggressive outbursts were not better accounted for by alternate disorders (First & Tasman). This broadened definition led to the disorder being more common than previously recognized (Coccaro et al.; Dell'Ossa et al., 2006). Today, IED can be seen as a prominent cause of violent behavior (McElroy, 1999). In particular, extreme cases of "road rage" have attracted not only considerable public attention, but psychiatric attention to determine whether a portion of these individuals meet criteria for IED. Research has found that 35% of court-referred aggressive drivers met criteria for IED vs. 0% in a control group of nonaggressive drivers (Galovski, Blanchard, & Veazey, 2002).

7.6.2   Diagnosis and Description

The DSM-IV TR currently defines IED as (a) the occurrence of recurrent, discrete
episodes of failure to resist aggressive impulses that result in serious verbal or
physical aggression toward another person or destruction of property; (b) the degree
of aggression during the episodes is grossly out of proportion with the precipitating
stressor; and (c) is not explained by other psychiatric disorders (e.g., g., antisocial,
BPD and conduct disorder), medical conditions, or effects of substances (e.g., a
drug of abuse or medication) that may cause the outbursts (APA, 2000). Research
criteria have additionally been proposed for IED to further operationalize the type,
frequency, and impairment of aggressive outbursts. These criteria suggest at least
two impulsive outbursts per week for more than 1 month, or three serious assaults
or destructions of property within 1 year to qualify for diagnosis (Coccaro, Schmidt,
Samuels, & Nestadt, 2004; McCloskey, Berman, Nobett, & Coccaro, 2006).
Aggressive episodes need to be impulsive rather than premeditated, and need to be
associated with significant impairment in psychosocial functioning (Coccaro, Lee,
& Kavoussi, 2009).

Given that aggressive episodes must be independent of other disorders, IED is
seen as a diagnosis of exclusion when impulsive aggression is not due to other
factors (First & Tasman, 2004). To date, there is still contention as to whether IED
is a separate psychiatric disorder, or whether impulsive aggression is a common
symptom that occurs across a wide range of disorders, and of which is exacerbated
by stressful situations (McElroy, 1999; McElroy, Soutullo, Beckman, Taylor, &
Keck, 1998; Ferguson, 2006). Moreover, some have debated that current diagnostic
criteria is too narrow given that it excludes those with some personality disorders
from receiving a diagnosis (Coccaro & Danehy, 2006; Caccoro et al., 2005;
McCloskey et al., 2006).

IED onset is thought to occur between childhood and early 20s (APA, 2000).
This disorder, however, tends to peak in mid-adolescence (13–18 years; Coccaro
et al., 2005; Grant & Potenza, 2010; Kessler, Coccaro, Fava, Jaeger, Jin, & Walters,
2006), and appears to become less common with age (Coccaro et al.; First & Tasman,
2004; Kessler et al., 2006; McElroy et al., 1998). Reliable epidemiological data on
IED is not currently available, which may in part be due to the differential criteria
used (i.e., diagnostic vs. research definitions; Coccaro & Danehy, 2006; Coccaro
et al.; Hollander et al., 2008). Some limited data has found lifetime and 1-month
prevalence estimates of 4–6% and 1–2%, respectively (Cocarro et al., 2004, 2005;
Kessler et al.). As high as 6–7% in individuals aged 18–29 year has been reported
(Adamec, 2008), and childhood prevalence remains unknown.

Some research has reported that IED prevalence does not differ based on socio-
demographic variables (e.g., occupational status, family income, ethnicity, education, marital status; Coccaro et al., 2005; Grant & Potenza, 2010; Kessler et al.,
2006; Ortega, Canino, & Alegria, 2008); though one epidemiological study found
that individuals with IED are significantly more likely to be high school drop outs
(Coccaro et al.). Furthermore, there is some debate as to whether or not IED occurs

more frequently in males than females (Coccaro & Danehy, 2006; Grant, 2008). Some have found that the gender prevalence is equal (e.g., Corraro et al., 2004), whereas others report that males are 2–3 times more likely than females to have the disorder (Grant & Potenza; Kessler et al.; McElroy et al., 1998). More consistently, onset of the disorder has been found to occur significantly earlier in males than females (i.e., 13 vs. 19 years; Corraro et al.).

In adolescents and adults, aggressive episodes are usually short in duration (i.e., generally 30 min or less; Grant & Potenza, 2010; McElroy, 1999); start and stop abruptly; occur frequently (e.g., multiple times per month; McElroy et al., 1998); and generally occur without forethought (APA, 2000). Prior to an episode, individuals may experience escalating automatic arousal (e.g., heart palpitations, tingling, racing thoughts), anxiety, irritability, tension, and/or anger, which is generally triggered by minor conflicts (APA; Coccaro & Danehy, 2006; McElroy, 1999). Similar to other ICDs, feelings of tension tend to increase until the explosive aggressive act, where arousal then temporarily decreases to below normal levels (Ferguson, 2006; McElroy). Temporary emotional relaxation and fatigue may then be accompanied and replaced by genuine remorse, bewilderment, and embarrassment (APA; First & Tasman, 2004). Aggression does not occur out of vengeance, self-defense, or as part of gang activities (First & Tasman). Most individuals with IED acknowledge that their aggressive outbursts are out of proportion to the provocation, dysfunctional, and uncontrollable (First & Tasman; McElroy). Research suggests that individuals with IED have a high co-occurrence of anxiety, mood, and substance abuse disorders (Coccaro et al., 2004; Grant, 2008; McElroy; McElroy et al., 1998; Olvera, 2002). In general, individuals with IED demonstrate significant functional impairment in social, academic, and occupational realms, and frequently encounter legal consequences for their actions (APA; Coccaro & Danehy; Grant & Potenza). In childhood, IED is generally presented as a history of frequent and severe temper tantrums, impaired attention, and hyperactivity (APA; Paone & Douma, 2009) which may lead to significant social and academic impairment. Co-occurring childhood disorders such as reactive attachment disorder, conduct disorder and ADHD have not been reported.

7.6.3 Etiology and Theoretical Frameworks

Although there is a scarcity of research on IED specifically, many researchers have investigated individuals with impulsive aggression and anger dyscontrol. This knowledge base may shed light on some of the elements of IED.

7.6.3.1 Biological Models

Genetics. McElroy and colleagues (1998) reported that almost one-third of first-degree relatives of those diagnosed with IED also had IED symptoms. Similarly,

Coccaro and Danehy (2006) reported on an existing controlled study (Coccaro, 2000) that found a morbid risk of IED of 26% in relatives of individuals diagnosed with IED, compared to 8% in a control group. Furthermore, Halperin and colleagues (2003) found that aggressive children have a two- to threefold increase in the incidence of aggressive behavior among relatives compared with psychiatric controls. Thus, these limited studies suggest a genetic component may be involved in the development of this disorder.

Neurobiological. Given that adolescence reflects a time of significant developmental change, changing neurological pathways may lead to increased risk-taking, which may contribute to biological contributions of IED onset in adolescence (Grant, 2008). In addition, some researchers have noted that an abnormality in metabolizing testosterone is implicated in individuals with IED (Adamec, 2008; Grant; Olvera, 2002). Thus, being male constitutes a risk factor for this disorder. This may also parallel the findings that males have a peak onset around puberty (Corraro et al., 2005; Kessler et al., 2006).

Research has further demonstrated that decreased metabolic activity in the prefrontal cortex is implicated in individuals with impulsive aggression (Coccaro & Danehy, 2006; Coccaro, McCloskey, Fitzgerald, & Phan, 2007; Coccoro et al., 2009). Specifically, dysfunctional responses appear to occur in the amygdala-prefrontal circuit, which may be responsible for deficits in social-emotional processing, as reflected in these individuals' difficulties in predicting consequences of their own aggressive behavior (Coccaro et al., 2007). Research has also reported that bilateral lesions and damage in this area is associated with chronic and impulsive aggressive behavior (First & Tasman, 2004; Swann & Hollander, 2002).

There is a high rate of family members of individuals with impulsive aggression who suffer from mood, substance, and other ICDs, which again may underscore the common link of serotonin dysfunction (Halperin, Schulz, McKay, Sharma, & Newcorn, 2003; Grant, 2008; McElroy, 1999; McElroy et al., 1998). Research has specifically reported low serotonergic responsiveness in the central serotonergic (5-HT) system is correlated with high scores of impulsive aggression (Coccaro, Lee, & Kavoussi, 2010; First & Tasman, 2004; Halperin et al., 2003). GABA, norepinephrine, and dopamine have also been connected to the ability to modulate impulsive aggression (Grant; Coccaro et al., 2010; Depue et al., 1994 as cited in Hollander et al., 2006; Swann & Hollander, 2002).

Finally, EEG studies have found that individuals with IED may have increased beta activity and decreased alpha activity in the brain (Koelsch, Sammler, Jentschke, & Siebel, 2008). This pattern is similarly implicated in children with ADHD and is related to an increased tendency for impulsive and disinhibited behavior, and a greater arousal and stress reaction to sensory stimuli (Koelsch et al., 2008).

7.6.3.2 Psychosocial Models

Information-Processing Theory. Researchers have suggested that IED is caused by cognitive distortions of environmental circumstances and deficits in social-emotional processing. That is, individuals with IED may attach distorted negative attributions to neutral events and people (Ferguson, 2006). Similarly, researchers have examined social information processing deficits in aggressive children. These children tend to misinterpret social cues and information (i.e., their own level of emotional arousal and the reactions of others as hostile) and then respond to these cues inappropriately due to difficulties with emotional regulation (Lemerise & Arsenio, 2000; Orobio de Castro, Veerman, Koops, Bosch, & Monshouwer, 2002).

Affective Regulation Theory. IED symptoms have been reported to generally occur prior to other co-morbid disorders, with the exception of anxiety disorders (Coccaro et al., 2005). Thus, anxiety may predispose individuals to develop IED, and co-occurring disorders then may reflect difficulties in coping and effectively expressing negative emotions in adaptive ways (Grant, 2008). Additional research is needed to better understand the nature of potential links between anxiety and the development of IED (Coccaro et al.), particularly in children and adolescents.

Early Life Experiences. Some posit that the effects of early life experiences and specifically childhood trauma impact the development of behavioral and emotional regulation, frustration tolerance, planning ability, and gratification delay; all of which are necessary components in the ability to inhibit impulsive aggressive outbursts (First & Tasman, 2004). Studies have found high proportions of PTSD in children and adolescents with impulsive aggression (Olvera et al., 2001). Others have proposed an inter-generational transmission of aggression from caregiver to child, where individuals who have witnessed and/or experienced aggression in childhood are at risk for the development of IED (Coccaro & Danehy, 2006; Conger, Neppl, Kim, & Scaramella, 2003; McCloskey, Noblett, Deffenbacher, & Gollan, 2008). Likewise, several lines of research have demonstrated that aggression in families is a highly salient risk factor for the persistence of childhood impulsive aggression to continue into adolescence and adulthood (Halperin et al., 2003).

7.6.4   Assessment

The majority of individuals with IED are thought to meet criteria for at least one other clinical disorder (Hollander, Berlin, & Stein, 2008; Kessler et al., 2006; McElroy, 1999; McElroy et al., 1998). Thus, as with other ICDs, the issue of co-morbidity can complicate the assessment of IED. Kessler and colleagues (2006) found that approximately 37% of adults with IED have a major depressive disorder, and 58% have anxiety disorders (i.e., social phobia and OCD). Conduct disorder (CD), oppositional defiant disorder (ODD), substance abuse disorders, other ICDs, and OCD are also commonly associated with impulsive aggression (Coccaro et al., 2005; Kessler et al.; McElroy et al.; Potenza et al., 2009). Thus, practitioners have the daunting task of attempting to rule out other disorders that may better account for impulsive outbursts. This involves distinguishing between impulsive and nonimpulsive types of aggression, and determining whether impulsive aggression is a secondary condition of another disorder or a distinct disorder on its own (Ferguson, 2006; First & Tasman, 2004). For instance, in adolescents, BPD and IED have notably overlapping clinical presentations, though IED does not generally have a pervasive pattern of intense instability in relationships and self-image (i.e., extremes of idealization and evaluation), that individuals with BPD characteristically exhibit (Ferguson; First & Tasman). Moreover, a diagnosis of conduct disorder (CD) in children and adolescents also requires aggressive acts that cause physical harm to others and damage to property (APA, 2000, p. 94). However, rather than a general pattern of antisocial behavior as seen in CD, aggressive outbursts and disregard for others and property are more episodic for those with IED. IED may also lack other behavioral features characteristic of CD (e.g., theft; deceitfulness; First & Tasman). In addition, remorse and guilt over aggressive actions, as characterized in IED rather than CD and BPD would also need to be assessed and determined.

Neurological testing is also appropriate prior to an IED diagnosis to ensure that factors such as traumatic brain injury and tumors that could be causing the impulsive aggression are ruled out (Ferguson, 2006; First & Tasman, 2004). In adolescents, to ensure that impulsive aggression is not due to substance intoxication or substance withdrawal, drug and urine drug screening is also informative (APA, 2000). In sum, precisely identifying alternative or co-occurring disorders is necessary, as it has important implications for appropriate intervention options. In addition, practitioners conducting assessment should also be knowledgeable of cultural factors that may influence impulsive aggression. For instance, APA (2000) notes that some individuals from traditional south-eastern Asian countries may have an episode of "acute, unrestrained violent behavior" called *Amok* (p. 665). Such rare cases can be distinguished from IED in that they are generally single episodes and have dissociative features (APA).

When assessing IED, practitioners need to consider DSM-IV TR criteria; the degree and frequency of failure to prevent aggressive outbursts; the extent that acts are premeditated; antecedents; and impairment in psychosocial functioning (Ferguson, 2006). The following scales have demonstrated utility for aiding practitioners in the assessment of IED with older children and adolescents:

- *The Interview Module for Intermittent Explosive Disorder (M-IED).* This scale assesses the frequency and level of aggressive episodes and functional impairment in individuals being assessed for IED (Coccaro, Kavoussi, Berman, & Lish, 1998). This measure has demonstrated reliability and validity in assessing children and adolescents for this purpose (Olvera et al., 2001).
- *The Novaco Anger Scale and Provocation Inventory (NAS; Novaco, 1975).* The NAS assesses anger from an information-processing perspective, through inquiry of cognitive (e.g., hostile attitudes and suspicion), arousal (e.g., feelings of tension and anxiety; anger intensity), and behavioral indices of aggression (e.g., physical and verbal; impulsive reaction). This scale also includes a provocation inventory, which identifies the kind of situations that induce anger. The NAS has been normed for children ages 9 and older, and may be particularly valuable in the assessment of IED (Ferguson, 2006).
- *The Aggression Questionnaire (AQ; Buss & Perry, 1992).* This screener instrument measures individuals' propensity for physical aggression, verbal aggression,

anger, hostility, and indirect aggression, It has demonstrated utility in children 9 years and older, and thus may be a helpful adjunct to screen for IED in older children and adolescents.

- *The Intermittent Explosive Disorder Diagnostic Questionnaire (IED-Q; Coccaro & McCloskey, 2010).* The IED-Q is a brief self-report that examines the frequency, severity, and distress associated with IED, and is consistent with current diagnostic and research criteria.
- *The Overt Aggression Scale (OAS; Yudofsky, Silver, Jackson, Endicott, & Williams, 1986 as cited in Silver & Yudofsky, 1991).* The OAS is a semistructured interview that assesses the severity and frequency of aggressive behavior in four areas: verbal aggression, physical aggression against objects, physical aggression against self, and physical aggression against others (Swann & Hollander, 2002). This measure has been validated on children with conduct disorder, though has also been suggested to be a useful measure of children and adolescents with impulsive aggression (Hollander et al., 2006).

7.6.5 Treatment and Intervention

7.6.5.1 Pharmacological Approaches

Although there has been few controlled pharmacological trials with children and adolescents with IED, in adults, SSRIs (e.g., fluoxetine), mood stabilizers, and antipsychotic medications have been shown to be moderately helpful in decreasing the frequency and severity of impulsive aggression, mood fluctuations, and hostility (Coccaro et al., 2010; Ferguson, 2006; Grant, 2008). Limited controlled studies with mood stabilizers (e.g., lithium) have demonstrated some evidence with children and adolescents with impulsive aggression, though not specifically with IED (Campbell, Adams, Small, et al., 1995; Connor & Steingard, 1996; Malone, Delaney, Luebbert, Cater, & Campbell, 2000). For instance, Malone and colleagues (2000) found in 28 aggressive children and adolescents (mean age 13 years) that treatment response to lithium was approximately 45%. Consistent with the other ICDs, a lack of pediatric trials limits the recommended use of these agents with children diagnosed with IED.

7.6.5.2 Psychosocial Approaches

Psychosocial interventions including CBT, group therapy, family therapy, and social skills training have demonstrated some efficacy for individuals' with anger dyscontrol and interpersonal aggression (Del Vecchio & O'Leary, 2004; Edmondson & Conger, 1996; Ferguson, 2006; Grant & Potenza, 2010). Limited research examining psychosocial approaches specifically with IED has been more equivocal, with some studies demonstrating only small improvement gains (Coccaro & Danehy,

2006; Grant, 2008). Attrition rates and general reluctance to seek treatment are further reported to be high for adults with IED (Coccaro et al., 2004; Ferguson; Grant), though not reported for child and adolescent samples. Aside from these potential treatment limitations, the following approaches may demonstrate some promise as IED intervention options for children and adolescents.

Insight-Oriented Psychotherapy. The aim of many psychotherapeutic approaches is to increase insight into individuals' aggressive outbursts. Specifically, such approaches may help individuals recognize physiological and external cues of escalation, behavioral consequences to their outbursts, and how to verbalize their negative affect appropriately (Grant, 2008). Some psychotherapeutic strategies also involve expressing and resolving fantasies surrounding rage (Lion, 1992 as cited in First & Tasman, 2004). Limited studies have reported some success with insight-oriented psychotherapy in small samples of adults with IED (McElroy et al., 1998). None have been reported with pediatric samples.

Cognitive-Behavioral Therapy. CBT approaches for IED aim to decrease the intensity and frequency of aggressive outbursts by (1) identifying, challenging, and modifying dysfunctional beliefs of the world, themselves, and others, and (2) increasing social problem-solving and social skills training, through identifying problems, considering consequences, and generating and practicing more adaptive ways to cope with negative emotions (Edmondson & Conger, 1996; Ferguson, 2006; Matson, Andrasik, & Matson, 2009; McCloskey et al., 2008). Both group- and individual-based CBT have been found to successfully reduce aggression, anger, hostile thinking, and depressive symptoms, and improve anger control in a randomized control trial on adults with IED (McCloskey et al.). This study further demonstrated that improvements were maintained after 3 months. Furthermore, RET may have some success for individuals with significant anger issues. This approach focuses on developing strategies to challenge irrational beliefs (i.e., perceiving a situation is threatening or unfair) that lead to the impulse aggressive acts (Ferguson, 2006). In sum, improvement does not seem to be dependent on the specific CBT approach utilized, though interventions that use multiple components (e.g., cognitive restructuring, relaxation, coping skills training) has the most empirical support (Del Vecchio & O'Leary, 2004; McCloskey et al.). No controlled research studies in IED with pediatric samples have been reported, and the ability to generalize these findings to IED specifically may be limiting as much of this literature fails to differentiate between anger problems and impulsive, pathological aggression (Coccaro & McCloskey, 2010).

Relaxation Therapy. Self-recognition of escalating anger and arousal and finding ways to prevent it is an important component of IED treatment. Relaxation therapy is based on the notion that arousal is reduced after pairing relaxation with antecedents for outbursts, so that eventually these triggers will prompt a relaxation response rather than an anger response (Deffenbacher & Stark, 1992; Ferguson, 2006). Self-monitoring in conjunction with progressive muscle relaxation, deep breathing, and other self-soothing strategies may also be taught to children and adolescents with IED. This may help them distinguish between relaxed vs. aroused states, and thus aid in preventing outbursts (Ferguson; McCloskey et al., 2008). In general, developing stress management skills is important given that difficulties may be in part due to their inability to tolerate negative emotion (Grant, 2008). Meta-analyses have found that relaxation training has a large positive effect on anger intensity (physiological arousal; Edmondson & Conger, 1996), though no empirical evidence has been found with pediatric IED samples.

Biofeedback Therapy. Limited researchers have proposed biofeedback to help individuals' combat impulsive aggression through learning to change their brainwave activity (Meyer, 1998; Raine & Hong Lui, 1998). This approach is based on operant conditioning principles, where individuals are taught to control and influence their physiological states such as muscle activity, brain waves, skin temperature, heart rate, and blood pressure (Firestone & Marshall, 2003). No studies have empirically examined the efficacy of this approach with children and adolescents diagnosed with IED, and in general, it is unclear whether biofeedback therapy reliably leads to lasting improvement of maladaptive behaviors (Firestone & Marshall).

Child-Centered Play Therapy. Play therapy has been a supported therapeutic approach for working with children with a variety of difficulties (Bratton, Ray, Rhine, & Jones, 2005). Evidence with children with IED, however, is currently limited to single case studies. Paone and Douma (2009) reported a case of a 9-year-old boy diagnosed with IED, who underwent 16 sessions of play therapy and showed significant behavioral improvement. This approach was generally nondirective, with emphasis on providing a safe environment, being sensitive to feelings, encouraging the child to solve personal problems and engaging in self-monitoring, self-directiveness and social skills training through play (Paone & Douma). Furthermore, parental involvement appears to enhance the effectiveness of play therapy (Bratton et al., 2005; Paone & Douma) and thus may be an important adjunct intervention component for children who meet criteria for this disorder.

7.6.6 Prognosis

Little systematic study has been completed on the course of IED, though behaviors appear to range from episodic to chronic in nature (APA, 2000; First & Tasman, 2004). In some cases, IED symptoms may naturally decrease or remit completely with age (Coccaro et al., 2004; Ferguson, 2006; First & Tasman). During its course, IED is generally associated with a substantial amount of lifetime co-morbidity and significant functional impairment (APA; Coccaro et al., 2005; Kessler et al., 2006). Individuals with IED frequently face legal difficulties, as they are charged with assault and destruction of property. IED may also result in significant social isolation due to embarrassment over the uncontrollable nature of their anger and subsequent avoidance of others (Ferguson). IED has also been found to be related to a myriad of physical health problems (e.g., coronary heart disease, hypertension, stroke, diabetes, arthritis, back/neck pain, ulcer, headaches, and other chronic pain; McCloskey, Kleabir, Berman, Chen, & Coccaro, 2010). Impulsivity and aggression has also been linked with increased rates of suicide (Hollander et al., 2006), although specific rates among children and adolescents with IED are not currently known.

In some studies, individuals who have engaged in treatment for IED behaviors have been shown to improve in their functional ability and perceived quality of life (Coccaro & Danehy, 2006; McCloskey et al., 2008). Individuals with IED however are more likely to seek help for anxiety, mood, or substance problems rather than their difficulties with aggression (Coccaro et al., 2005, Coccaro, Lee, & Kavoussi, 2009; Kessler et al., 2006), which suggests that IED symptoms goes relatively untreated. Co-morbid substance abuse difficulties are known to complicate treatment and intervention, making prognosis poor (Grant, 2008). Finally, given the early onset of IED and its explicit symptoms, early detection and immediate treatment may alter the course of the disorder and promote positive outcomes by adulthood (Coccaro, 2000; Paone & Douma, 2009). Thus, treating the disorder early may lead to better long-term prognosis for these individuals.

7.7 Impulse Control Disorders: A Global Perspective

As discussed in the above sections, ICDs are extremely complex and at present there is a limited understanding of their complexities. Research has been hindered due to low prevalence rates, significant variation between and within ICDs, an over-reliance on single case reports and studies with small sample sizes, and due to the secrecy of the disorder. ICDs are most notably understudied in childhood and adolescence, which is surprising given that many ICDs often begin before adulthood (APA, 2000; Bloch, 2009; Bohne, 2010; Grant, 2008; Grant & Kim, 2002c).

The limited data available suggests that up to 8–10% of the total population meet diagnostic criteria for any ICD (Grant, 2008). Prevalence in pediatric populations has yet to be reported for this diagnostic group, though Bohne (2010) found a lifetime ICD rate of 3.5% in college students. Moreover, it has been consistently noted that individuals with ICDs are generally reluctant to disclose, and may actively attempt to hide their behaviors due to feelings of shame, guilt, and fear of social stigma and often legal consequences (Adamec, 2008; APA, 2000; First & Tasman, 2004; Grant). As a result, individuals may not be diagnosed or may be misdiagnosed with alternative disorders; in both cases, the ICD is not appropriately treated (Grant). This poor understanding of ICDs in general and ICDs in pediatric populations specifically has subsequent implications for appropriate prevention, classification, diagnosis, and intervention options for this group.

As summarized above, there is evidence to suggest the multiple "subtypes" of ICDs share homogenous characteristics although there are unique factors that related to subtypes as outlined in the sections above. There is a belief among some researchers that ICDs share many common features with OCD (Grant, 2008). Furthermore, similar neurological elements have been found in subjects with ICDs, substance-related addictions (i.e., drugs and alcohol), and even Anorexia Nervosa (Fassino et al., 2002; Grant; Potenza et al., 2009). This neurological link may explain the high co-morbidity rates found between ICDs, OCD, eating disorders, and substance use disorders (Aboujaoude et al., 2004; Adamec, 2008; Grant; Potenza et al.).

Thus, individuals with "behavioral addictions" including those with ICDs may have neurocircuit deficiencies that implicate reward pathways in the brain (Miller, 2010).

7.7.1 DSM-V

The commonalities of ICDs and OCD have led the lead researchers of the upcoming DSM-V to consider broadening the scope of OCD to include multiple disorders such as Tourette's, tic disorders, Sydenham's, and other PANDAS (pediatric auto-immune neuropsychiatric disorders associated with streptococcal infections), body dysmorphic disorder, hypochondriasis, autism, eating disorders, Huntington's and Parkinson's diseases, impulse control disorder (e.g., kleptomania and trichotilloma-nia), and substance addictions (First, 2006). Thus, the nosology of ICDs continues to be a matter of debate and the DSM-V will provide the next phase of theories related to the classification of these disorders. Technological advanced such as fMRI's and diffusion tensor imaging (DTI) may be helpful in furthering the science that explains the etiologies of ICDs.

7.8 Future Directions

Research on ICDs is in its infancy and requires greater empirical scrutiny. The etiology and classification of ICDs are complicated given the heterogeneity between and even within each ICD profile. There is debate regarding whether ICDs may be better viewed as part of the OCD spectrum, or if they should be classified as an affective or behavioral disorder due to overlapping impulsive features and high rates of co-morbidity between ICDs and these other spectrum disorders (Bayle et al., 2003; Dannon et al., 2006; Grant, 2008; Grant & Potenza, 2010; McElroy et al., 1992). Additional research in this area will be clarifying and may implicate the way we research, assess, diagnose, and treat ICDs.

A common theme repeated throughout this chapter was that robust ICD studies are still lacking with pediatric samples. This limits practitioners from making evidence-based treatment recommendations. Accordingly, studies that compare the efficacy of different treatment approaches to best manage ICD behaviors in children and adolescents are still desperately needed. Furthermore, future emphasis on relapse prevention is warranted given that this may be the key component for effective long-term treatment of ICDs.

Continued improvement in screening and identifying ICDs and increasing familiarity among practitioners is also necessary to facilitate correct diagnosis in the future. This should be particularly underscored since individuals with ICDs are frequently referred to mental health services for other difficulties. The influence of cultural factors and attitudes as it pertains to ICD behaviors is also a needed future research area. This understanding will aid assessment and diagnostic considerations (Potenza et al., 2009).

Children and adolescents with ICDs represent a significant challenge to practitioners. New research in this field will yield a better understanding of ICD features and underlying mechanisms and will ultimately inform decisions about effective treatments in order to best support those diagnosed and well as those charged with the management of their care (i.e., teachers, parents, practitioners).

References

Aboujaoude, E., Gamel, N., & Koran, L. M. (2004). Overview of Kleptomania and phenomenological description of 40 patients. *Primary Care Companion Journal of Clinical Psychiatry, 6*, 244–247.

Adamec, C. (2008). *Impulse control disorders*. New York: Chelsea House.

American Psychiatric Association. (1994). *Diagnostic and statistical manual of mental disorders* (4th ed.). Washington, DC: Author.

American Psychiatric Association. (2000). *Diagnostic and statistical manual of mental disorders* (4th Text Rev. ed.). Washington, DC: Author.

American Psychiatric Association (APA). (2010). DSM-V development: The future of psychiatric diagnosis. Accessed from http://www.dsm5.org/Pages/Default.aspx.

Bayle, F. J., Caci, H., Millet, M., Richa, S., & Olie, J. (2003). Psychopathology and comorbidity of psychiatric disorders in patients with kleptomania. *The American Journal of Psychiatry, 160*, 1509–1513.

Bloch, M. (2009). Trichotillomania across the life span. *Journal of the American Academy of Child and Adolescent Psychiatry, 48*(9), 879–883.

Bohne, A. (2010). Impulse-control disorders in college students. *Psychiatry Research, 176*(1), 91–102.

Bratton, S. C., Ray, D., Rhine, T., & Jones, L. (2005). The efficacy of play therapy with children: A meta-analytic review of treatment outcomes. *Professional Psychology: Research and Practice, 36*, 376–390.

Buss, A. H., & Perry, M. (1992). The aggression questionnaire. *Journal of Personality and Social Psychology, 59*, 73–81.

Campbell, M., Adams, P. B., Small, A. M., Kafantaris, V., Silva, R. R., Shell, J., et al. (1995). Lithium in hospitalized aggressive children with conduct disorder: A double blind and placebo controlled study. Journal of the American Academy of Child and Adolescent Psychiatry, 34 , 445–453.

Chamberlain, S. R., Menzies, L., Fineberg, N., Del Campo, N., Suckling, J., Craig, K., et al. (2008). Grey matter abnormalities in trichotillomania: Morphometric magnetic resonance imaging study. *The British Journal of Psychiatry, 193*, 216–221.

Chamberlain, S. R., Menzies, L., Sahakian, B., & Fineberg, N. (2007). Lifting the veil on trichotillomania. *The American Journal of Psychiatry, 164*(4), 568–574.

Chamberlain, S. R., Odlaug, B., Boulougouris, V., Fineberg, N., & Grant, J. (2009). Trichotillomania: Neurobiology and treatment. *Neuroscience and Biobehavioral Reviews, 33*, 831–842.

Christensen, G. A., Pyle, R. L., & Mitchell, J. E. (1991). Estimated lifetime prevalence of trichotillomania in college students. *The Journal of Clinical Psychiatry, 52*, 415–417.

Christenson, G. A. (1995). Trichotillomania: From prevalence to comorbidity. *Psychiatric Times, 12*, 44–48.

Christenson, G. A., Mackenzie, T. B., & Mitchell, J. E. (1991). Characteristics of 60 adult chronic hair-pullers. *The American Journal of Psychiatry, 148*, 365–370.

Christenson, G. A., & Mackenzie, T. B. (1994). Trichotillomania. In M. Hersen & R. T. Ammerman (Eds.), Handbook of prescriptive treatment for adults (pp. 217–235). New York: Plenum.

Christenson, G. A., & Mansueto, C. S. (1999). Trichotillomania: Descriptive characteristics and phenomenology. In D. J. Stein, G. A. Christenson, & E. Hollander (Eds.), *Trichotillomania* (pp. 1–41). Washington, DC: American Psychiatric Press.

Coccaro, E. F. (2000). Intermittent explosive disorder. *Current Psychiatry Reports, 2*(1), 67–71.

Coccaro, E. F., & Danehy, M. (2006). Intermittent explosive disorder. In E. Hollander & D. J. Stein (Eds.), *Clinical manual of impulse control disorders* (pp. 19–37). Washington, DC: American Psychiatric Publishing.

Coccaro, E. F., Kavoussi, R. J., Berman, R. E., & Lish, J. D. (1998). Intermittent explosive disorder-revised: Development, reliability and validity of research criteria. *Comprehensive Psychiatry, 39*(5), 368–376.

Coccaro, E. F., Lee, R., & Kavoussi, R. (2009). A double-blind, randomized, placebo-controlled trial of fluoxetine in patients with intermittent explosive disorder. *The Journal of Clinical Psychiatry, 70*, 653–662.

Coccaro, E. F., Lee, R., & Kavoussi, R. (2010). Inverse relationship between numbers of 5-HT transporter binding sites and life history of aggression and intermittent explosive disorder. *Journal of Psychiatric Research, 44*, 137–142.

Coccaro, E. F., & McCloskey, S. (2010). Intermittent explosive disorder: Clinical aspects. In E. Aboujauode & L. Koran (Eds.), *Impulse control disorders* (pp. 221–232). New York: Cambridge University Press.

Coccaro, E. F., McCloskey, M. S., Fitzgerald, D., & Phan, K. L. (2007). Amygala and orbitofrontal reactivitity to social threat in individuals with impulsive aggression. *Biological Psychiatry, 62*, 168–178.

Coccaro, E. F., Posternak, M., & Zimmerman, M. (2005). Prevalence and features of intermittent explosive disorder in a clinical setting. *The Journal of Clinical Psychiatry, 66*(10), 2221–2228.

Coccaro, E. F., Schmidt, C. A., Samuels, J. F., & Nestadt, G. (2004). Lifetime and 1-month prevalence rates of intermittent explosive disorder in a community sample. *The Journal of Clinical Psychiatry, 65*(6), 820–824.

Cohen, L. J., Stein, D., Simeon, D., Spadaccini, E., Rosen, J., Aronoitz, B., et al. (1995). Clinical profile, comorbidity and treatment history of 123 hair pullers: A survey study. *The Journal of Clinical Psychiatry, 56*, 319–326.

Conger, R. D., Neppl, K., Kim, K., & Scaramella, L. (2003). Angry and aggressive behavior across three generations: A prospective longitudinal study of parents and children. *Journal of Abnormal Child Psychology, 31*, 143–160.

Connor, D. F., & Steingard, R. J. (1996). A clinical approach to the pharmacotherapy of aggression in children and adolescents. *Annals of the New York Academy of Sciences, 794*, 290–307.

Dannon, P. (2002). Kleptomania: An impulse control disorder? *International Journal of Psychiatry in Clinical Practice, 6*, 3–7.

Dannon, P., Aizer, A., & Lowengrub, K. (2006). Kleptomania: Differential diagnosis and treatment modalities. *Current Psychiatry Reviews, 2*, 281–283.

Dannon, P., Lowengrub, K., Iancu, I., & Kotler, M. (2004). Kleptomania: Comorbid psychiatric diagnosis in patients and their families. *Psychopathology, 37*, 76–80.

De Sousa, A. (2008). An open-label pilot study of naltrexone in childhood-onset trichotillomania. *Journal of Child and Adolescent Psychopharmacology, 18*, 30–33.

Deffenbacher, J. L., & Stark, R. (1992). Relaxation and cognitive-relaxation treatments for general anger. *Journal of Counselling Psychology, 39*, 158–167.

Del Vecchio, T. D., & O'Leary, K. D. (2004). Effectiveness of anger treatments for specific anger problems: A meta-analytic review. *Clinical Psychology Review, 24*, 15–34.

Dell'Osso, B., Altamura, C., Allen, A., Marazziti, D., & Hollander, E. (2006). Epidemiologic and clinical updates on impulse control disorders: A critical review. *European Archives of Psychiatry and Clinical Neuroscience, 256*, 464–475.

Diefenbach, G. J., Mouton-Odum, S., & Stanley, M. A. (2002). Affective correlates of trichotillomania. *Behaviour Research and Therapy, 40*, 1305–1315.

Diefenbach, G. J., Tolin, G., Hannan, S., Crocetto, J., & Worhunsky, P. (2005). Trichotillomania: Impact on psychosocial functioning and quality of life. *Behaviour Research and Therapy, 43*, 869–884.

Diefenbach, G. J., Tolin, D. F., Meunier, S., & Worhunsky, P. (2008). Emotion regulation in trichotillomania: A comparison of clinical and non clinical hair-pulling. *Journal of Behavioral Therapy and Experimental Psychiatry, 49*, 32–41.

Doughterty, D., Loh, R., Jenike, M., & Keuthen, N. (2006). Single modality versus dual modality treatment for trichotillomania, sertanline, behavioural therapy or both? *The Journal of Clinical Psychiatry, 67*(7), 1086–1092.

Duke, D., Keeley, M., Geffken, G., & Storch, E. (2009). Trichotillomania: A current review. *Clinical Psychology Review, 10*(1016), 1–13.

Edmondson, C. B., & Conger, J. C. (1996). A review of treatment efficacy for individuals with anger problems: Conceptual, assessment and methodological issues. *Clinical Psychology Review, 16*, 251–275.

Ellis, A. (1994). *Anger: How to live with and without it.* New York: Carol Publishing Group.

Fassino, S., Piero, A., Daga, G. A., Leombruni, P., Mortara, P., & Rovera, G. G. (2002). Attentional biases and frontal functioning in anorexia nervosa. *The International Journal of Eating Disorders, 31*, 274–283.

Ferguson, K. E. (2006). Intermittent explosive disorder. In J. E. Fisher & W. O'Donohue (Eds.), *Practitioner's guide to evidence-based psychotherapy* (pp. 335–351). New York: Springer.

Firestone, P., & Marshall, W. L. (2003). *Abnormal psychology* (2nd ed.). Toronto, ON: Prentice Hall.

First, M. B. (2006). Obsessive compulsive spectrum disorders. Retrieved November 1, 2010 from http://www.dsm5.org/research/pages/obsessivecompulsivespectrumdisordersconference(jun e20-22,2006).aspx.

First, M. B., Frances, A., & Pincus, H. A. (2004). *DSM-IV-TR guidebook.* Washington, DC: American Psychiatric Publication.

First, M. B., & Tasman, A. (2004). *DSM-IV-TR mental disorders: Diagnosis, etiology and treatment.* Noboken, NJ: Wiley.

Flessner, C., Woods, D., Franklin, M., Keuthen, N., & Piacentini, J. (2008). Styles of pulling in youths with trichotillomania: Exploring differences in symptom severity, phenomenology, and comorbid psychiatric symptoms. *Behaviour Research and Therapy, 46*, 1055–1061.

Flessner, C. A., Woods, D. W., Franklin, M. E., Keuthen, N. J., Piacentini, J. C., Cashin, S. E., et al. (2007). The Milwaukee Inventory for Styles of Trichotillomania-Child Version (MIST-C): The assessment of pulling subtypes in children and adolescents. *Behavior Modification, 31*, 896–918.

Franklin, M., Flessner, C., Woods, D., Piacentini, J., Moore, P., Stein, D., et al. (2008). The Child and adolescent trichotillomania impact project: Descriptive psychopathology, comorbidity, functional impairment, and treatment utilization. *Journal of Developmental and Behavioral Pediatrics, 29*(6), 493–500.

Franklin, M. E., & Tolin, D. F. (2007). *Treating trichotillomania: Cognitive-behavioral therapy for hair-pulling and related problems.* New York: Springer.

Franklin, M. E., Tolin, D., & Diefenbach, G. J. (2006). Trichotillomania. In E. Hollander & D. J. Stein (Eds.), *Clinical manual of impulse control disorders* (pp. 149–173). Arlington, VA: American Psychiatric Publishing.

Fullerton, R. A., & Punj, G. N. (2004). Shoplifting as moral insanity: Historical perspectives on kleptomania. *Journal of Macromarketing, 24*(1), 8–16.

Galovski, T., Blanchard, E. B., & Veazey, C. (2002). Intermittent explosive disorder and other psychiatric comorbidity among court-referred and self-referred aggressive drivers. *Behaviour Research and Therapy, 40*, 641–651.

Gershuny, B. S., Keuthen, N. J., Gentes, E. L., Russo, A. R., Emmott, E. C., Jameson, M., et al. (2006). Current posttraumatic stress disorder and history of trauma in trichotillomania. *Journal of Clinical Psychology, 62*, 1521–1529.

Glosscock, S. G., Rapoff, M. A., & Christerpherson, E. R. (1988). Behavioral methods to reduce shoplifting. *Journal of Business and Psychology, 2*(3), 272–278.

Goldman, M. J. (1991). Kleptomania: Making sense of the nonsensical. *The American Journal of Psychiatry, 148*, 986–996.

Goldman, M. J. (1992). Kleptomania: An overview. Psychiatry Annals, 22, 68–71.

Grant, J. E. (2004). Co-occurrence of personality disorders in persons with kleptomania: A preliminary investigation. *Journal of American Academy of Psychiatry, 32*, 395–398.

Grant, J. E. (2006). Understanding and treating kleptomania: New models and new treatments. *The Israel Journal of Psychiatry and Related Sciences, 43*(2), 81–87.

Grant, J. E. (2008). *Impulse control disorders*. New York: Norton and Company.

Grant, J. E., & Kim, S. W. (2002a). Clinical characteristics and associated psychopathology of 22 patients with kleptomania. *Comprehensive Psychiatry, 43*, 378–384.

Grant, J. E., & Kim, S. W. (2002b). Temperament and early environmental influences in kleptomania. *Comprehensive Psychiatry, 43*(3), 223–228.

Grant, J. E., & Kim, S. (2002c). Adolescent kleptomania treated with naltrexone: A case report. *European Child & Adolescent Psychiatry, 11*, 92–95.

Grant, J. E., & Kim, S. W. (2002d). Open-label study of naltrexone in the treatment of kleptomania. *The Journal of Clinical Psychiatry, 63*, 349–356.

Grant, J. E., Kim, S. W., & Grosz, R. (2003). Perceived stress in kleptomania. *The Psychiatric Quarterly, 74*(3), 251–258.

Grant, J. E., Kim, S. W., & McCabe, J. (2006). Structured clinical interview for kleptomania (SCI-K): Preliminary validity and reliability testing. *International Journal of Methods in Psychiatric Research, 15*, 83–94.

Grant, J. E., Mancebo, M., Eisen, J., & Rasmussen, S. (2010). Impulse control disorders in children and adolescents with obsessive-compulsive disorder. *Psychiatry Research, 75*, 109–113.

Grant, J. E., Odlaug, B. L., Davis, A., & Kim, S. (2009). Legal consequences of kleptomania. *Psychiatry Quarterly, 80*, 251–259.

Grant, J. E., Odlaug, B. L., & Woznik, J. (2007). Neuropsychological functioning in kleptomania. *Behaviour Research and Therapy, 45*, 1663–1670.

Grant, J. E., & Potenza, M. (2008). Gender-related differences in individuals seeking treatment for kleptomania. *CNS Spectrum, 13*(3), 235–245.

Grant, J. E., & Potenza, M. (2010). Impulse control disorder. In J. E. Grant & M. Potenza (Eds.), *Young adult mental health* (pp. 335–351). New York: Oxford University Press.

Grant, J. E., Williams, K., & Potenza, M. (2007). Impulse control disorders in adolescent psychiatric inpatients: Co-occurring disorders and sex differences. *The Journal of Clinical Psychiatry, 68*, 1584–1592.

Halperin, J. M., Schulz, K. P., McKay, K. E., Sharma, V., & Newcorn, J. H. (2003). Familial correlates of central serotonin function in children with disruptive behavior disorders. *Psychiatry Research, 119*, 205–216.

Hanna, G. L. (1997). Trichotillomania and related disorders in children and adolescents. *Child Psychiatry and Human Development, 27*, 255–268.

Hollander, E., Baker, B. R., Kahn, J., & Stein, D. J. (2006). Conceptualizing and assessing impulse control disorders. In M. D. Hollander & D. J. Stein (Eds.), *Clinical manual of impulse-control disorders* (pp. 1–18). Arlington, VA: American Psychiatric Publishing.

Hollander, E., Berlin, H. A., & Stein, D. J. (2008). Impulse control disorders not elsewhere classified. In R. E. Hales, G. O. Gabbard, & S. C. Yudofsky (Eds.), *The American psychiatric publishing textbook of psychiatry* (5th ed., pp. 777–820). Arlington, VA: American Psychiatric Publishing.

Kessler, R. C., Coccaro, E. F., Fava, M., Jaeger, S., Jin, R., & Walters, E. (2006). The prevalence and correlates of DSM-IV intermittent explosive disorder in the national comorbidity survey replication. *Archives of General Psychiatry, 63*, 669–678.

Keuthen, N. J., Makris, N., Schlerf, J. E., Martis, B., Savage, C. R., McMullin, K., et al. (2007). Evidence for reduced cerebellar volumes in trichotillomania. *Biological Psychiatry, 61*, 374–381.

King, R. A., Scahill, L., Vitulano, L. A., Schwab-Stone, M., Tercyak, K. P., Jr., & Riddle, M. A. (1995). Childhood trichotillomania: Clinical phenomenology, comorbidity, and family genetics. *Journal of the American Academy of Child and Adolescent Psychiatry, 34*, 1451–1459.

Koelsch, S., Sammler, D., Jentschke, S., & Siebel, W. (2008). EEG correlates of moderate intermittent explosive disorder. *Clinical Neurophysiology, 119*, 151–162.

Kohn, C. S. (2006). Conceptualization and treatment of kleptomania behaviors using cognitive and behavioral strategies. *The International Journal of Behavioral Consultation and Therapy, 2*(4), 553–559.

Kohn, C. S., & Antonuccio, D. (2002). Treatment of Kleptomania using cognitive and behavioural strategies. *Clinical Case Studies, 1*(25), 25–38.

Koran, L. M., Bodnik, D., & Dannon, P. H. (2010). Kleptomania: Clinical aspects. In E. Aboujaoude
& L. M. Koran (Eds.), *Impulse control disorders* (pp. 34–44). New York: Cambridge
University Press.

Kozian, R. (2001). Kleptomania in frontal lobe lesion. *Psychiatry Praxis, 28,* 98–99.

Lejoyeux, M., Arbaretaz, M., Mcloughlin, M., & Ades, J. (2002). Impulse control disorders and
depression. *The Journal of Nervous and Mental Disease, 190*(5), 310–314.

Lemerise, E. A., & Arsenio, W. F. (2000). An integrated model of emotion processes and cognition
in social information processing. *Child Development, 71,* 107–118.

Lenane, M. C., Swedo, S. E., Rapoport, J. L., Leonard, H., Sceery, W., & Guroff, J. J. (1992). Rates
of obsessive compulsive disorder in first degree relatives of patients with trichotillomania:
A research note. *Journal of Child Psychology and Psychiatry, 33*(5), 925–933.

Lerner, J., Franklin, M., Meadows, E., Hembree, E., & Foa, E. B. (1998). Effectiveness of a cognitive behavioural treatment program for trichotillomania: An uncontrolled evaluation. *Behavior
Therapy, 29,* 157–171.

Lewin, A., Piacentini, J., Flessner, C., Woods, D., Franklin, M., Keuthen, N., et al. (2009).
Depression, anxiety, and functional impairment in children with trichotillomania. *Depression
and Anxiety, 26,* 521–527.

Lion, J. (1992). The intermitten explosive disorder. *Psychiatry Annals, 2,* 64–66.

Lopez, V. C. (1998). Treating pathological gambling. In W. Miller & N. Heather (Eds.), *Treating
addictive behaviours* (2nd ed., pp. 259–271). New York: Plenum.

Malone, R. P., Delaney, M. A., Luebbert, J. F., Cater, J., & Campbell, M. (2000). A double blind
and placebo controlled study of lithium in hospitalized aggressive children and adolescents
with conduct disorder. *Archives of General Psychiatry, 57,* 649–654.

Mancini, C., Van Ameringen, M., Patterson, B., Simpson, W., & Truong, C. (2009). Trichotillomania
in youth: A retrospective case series. *Depression and Anxiety, 26,* 661–665.

Mansueto, C. S., Ninan, P. T., Rothbaum, B. O., & Reeve, E. (2010). Trichotillomania and its treatment in children and adolescents: A guide for clinicians. http://www.trich.org/articles/view_
default.asp?aid=27&yd=about_ttm_medications.

Matson, J. L., Andrasik, F., & Matson, M. (Eds.). (2009). *Treating childhood psychopathology and
developmental disabilities.* New York: Springer.

McCloskey, M. S. (2006). Intermittent explosive disorder-integrated research diagnostic
criteria: Convergent and discriminant validity. *Journal of Psychiatric Research, 40*(3), 231–242.

McCloskey, M. S., Berman, M., Nobett, K., & Coccaro, E. (2006). Intermittent explosive disorder-
integrated research diagnostic criteria: Convergent and discriminant validity. *Journal of
Psychiatric Research, 40,* 231–242.

McCloskey, M. S., Kleabir, K., Berman, M. E., Chen, E. Y., & Coccaro, E. F. (2010). Unhealthy
aggression: Intermittent explosive disorder and adverse physical health outcomes. *Health
Psychology, 29*(3), 324–332.

McCloskey, M. S., Noblett, K., Deffenbacher, J., & Gollan, J. (2008). Cognitive-behavioral therapy for intermittent explosive disorder: A pilot randomized clinical trial. *Journal of Counselling
and Clinical Psychology, 76*(3), 876–886.

McElroy, S. L. (1999). Recognition and treatment of DSM-IV intermittent explosive disorder. *The
Journal of Clinical Psychiatry, 60*(15), 12–16.

McElroy, S. L., Hudson, J. I., Pope, H., & Keck, P. E. (1991). Kleptomania: Clinical characteristics
and associated psychopathology. *Psychological Medicine, 21,* 93–108.

McElroy, S. L., Hudson, J., Pope, H., Keck, P., & Aizley, H. G. (1992). The DSM-III-R impulse
control disorders not elsewhere classified: Clinical characteristics and relationship to other
psychiatric disorders. *The American Journal of Psychiatry, 149,* 318–327.

McElroy, S. L., Pope, H. G., Hudson, J., Keck, P., & White, K. (1991). Kleptomania: A report of
20 cases. *The American Journal of Psychiatry, 148,* 652–657.

McElroy, S. L., Soutullo, C. A., Beckman, D. A., Taylor, P., Jr., & Keck, P. E., Jr. (1998). DSM-IV intermittent explosive disorder: A report of 27 cases. *The Journal of Clinical Psychiatry, 69,* 203–210.

Meunier, S., Tolin, D., & Franklin, M. (2009). Affective and sensory correlates of hair-pulling in
pediatric trichotillomania. *Behavior Modification, 33*(3), 396–407.

Meyer, R. C. (1998). *The third edition clinician's handbook: Integrated diagnostics, assessment and intervention in adult and adolescent psychotherapy*. Needham Heights, MA: Allyn and Bacon.

Miller, R. (2010). The feeling-state theory of impulse control disorders and the impulse-control disorder protocol. *Traumatology, 16*(3), 2–10.

Miller, D., & McMichael, A. (2010). Trichotillomania: The view from dermatology. In E. Aboujaoude & L. M. Koran (Eds.), *Impulse control disorders* (pp. 111–117). New York: Cambridge University Press.

Ninan, P. T., Rothbaum, B. O., Marsteller, F. A., Knight, B. T., & Eccard, M. B. (2000). A placebo-controlled trial of cognitive-behavioral therapy and clomipramine in trichotillomania. *The Journal of Clinical Psychiatry, 61*(1), 47–50.

Norberg, M. M., Wetterneck, C. T., Woods, D. W., & Conelea, C. A. (2007). Experiential avoidance as a mediator of relationships between cognitions and hair-pulling severity. *Behavioral Modification, 31*, 367–381.

Novak, B. (2010). Kleptomania and the law. In E. Aboujaoude & L. M. Koran (Eds.), *Impulse control disorders* (pp. 45–50). New York: Cambridge University Press.

Novak, C. E., Keuthen, N. J., Stewart, E. S., & Pauls, D. L. (2009). A twin concordance study of trichotillomania. *American Journal of Medical Genetics, 150*, 944–949.

Novaco, R. W. (1975). *Anger control: The development of experimental treatment*. Lexington, KY: Lexington.

O'Sullivan, R., Keuthen, N., Christenson, G., Mansueto, C., Stein, D., & Swedo, S. (1997). Trichotillomania: Behavioral symptom or clinical syndrome? *The American Journal of Psychiatry, 154*(10), 1442–1449.

O'Sullivan, R. L., Rauch, S., Breiter, H., Grachev, I. D., Baer, L., Kennedy, D. N., et al. (1997). Reduced basal ganglia volumes in trichotillomania measured via morphometric magnetic resonance imaging. *Biological Psychiatry, 42*, 39–45.

Olvera, R. L. (2002). Intermittent explosive disorder: Epidemiology, diagnosis and management. *CNS Drugs, 16*, 517–526.

Olvera, R. L., Pliszka, S., Konyecsni, W., Hernandez, Y., Farnum, S., & Tripp, R. (2001). Validation of the interview module of intermittent explosive disorder in children and adolescents: A pilot study. *Psychiatry Research, 101*, 259–267.

Orobio de Castro, B., Veerman, J. W., Koops, W., Bosch, J. D., & Monshouwer, H. J. (2002). Hostile attribution of intent and aggressive behavior: A meta-analysis. *Child Development, 73*, 916–934.

Ortega, A. N., Canino, G., & Alegria, M. (2008). Lifetime and 12-month intermittent explosive disorder in latinos. *The American Journal of Orthopsychiatry, 78*(1), 133–139.

Palmer, C., Yates, W., & Trotter, L. (1999). Childhood trichotillomania: Successful treatment with fluoxemine following an SSRI failure. *Psychosomatics, 40*(6), 526–528.

Paone, T. R., & Douma, K. (2009). Child-centered play therapy with a seven-year-old boy diagnosed with intermittent explosive disorder. *International Journal of Play Therapy, 18*(1), 31–44.

Potenza, M., Koran, L., & Pallanti, S. (2009). The relationship between impulse-control disorders and obsessive-compulsive disorder: A current understanding and future research directions. *Psychiatry Research, 170*, 22–31.

Raine, A., & Hong Lui, J. (1998). Biological predispositions to violence and their implications for biosocial treatment and prevention. *Psychology, Crime and Law, 4*(2), 107–125.

Rapp, J. T., Miltenberger, R., Long, E., Elliot, A., & Lumley, V. (1998). Simplified habit reversal treatment for chronic hair-pulling in three adolescents: A clinical replication with direct observation. *Journal of Applied Behavioral Analysis, 31*, 299–302.

Reeve, E. (1999). Hair-pulling in children and adolescents. In D. J. Stein, G. Christenson, & E. Hollander (Eds.), *Trichotillomania* (pp. 201–224). Washington, DC: American Psychiatric Press.

Reynolds, W. M. (2002). *Reynolds Adolescent Depression Scale – 2nd Edition. Professional manual*. Odessa, FL: Psychological Assessment Resources.

Shusterman, A., Feld, L., Baer, L., & Keuthen, N. (2009). Affective regulation in trichotillomania: Evidence from a large-scale internet survey. *Behavior Research and Therapy, 47*, 637–644.

Silver, J. M., & Yudofsky, S. C. (1991). The Overt Aggression Scale: Overview and guiding principles. *Journal of Neuropsychiatry, 3*(2), S22–S29.

Smith, A., Cardillo, J. E., Smith, S. C., & Amezaga, A. M. (1998). Improvement scaling (rehabilitation version): A new approach to measuring progress of patients in achieving their individual rehabilitation goals. *Medical Care, 36*, 333–347.

Swann, A. C., & Hollander, E. (2002). *Impulsivity and aggression: Diagnostic challenges for the clinician. A monograph for continuing medical education credit.* Arlington Heights, IL: ACCESS Medical Group. Accessed from http://www.cene.com/PDFs/D11-1_Impulsivity.pdf.

Swedo, S. E., & Leonard, H. L. (1992). Trichotillomania: An obsessive compulsive spectrum disorder? *The Psychiatric Clinics of North America, 15*, 777–790.

Trainor, K., Chamberlain, S., & Heyman, I. (2007). Treating trichotillomania in children and adolescents: CBT versus medication. *The American Journal of Psychiatry, 164*(10), 1610–1612.

Tolin, D. F., Diefenbach, G. J., Flessner, C. A., Franklin, M. E., Keuthen, N. J., Moore, P., et al. (2008). The Trichotillomania Scale for Children: Development and validation. *Child Psychiatry and Human Development, 39*, 331–349.

Tolin, D. F., Franklin, M. E., Dienfenbach, G., Anderson, E., & Meunier, S. A. (2007). Paediatric trichotillomania: Descriptive psychopathology and an open trial of cognitive behavioral therapy. *Cognitive Behavioral Therapy, 36*, 129–144.

van Minnen, A., Hoogduin, K., Keijsers, G., Hellenbrand, I., & Hendriks, G. (2003). Treatment of trichotillomania with behavioral therapy or fluoxetine: A randomized, waiting-list controlled study. *Archives of General Psychiatry, 60*, 517–522.

Vitulano, L. A., King, R. A., Scahill, L., & Cohen, D. J. (1992). Behavioral treatment of children and adolescents with trichotillomania. *Journal of the American Academy of Child and Adolescent Psychiatry, 31*, 139–146.

Walther, M., Tucker, B., & Woods, D. (2010). Trichotillomania: Clinical aspects. In E. Aboujaoude & L. M. Koran (Eds.), *Impulse control disorders* (pp. 97–110). New York: Cambridge University Press.

Woods, D. W., Flessner, C., Franklin, M., Wetterneck, C., Walther, M., Anderson, E., et al. (2006). Understanding and treating trichotillomania: What we know and what we don't know. *The Psychiatric Clinics of North America, 29*, 487–501.

Yong-Kwang, T., Levy, M., & Metry, D. (2004). Trichotillomania in childhood: Case series and review. *American Academy of Pediatrics, 113*, 494–498.

Chapter 8
Selective Mutism

with
Andrea Krol

There are times when silence has the loudest voice.

–Leroy Brownlow (1914–2002)

8.1　Overview

Selective mutism (SM) is a rare and unique condition in which a child does not speak in selective environments. In many cases, these children are brought to the attention of medical personnel after a school teacher reports their apparent inability to speak in the classroom. Although SM typically emerges prior to the age of 5, many children are not referred for assessment until after they begin school. This is because most children with SM do not show a significant level of impairment prior to beginning school (Spasaro & Schaefer, 1999). The emerging change in expressive communication patterns is extremely perplexing for parents, teachers, and peers, often leading to amassed speculation about the causes of the child's mutism. In many cases, the child is wrongfully understood and given labels relating to oppositional behavior.

In recent years, there have been several pop culture references to selective mutism not only within popular film but also within music lyrics and literature. Paul McCartney composed a song in 2001 titled, "She's Given Up Talking" that depicts a young girl with selective mutism. The child speaks at home but is mute at school. The lyrics, "when she comes home it's a yap yap yap, words are running freely like water from a tap" illustrate the child's behaviors to be consistent with selective mutism. Other pop culture references to selective mutism include the young boy character featured in Jumanji – a Disney film released in 1995. The young boy in the film refuses to speak to anyone except his sister. Furthermore, a contemporary television sitcom, The Big Bang Theory, depicts the character Rajesh Koothrappali as suffering from selective mutism. Rajesh's social anxiety precludes him from speaking with women unless they are family members. Although selective mutism

S.C. Dombrowski et al., *Assessing and Treating Low Incidence/High Severity Psychological Disorders of Childhood*, DOI 10.1007/978-1-4419-9970-2_8,
© Springer Science+Business Media, LLC 2011

has become a popular plot in stories and movies, the portrayal of this disorder has varied dramatically, with some characterizations being erroneous and deceptive.

The rarity of SM has rendered this disorder difficult to study and as a consequence there are many differing opinions regarding its classification and etiology (Sharp, Sherman, & Gross, 2007). Children with SM also represent a very heterogeneous group, making the assessment, diagnosis, and treatment of this disorder challenging. As more large-scale studies are conducted and more information about this unique disorder is obtained, it is hoped that there will become a clearer understanding of this disorder in addition to increased awareness among parents, teachers, caregivers, and clinicians. The following chapter reviews the clinical conceptualization of SM, including diagnostic classification, historical context, etiological hypotheses, assessment, treatment, outcome, and areas for future research.

8.2   Historical Context

Clinical cases of SM have been documented since around the time of 1877. A German physician by the name of Kussmaul was the first to label the disorder, referring to the pattern of symptoms as *aphasia voluntaria* (Spasaro & Schaefer, 1999; Steinhausen, Wachter, Laimbock, & Winkler Metzke, 2006). It was not until 1934 when a renowned child psychiatrist by the name of Moritz Tramer coined the term *elective mutism* for children presenting with marked and consistent selectivity in speaking (Spasaro & Schaefer; Steinhausen et al., 2006). The term *elective mutism* was chosen to describe this disorder because of the understanding that these children were *electing* not to speak (Spasaro & Schaefer). At this time, children with elective mutism were portrayed as oppositional and defiant and were often described as manipulative, dominating, negative, stubborn, and/or aggressive (Sharp et al., 2007). Over the last two decades, the etiological understanding of this disorder has changed. In the revision of the diagnostic and statistical manual (DSM) in 1994, the term *elective mutism* was changed to *selective mutism*. The impetus behind the change was to emphasize the fact that these children do not simply refuse to speak but rather they do not speak in selective situations (Krysanski, 2003; Viana, Beidel, & Rabian, 2009). The term SM is more congruent with new etiological theories that focus on anxiety rather than on oppositional behavior (Spasaro & Schaefer). Although there has been a shift in the understanding of this disorder, it is important to note that other diagnostic systems such as the ICD-10 have retained the label of "elective mutism."

8.3   Description and Diagnostic Classification

Selective mutism, a disorder of childhood, is characterized by a complete lack of speech in at least one particular social situation (i.e., in the classroom), despite the ability to speak in other situations (American Psychiatric Association, 2000;

Viana et al., 2009). The diagnostic criteria for SM in the DSM-IV TR are as follows (American Psychiatric Association):

- Consistent failure to speak in specific social situations (in which there is an expectation for speaking, e.g., at school) despite speaking in other situations.
- The disturbance interferes with educational or occupational achievement or with social communication.
- The duration of the disturbance is at least 1 month (not limited to the first month of school).
- The failure to speak is not due to a lack of knowledge of, or comfort with, the spoken language required in the social situation.
- The disturbance is not better accounted for by a communication disorder (e.g., stuttering) and does not occur exclusively during the course of a pervasive developmental disorder, schizophrenia, or other psychotic disorder.

At present, SM is categorized in the section of the DSM-IV TR titled, "Other disorders of Infancy, Childhood and Adolescence." SM, and even its diagnostic predecessor, elective mutism have always been classified in the miscellaneous section of the DSM. However, more recently, the inclusion of SM in the miscellaneous section of the DSM-IV TR has led to much debate among researchers and clinicians (Dummit, Klein, Tancer, & Asche, 1997; Sharp et al., 2007). It has been argued that SM should not be included in the miscellaneous section of the DSM-IV TR as it implies that SM is separate from other widespread conditions (Dummit et al., 1997; Sharp et al.).

Since the first conceptualization of this disorder, numerous different etiologies have been proposed which have led to confusion and uncertainty regarding SM's classification. While some have suggested that SM is a variant of an anxiety disorder, others propose that SM is more complicated. Researchers have hypothesized that SM may be due to psychodynamic factors, family dysfunction, neurodevelopmental problems, oppositional behavior, trauma, and in some cases the manifestation of a dissociative identity disorder (Anstendig, 1999; Krysanski, 2003; Sharp et al., 2007). With an increase in large-scale studies in children with SM over the last two decades, it is anticipated that there will be an improved understanding of this disorder including the diagnostic criteria used to identify it.

8.3.1 Prevalence

The overall prevalence of SM in childhood is rare and is estimated to occur in less than 1% of individuals in mental health settings (American Psychiatric Association, 2000). In a recent review of the literature, Viana et al., (2009) examined seven different large-scale studies from 1996 to 2004 and found the prevalence rate of SM to range from 0.47% to 0.76% in the general population. These were collected using the diagnostic criteria from the ICD-10, DSM-III, or the DSM-IV. SM is also seen to occur slightly more frequently in females than males with a ratio ranging from

2.6:1 to 1.5:1 (Kumpulainen, Rasanen, Raaska, & Somppi, 1998; Sharp et al., 2007). It has been hypothesized that the gender difference in SM may reflect a more general trend between gender and anxiety-related conditions, as females have been reported to experience more symptoms of anxiety than males (Sharp et al.; Standart & Le Couteur, 2003).

8.3.2   Age of Onset

According to the DSM-IV TR, the onset of SM typically occurs before the age of 5 and the mean age of onset ranges from 2.7 to 4.1 years (American Psychiatric Association, 2000; Viana et al., 2009). However, SM is often not recognized or diagnosed until a child enters school (Giddan, Ross, Sechler, & Becker, 1997). Researchers have noted that there is often a delay from when a child first enters school until they are formally referred for an assessment. This lag time can vary but the research suggests that the average age of assessment for SM ranges from 6.5 to 9 years of age (Kumpulainen et al., 1998; Standart & Le Couteur, 2003). The delay in identification could be that families fail to recognize the need for assessment because of normal speech presentation in the home environment (Sharp et al., 2007). In any case, there is a need for better screening and identification of children with SM in the school systems in order to prevent or limit functional impairment (Sharp et al.).

8.3.3   Ethnicity

Research shows a higher incidence of SM in ethnic minority and immigrant groups (Cline & Baldwin, 2004; Elizur & Perednik, 2003). One of the first studies conducted with an immigrant population not only found a higher incidence of SM but they also found a family background of migration to be a common risk factor in the development of this disorder (Bradley & Sloman, 1975; Elizur & Perednik). Large population studies have continued to demonstrate a higher incidence of SM in immigrant and language minority children compared to native born populations (Toppelberg, Tabors, Coggins, Lum, & Burger, 2005). For example, in a study conducted by Elizur and Perednik, the prevalence of SM found in the general child population in Israel was 7.6 per 1,000 compared to a prevalence rate of 22 per 1,000 for those children of immigrant background. Similarly, in a large case analysis conducted with children from Switzerland and Germany, out of 100 children with SM, 28 were immigrants (Steinhausen & Adamek, 1997; Steinhausen & Juzi, 1996). Although more research is needed, the high proportion of immigrant children should be regarded as a risk factor in the development of SM (Steinhausen & Juzi).

8.3.4   Socioeconomic Status

The occurrence of SM is reported in all social strata, with no evidence to suggest that SM occurs more frequently in some socioeconomic groups compared to others (Steinhausen & Juzi, 1996).

8.4   Etiological Hypotheses

Etiological explanations for SM have varied considerably since the first descriptions of this disorder in the late nineteenth century (Cohan, Chavira, & Stein, 2006; Cohan, Price, & Stein, 2006; Spasaro & Schaefer, 1999). A plethora of etiological hypotheses have been proposed but to date, there is no known single cause for SM (Viana et al., 2009). Rather, this disorder is best explained as one which results from an interaction of various environmental and genetic factors.

8.4.1   Psychodynamic Theory

Within a psychodynamic tradition, SM is explained as unresolved internal conflict within a child (Viana et al., 2009). SM is thought to be a protective mechanism for a child. For example, it is argued that children with SM have hostile feelings toward their mother but are unable to express them directly because of their mothers' personal rejection of them (Cline & Baldwin, 2004). Since the child fears abandonment and separation from the parent, the child then directs their hostility and anger toward third parties such as teachers or other adult figures (Cline & Baldwin; Giddan et al., 1997). The primary psychological gain for the child is that their hostility and anger toward the parent is lessened. In addition, the child is able to remain dependent and receive increased attention as a result of their behavior (Cline & Baldwin). It is important to note that there are differences in the conceptualization of this disorder among theorists within the psychodynamic tradition. The psychodynamic theory, while important to review, is losing popularity to more empirically sound theories (Krysanski, 2003).

8.4.2   Behavioral Theory

Within a behavioral tradition, SM is thought to occur as a result of negatively reinforced behavior (Krysanski, 2003). More explicitly, the child perceives the consequences of not speaking as positive. For example, the child may experience a reduction in anxiety and fear (negative reinforcement) and/or they may obtain privileges and attention as a result of their behavior (positive reinforcement) (Krysanski). Behaviorists view SM as a disorder that exists because of the interaction between the child and his or her environment (Krysanski). From this theoretical understanding, SM is something that is functional for a child and is reinforced by the child's environmental surroundings (Anstendig, 1999). For example, if adults begin to accept nonverbal communication from a child with SM, or if other children begin speaking for a child with SM, the behavior is reinforced and maintained.

8.4.3 Family Dynamics

Other theories of SM point to dysfunctional family relationships as the root cause of this disorder (Anstendig, 1999; Krysanski, 2003). In this theory, the family's involvement in the development of SM may be related to either (a) parent mutest modeling, (b) family cultural tradition, (c) symbiotic attachment, (d) separation anxiety, or (e) poor marital adjustment (Krysanski; Spasaro & Schaefer, 1999). In mutest modeling, it is hypothesized that a child's SM results from witnessing one or both parents using silence as a way of coping with stress (Spasaro & Schaefer). The silence then becomes modeled and reinforced in the children (Spasaro & Schaefer). In other situations, children may be taught by their families that the outside world is unsafe. In this context, children with SM may have learned through observation that people outside of the family are a danger to their well-being (Anstendig). This is often common with immigrant and refugee families who are of a different culture and who may be experiencing distrust of the dominant cultural group (Krysanski; Spasaro & Schaefer). Symbiotic attachment refers to an intense attachment that a child may have with another family member (often the mother) (Anstendig; Spasaro & Schaefer). This enmeshment can disrupt the child's individual growth and development and the child may develop SM as a result of this dependent relationship (Spasaro & Schaefer). Finally, SM may be a result of martial conflict in the home where the child often absorbs heightened levels of stress (Spasaro & Schaefer). More specifically, it has been suggested that in homes where marital discord is present, family coping mechanisms are often poor or nonexistent (Elizur & Perednik, 2003). Overwhelming stress in the home, in conjunction with limited coping resources can sometimes lead children to adopt defensive mechanisms (i.e., SM) which are dysfunctional and problematic. In sum, marital discord is a general stress factor, known to affect parent–child relationships and family coping and can increase a child's vulnerability to SM (Elizur & Perednik).

8.4.4 Trauma

Traumatic experiences have also been implicated in the development of SM (Brix Andersson & Hove Thomsen, 1998; Dummit et al., 1997). However, to date, there has been little evidence to support this etiological hypothesis. In a study conducted by Black and Uhde (1995), only 4 out of the 30 children with SM were reported to have experienced significant early trauma. Even then, the onset of SM for these children was not temporally or causally related to a traumatic event. Black and Uhde were unable to identify any clear precipitants to the onset of SM in the 30 children that they studied. Furthermore, Steinhausen and Juzi (1996) found similar results in a study which examined 100 nonreferred and referred children with SM. These children demonstrated low rates of psychological trauma which either preceded or followed the onset of SM (Steinhausen & Juzi). Similar findings have also been corroborated by Dummit, Klein, Tancer, Asche, Martin, and Fairbanks (1997). However, some research has suggested that a child's reaction to trauma, namely, frequent moves and/or changes of kindergarten or school, may be a potential risk factor in the development of SM (Kristensen, 2000).

8.4.5 Genetic Vulnerabilities

Research has suggested that children with SM may have a genetic predisposition to the disorder (Cline & Baldwin, 2004; Viana et al., 2009). Black and Uhde (1995) found a high familial prevalence of SM and an even higher prevalence of avoidant disorder in a sample of 30 children with SM. More explicitly, the first degree family history of SM and social phobia among participants in the study was 37% and 70%, respectively. Overall, the results from this study highlight the increased prevalence of social phobia and SM among family members of children with SM. In another similar study, researchers found a history of SM or mutistic reactions in 27 % (12 of 45) parents (Remschmidt, Poller, HerpertzDahlmann, Hennighausen, & Gutenbrunner, 2001). The prevalence of other speech and language disorders was also found to be high among family members. Taciturnity (minimal speech) was present in 51% of the fathers and 44% of the mothers (Remschmidt et al., 2001). Other language and communication disorders including stuttering, cluttering, and articulative problems were present in 9% of the families (Remschmidt et al.). A high proportion (58%) of the mothers and fathers also revealed severe psychopathological symptoms at measured by a standardized psychological questionnaire at the time of the study (Remschmidt et al.). Taken as a whole, there appears to be a high prevalence rate of communication deficits and psychopathological disorders within families of children with SM (Remschmidt et al.).

In an effort to examine the personality traits and symptom traits in parents of children with SM, Kristensen and Torgersen (2001) studied a group of 54 children with SM and their families in addition to a control group. Using the Millon Clinical Multiaxial Inventory (MCMI-II), the parents of children with SM and the control group completed the self-report inventory to obtain data on parental personality features (Kristensen & Torgersen). Results obtained support the hypothesis that SM is familial. The mothers of SM children showed higher scores on the Avoidant and Schizotypal scales of the MCMI-II, whereas fathers demonstrated higher scores on the anxiety scales in comparison to the control groups (Kristensen & Torgersen). These results underscore the fact that social anxiety is a significant factor in SM and has a heritable component. Although the intent of this study was not to determine how personality traits associated with social anxiety and SM is transmitted, it is likely that both genetic and environmental factors are involved in the transference of this disorder (Kristensen & Torgersen). In addition, the researchers found differences among the group of SM with co-morbid communication disorders compared to the group of SM without communication disorders. More specifically, it was found that only the mothers of children who had SM without communication disorders displayed elevated scores on the MCMI-II avoidant, schizoid, schizotypal, and dysthymia scales (Kristensen & Torgersen). These results suggest that in children with SM (without a communication disorder), the development of the disorder is more attributable to parental personality traits and symptom traits. Research shows that communication disorders are often associated with shyness, aloofness, and anxiety and thus, SM in these children may be secondary to a language disorder (Paul & Kellogg, 1997). More research in this domain is clearly warranted.

A subsequent study was conducted using the Structured Clinical Interview for DSM-IV (First, Spitzer, Gibbon, & Williams, 2002) and the NEO Personality Inventory (Costa & McCrae, 1985) to examine the prevalence of psychiatric disorders in parents of children with SM (Chavira, ShiponBlum, Hitchcock, Cohan, & Stein, 2007). This study specifically sought to examine the relation of SM to the different subtypes of social phobia (SP). The generalized subtype of SP is characterized by the fear of most social situations, whereas the nongeneralized type refers to the fear of circumscribed situations, usually performance related (Chavira et al., 2007). Overall, it was found that the parents of children with SM had an incidence of generalized social phobia and avoidant personality disorder three to four times greater than controls (Chavira et al.). Interestingly, it was also found that the severity of child SM also predicted parent SP (generalized type) (Chavira et al.). Generalized social phobia has been thought of as a more severe form of social anxiety and researchers have hypothesized that SM may be an early onset form of this disorder (Chavira et al.). Parents of children with SM also demonstrated higher levels of neuroticism, which is a known risk factor for the development of anxiety (Jylha & Isometsa, 2006). Taken together, the results from this study highlight the link between SM and social phobia (generalized subtype) as well as SM and later psychopathology (Chavira et al.).

In sum, while more research is needed to discern the hereditability of SM, family history of SM, communication disorders, and/or psychopathological disorders (social phobia, avoidant personality disorder) are primary risk factors for the development of this disorder.

8.4.6   Externalizing (Oppositional) Behavior

In the literature on SM, there have been several different descriptions of these children's behavior. While some of the children with SM are described as submissive, sensitive, shy, weepy, and sulky, in other cases, these children are also depicted as aggressive, stubborn, anxious, immature, and dominating (Cohan, Price, et al., 2006;

Cohan et al., 2008; Kumpulainen et al., 1998). Some studies have provided evidence that children with SM also display oppositional behavior and in some cases meet the diagnostic criteria for oppositional defiant disorder (ODD) (Kristensen & Torgersen, 2001; Manassis et al., 2007; Steinhausen & Juzi, 1996; Yeganeh, Beidel, & Turner, 2006). For example, in a study conducted by Steinhausen and Juzi (1996), oppositional defiant and/or aggressive behavior was found in 20% of the children with SM. In addition, another study found the prevalence of ODD to be 29% in a group of children with SM and co-morbid social phobia, but only 5% in a group of children with social phobia alone (Yeganeh et al., 2006). However, in other studies, the presence of oppositional behavior is low, suggesting that the presence of externalizing disorders among children with SM is not common (Bergman, Piacentini, & McCracken, 2002; Cunningham, McHolm, & Boyle, 2006; Vecchio & Kearney, 2005). It is clear that the literature on externalizing disorders within a SM population is mixed. Given that oppositional behaviors have also been described in children with anxiety disorders, more research is warranted in order to better understand how oppositional behavior may play a role in SM (Viana et al., 2009). Some researchers have suggested that the avoidant behavior exhibited by children with SM may be interpreted as oppositional or devious; however, a more likely explanation for the behavior is because of the remarkable anxiety these children face (Cohan et al.).

8.4.7 Anxiety

Research continues to find a strong association between SM and social anxiety (Black & Uhde, 1995; Chavira et al., 2007; Cohan et al., 2008). Early hypotheses suggested that SM may be a variant of social phobia. However, until 1995, no studies empirically validated these ideas (Black & Uhde). One of the first studies to examine the characteristics of children with SM using comprehensive evaluations and diagnostic interviews was done by Black and Uhde. Results of this study found that of 30 SM participants, 29 (97%) also met the diagnostic criteria for either social phobia, avoidant disorder, or both (Black & Uhde). Other studies have found equally high rates of social phobia and other co-morbid anxiety disorders in SM populations. For example, one study which sought to examine a group of children with SM in relation to other youth with and without anxiety disorders found that all of the children with SM met the diagnostic criteria for social phobia using the DSM-IV criteria and 53% also met the criteria for an additional anxiety disorder (Vecchio & Kearney, 2005). Similarly, in another study, 74.1% of children with SM also met the criteria for another anxiety disorder (Kristensen, 2000; Kristensen & Torgersen, 2001). Of these 74.1% of children, 67.9% had social phobia and 31.5% had separation anxiety (Kristensen). These results were further corroborated by Manassis et al. (2007), who found that 27 of 44 (61.4%) children with SM were also afflicted with social phobia. In addition to these studies, there are a plethora of others which demonstrate a strong relationship between SM and anxiety (Bergman et al., 2002; Cunningham, McHolm, Boyle, & Patel, 2004; Cunningham et al., 2006; Manassis et al., 2003).

Due to the high rates of co-morbidity between SM and social phobia, many researchers have proposed that SM may be better explained as a variant of social phobia and classified as an anxiety disorder (Anstendig, 1998, 1999; Sharp et al., 2007). Because of the varied etiological explanations for SM since its inception, SM is currently a diagnostic category of other disorders of infancy, childhood, and adolescence. However, with a recent increase in research that shows a parallel between SM and anxiety disorder symptomatology, some researchers are debating whether SM would be better categorized as an anxiety disorder rather than a separate diagnostic entity as it is now (Anstendig, 1999). Although there is strong evidence to support SM as a variant of anxiety, not all researchers are in favor of changing the diagnostic category of this disorder. Cohan et al. (2008) are concerned with changing the classification of SM as it is felt that a new diagnostic category would obscure important differences in the profiles of children affected with this disorder (Cohan et al.). The authors argue that results from their study found that while anxiety is a prominent feature of SM, children with SM also often present with communication delays and/or mild behavior problems. If SM was reclassified to be an anxiety disorder, other additional features of this disorder such as communication deficits and behavior problems may be disregarded (Cohan et al.). It has been proposed that within the diagnostic category of SM, subgroups or diagnostic specifiers be created in order to capture the communication deficits and/or behavior problems that may also be present in this population (Cohan et al.).

Taken together, the abovementioned studies highlight the fact that children with SM often face significant anxiety. Although it is undeniable that anxiety plays a significant role in SM, there is also evidence to suggest that other factors (communication deficits and/or behavior problems) may be involved (Cline & Baldwin, 2004; Cohan et al., 2008; Fisak, Oliveros, & Ehrenreich, 2006). It is of utmost importance that those clinicians, parents, therapists, caregivers, and others working with children with SM consider all variables that may be involved in the development and maintenance of this disorder in order to effectively implement intervention and treatment (Cline & Baldwin).

8.5 Assessment

The assessment of SM requires a comprehensive evaluation in order to rule out any other reasons that might explain the disturbance in language use (Krysanski, 2003). A comprehensive assessment also allows a clinician to evaluate for any co-morbid conditions that may be present (Krysanski). In majority of cases, a clinician will begin by conducting an interview with the child's parents, as the nature of the disorder precludes a child from being the primary source of information (Krysanski; Viana et al., 2009). One semistructured interview schedule that has been recommended for use with a SM population is *The Anxiety Disorders Interview Schedule for Children and Parents* (Silverman, Saavedra, & Pina, 2001). This interview schedule assesses for SM in addition to many other disorders (Silverman et al., 2001; Viana et al.).

Whether or not a clinician chooses to use a specific interview schedule, it is essential that information regarding the child's symptom history (specifically onset), any neurological difficulties, atypical speech and language difficulties, and history of treatment is obtained. In addition, it is important to learn about the conditions under which the mutism occurs (i.e., school, peers, etc.) as well as whether or not the child engages in any form of communication (i.e., smiling, nodding, eye contact) (Viana et al.).

It is also important to assess for psychiatric conditions as other disorders can be characterized by a lack of speech. These disorders may include autism, aphasia, mental retardation, and schizophrenia, to name a few. Information regarding a child's developmental history including prenatal and perinatal complications, medical history including auditory concerns, neurological status, as well as history of family psychiatric problems and shyness is essential (Krysanski, 2003). Before a diagnosis of SM can be made, clinicians must rule out other conditions which may better account for a child's lack of speech. Therefore, a comprehensive assessment which reviews all of the abovementioned components is vital.

It is recommended that the child's school teacher be involved in the assessment of SM (Cline & Baldwin, 2004). A teacher often has key information about the child's behavior in a large group setting that a parent may not have. For example, a teacher is able to describe the child's communication behavior among peers. More specifically, does the child speak to anyone in particular? Does the child use nonverbal communication with peers? A teacher may also have insight into whether there are specific situations where the child may be more inclined to speak and whether or not there any specific strategies that are effective for the child (Cline & Baldwin; Viana et al., 2009). In some cases, it may be appropriate to have the child with SM undergo a psychoeducational assessment whereby report cards are reviewed and a standardized cognitive ability test is administered (although these tests require a child to respond verbally which could prove challenging in cases of SM). Tests such as the Wechsler Intelligence Scale for Children (WISC), the Standford Binet Test of Intelligence (SB), or the Wechsler Preschool and Primary Scale of Intelligence (WWPSI) may be administered and interpreted by a qualified psychologist (Krysanski, 2003).

Finally, a child with SM should undergo a comprehensive speech and language assessment in order to evaluate their fluency, pitch, rhythm, inflection, tone, and quality of speech. In some cases, children who speak English as a second language may have had limited exposure to the dominant language which may be contributing to the SM. In other cases, a child with SM may have an undetected speech problem which may be the leading cause of the mutism. In any case, a child with SM should be evaluated by a speech language pathologist (Cleator & Hand, 2001).

8.6 Treatment

SM is a disorder that is challenging to treat (Blum et al., 1998; Jackson, Allen, Boothe, Nava, & Coates, 2005). Different treatment approaches for SM have been identified in the literature; however, due to the rarity of this disorder little is known about their efficacy (Cohan, Chavira, et al., 2006; Cohan, Price, et al., 2006; Pionek Stone, Kratochwill, Sladezcek, & Serlin, 2002; Spasaro & Schaefer, 1999). Many of the treatments for SM are chosen by clinicians in accord with their theoretical understanding of the disorder (i.e., behavioral and psychodynamic) and their assumptions regarding the etiology and maintenance of it (Spasaro & Schaefer). While it is apparent that more research is needed in order to determine what treatments are the most efficacious, it is difficult to conduct empirical studies when the prevalence rate of this disorder is so low (Spasaro & Schaefer). The next section reviews the treatment approaches for SM as discussed in the literature, however, it is important to keep in mind that many of the studies on the treatment of SM are case studies which limit their generalizability.

8.6.1 Behavioral Interventions

Behavioral theory of SM perceives the disorder as one that is learned (Cohan, Chavira, et al., 2006; Cohan, Price, et al., 2006; Pionek Stone et al., 2002). That is, according to this theory SM exists because of a series of conditioning events that have led to the behavior. SM is subsequently maintained because there is often a secondary gain for the child (i.e., decreased anxiety and increased attention). Behavioral treatments for SM utilize techniques such as contingency management, shaping and stimulus fading, systematic desensitization, social skills training, as well as modeling (Cohan, Chavira, et al.). In recent years, there has been a shift in the use of behavioral interventions. It is now more common for therapists to use multimodal interventions where behavioral techniques are used in conjunction with an analysis of the child and his or her family (Jackson et al., 2005). Research continues to suggest that behavioral interventions are the most widely used in the treatment of SM and appear to be very effective (Jackson et al.).

8.6.1.1 Contingency Management

Contingency management is a reinforcement strategy whereby a child with SM is reinforced for verbal behavior (Krysanski, 2003). Reinforcement begins for any close approximation to the targeted verbal behavior (i.e., mouthing words, whispering, etc.) and later for normal speech (Cohan, Chavira, et al., 2006; Cohan, Price, et al., 2006). Although some research has provided positive outcomes using contingency management in the treatment of SM (Beare, Torgerson, & Creviston, 2008), the long-term outcome using this approach is still unclear (Cohan, Chavira, et al.). Stimulus fading techniques have also proved to be beneficial in addition to contingency management regimes (Cohan, Price, et al.). With stimulus fading, a child with SM is gradually introduced to a larger group environment where he or she must speak (Viana et al., 2009). At first, the child may be reinforced for speaking in front of one stranger. Over time, the child will get reinforced for speaking to a larger group of people and/or in numerous different settings (Cohan, Chavira, et al.).

8.6.1.2   Systematic Desensitization

Systematic desensitization is another type of behavioral intervention that involves the use of relaxation strategies while an individual is exposed to anxiety provoking scenarios (Cohan, Chavira, et al., 2006). Research shows that while systematic desensitization can be very beneficial for older children with SM (Rye & Ullman, 1999), this technique is more difficult for younger children as they often struggle with the progressive muscle relaxation and imagery exercises (Compton et al., 2004).

8.6.1.3   Self-Modeling

Self-modeling is a unique behavioral intervention that has been successfully used with SM children (Blum et al., 1998). It involves making a video which depicts the child speaking in a situation with which they are normally mute (Blum et al.). The tapes are then repeatedly played back to the child during treatment. The idea behind self-modeling is that the child will become accustomed to hearing themselves speak in anxiety provoking situations and will gain confidence for speaking later on in similar circumstances (Cohan et al., 2006). A case study conducted by Blum et al. examined three girls aged 6–9 who had histories of inhibited speech in the school and community for a period of at least one and a half years. In all three of these children, an audio feedforward intervention proved to be successful and the behavior change in these children appeared to be rapid. It was also noted that these children had previously been resistant to other treatment methods. While self-modeling remains a promising behavioral intervention technique, more research is needed to determine its effectiveness across many different contexts. This is due to the fact that self-modeling has only been used in conjunction with other behavioral interventions (positive reinforcement and stimulus fading) and never as a technique in isolation (Cohan, Chavira, et al.).

8.6.2   Cognitive-Behavioral Intervention

Although the majority of the interventions used for SM focus on behavioral modification, there has been some research which has examined the effectiveness of cognitive-behavioral therapies (CBTs) with this disorder (Fung, Manassis, Kenny, & Fiksenbaum, 2002). CBT focuses on cognitive restructuring and has been reported to be effective for children with anxiety disorders (Fung et al., 2002; Kendall, 1994). In a study conducted by Fung et al., a CBT Web-based intervention was administered to a 7-year-old child with a diagnosis of SM. The intervention was 14 weeks long and included a child workbook as well as a parent/teacher manual which focused on psychoeducation (Fung et al.). The aim of the workbook was to teach the child with SM how to recognize the signs of anxiety associated with speaking and how to use appropriate management strategies (Fung et al.). An additional component of the intervention included using a computer program which encouraged the child to record short messages. The recorded messages could then be played back to the child throughout the sessions with an expectation that the child would become desensensitized to hearing his or her own voice and speaking in different situations (Fung et al.). Results from this study are encouraging. The child with SM showed significantly lower ratings of anxiety evaluated in a pretreatment, posttreatment design by the child, the child's parents, and the classroom teacher (Fung et al.). Since this research study was only based on the results from one child, further research is clearly warranted. It would be interesting to see if the results of this study would hold true in a controlled research design.

To date, there is not much research conducted on the use of CBT in the treatment of SM. One of the reasons could be because, in general, cognitive therapies are better suited for older children, whereas the majority of cases of SM occur in young children (Cohan, Chavira, et al., 2006).

8.6.3   Family Therapy Intervention

In some cases of SM, a family systems approach to therapy may be beneficial for both the child and his or her family (Cohan, Chavira, et al., 2006). Family therapy is not conducted as frequently as other types of therapy but is appropriate in specific cases of SM (Anstendig, 1999). Family therapy may be considered when a child's mute symptomatology is thought to occur because of dysfunctional family patterns (Anstendig; Krysanski, 2003). Family therapy seeks to identify faulty family relationships and patterns of communication that may have caused the selectively mute behavior and/or maintained it (Cohan, Chavira, et al.). Therapy using this approach often incorporates the child, the child's parents, as well as any other family members who might be relevant. The therapist may use many different approaches to gain insight on how the family operates and what key variables might be associated with the child's mutism (i.e., communication, stress, support, etc.). Overall, the goal of therapy using the family systems approach is to resolve any faulty systems that may be operating in the home. The therapist works to improve the family's functioning with the hope that doing so will alleviate the child's mutism (Cohan, Chavira, et al.).

The research on family therapy for the treatment of SM is scant. The research that has been conducted has been based upon case studies which lack external validity (Cohan, Chavira, et al., 2006). However, the role of families in the treatment of SM should not be disregarded. Future research is warranted in order to better understand how family therapy can be used most effectively in the treatment of this rare disorder.

8.6.4   Pharmacotherapy

The treatment of SM has been focused primarily on psychosocial and behavioral approaches until recently, when researchers and clinicians have turned their attention to different options within pharmacology. Since the pharmacological treatment of

SM is still relatively new, more research is still needed. However, the results obtained so far have been promising (Carlson, Mitchell, & Segool, 2008).

Most of the pharmacological studies of SM report on the use of selective serotonin reuptake inhibitors (SSRIs) (Carlson et al., 2008). One of the first studies to report on the effectiveness of SSRIs in the treatment of SM was conducted by Black and Uhde (1994), in a placebo controlled, double blind study using fluoxetine. The six children with SM enrolled in this study showed improvement in 24 out of 28 measures. These measures looked at ratings of mutism, anxiety, and social anxiety by the child's clinician, parents, as well as teachers. More specifically, the measures looked at mutism change, anxiety change, and shyness change. In addition, factors from a psychiatric and behavior rating scale were used. These factors further examined anxiety, conduct problems, social anxiety, depression, and overall problem severity. However, it should be noted that similar results were also found for children in the placebo group. Overall, there were only three measures that the children treated with fluoxetine showed significant improvement when compared to the placebo group (Black & Uhde). In another similar study, researchers conducted a 9-week open trial study using fluoxetine to treat children with SM and co-morbid social anxiety disorders who had failed to respond to psychosocial treatment (Dummit, Klein, Tancer, & Asche, 1996; Dummit et al., 1997). Following the 9-week study, 76% of the children were rated by their treating psychiatrists to have either made some improvement, much improvement, or complete recovery, and children who were under the age of 11 made larger treatment gains than those who were older (Dummit et al., 1996). There have been numerous other studies which have also reported improvement in children with SM using fluoxetine treatment. However, since these research reports utilized case study designs, the results are difficult to generalize (Boon, 1994; Guna-Dumitrescu & Pelletier, 1996; Harvey & Milne, 1998; Kehle, Madaus, Baratta, & Bray, 1998). In addition to fluoxetine, researchers have also conducted studies using other SSRIs, such as sertaline, citalopram, fluvoxamine, and paroxetine and similar results have been found. SSRIs, which alter the serotonin levels in a human brain, appear to be a potentially useful medication in the treatment of SM, especially in cases when psychosocial treatments may not be effective (Carlson et al., 2008). There have been a few reports published by researchers and clinicians using medications (i.e., monoamine oxidase inhibitors (MOAIs), depressants) other than SSRIs in the treatment of SM, but the results have been mixed and the research in each of these reports have single case studies with few patients (Golwyn & Sevlie, 1999; Maskey, 2001; Steffen & van Waes, 1999). Further research is warranted in the pharmacological treatment of SM.

8.7 Outcome and Prognosis

The rarity of SM has rendered this disorder difficult to study, especially in longitudinal research designs. For this reason, there is a paucity of studies which have examined the long-term outcome of individuals with SM. However, it is clear that

SM has a variable course. In some cases of SM, patients go through extensive treatment with unyielding results, whereas in other cases patients go through spontaneous remission (Steinhausen et al., 2006). In the long-term outcome studies that have been conducted, complete remission has been observed in 39–100% of SM patients (Steinhausen et al.). It has been noted that even after a complete resolution of the core symptoms of SM, these individuals often continue to exhibit deficits in communication (i.e., being afraid of unknown situations, talking to strangers, being afraid of using the telephone), they are socially withdrawn and they show psychosocial impairment affecting their ability to function on a day-to-day basis (Remschmidt et al., 2001; Steinhausen et al.). Some research has even reported a higher rate of unemployment among adults with a history of SM (Remschmidt et al.). Overall, this suggests that while the core symptoms of SM may resolve; this disorder is likely to persist and there is a tendency for a poor outcome (Remschmidt et al.). Of the many factors that impact the course of SM, researchers have revealed that mutistic behavior within the core family (i.e., the child refusing to speak to his/her mother, father, or siblings) is the most predictive of poor outcome (Remschmidt et al.). These results highlight the fact that family psychopathology is an important variable in the diagnosis, treatment, and outcome of children with SM. The implications of this research suggest that even despite the resolution of symptoms, many individuals' with SM continue to experience debilitating anxiety throughout their lives. Therefore, it is important for clinicians to recognize that, in many cases, SM is a lifelong disorder which can continue to affect the lives of those individuals even long after the resolution of mute behavior.

8.8 Future Directions

While there has been much progress over the last two decades in SM research, clinicians are still in dire need of knowledge regarding the etiology, course, and treatment of this rare disorder. SM is a serious disorder of childhood that has significant implications if left untreated. However, in order for children with SM to receive appropriate treatment, there must be an awareness and understanding among parents, teachers, and clinicians with regard to this disorder and the significance of it. There needs to be a greater effort at SM knowledge dissemination within schools, community centers, and medical facilities so that more children with this disorder can be identified, assessed, and treated early.

Many of the research studies that have been published on SM lack strong methodology and often consist either of retrospective chart reviews, uncontrolled case studies, or small single-participant experiments (Cohan, Chavira, et al., 2006). This is especially true of the research on the treatment of SM. For example, while the research on the use of SSRIs with SM appears quite promising, studies with a much larger sample size are needed before more definite conclusions can be drawn. Therefore, one recommendation for future research with SM is to implement large-scale randomized, controlled treatment studies. While there are a range of different treatments for SM, there is little empirical evidence regarding the efficacy of the treatments. It is not an easy task to conduct large-scale studies on rare disorders such as SM; however, it is imperative if progress is to be made in this area.

There continues to be a debate regarding the role of anxiety in SM. While there is strong evidence to suggest SM and social anxiety may be etiologically linked, researchers and clinicians are still uncertain about how to best classify this disorder (Sharp et al., 2007). There is a strong push by many researchers to reclassify SM as an anxiety disorder. It is felt that by doing so, the ambiguity of this disorder will dissipate and clinicians can focus their attention on developing appropriate assessment tools and treatment techniques. It is likely that until a unanimous decision regarding the taxonomy of SM is reached, progress in this field will be slow. Therefore, more research and, in particular, longitudinal research is needed in order to determine SM's relationship to anxiety.

8.9 Summary

SM is a rare, socially debilitating disorder which has puzzled clinicians, researchers, and medical personnel since its first clinical description in the early 1930s. This highly complex disorder has been difficult to classify, assess, and treat due to the various other developmental and behavioral disorders that often accompany it. Although many etiological explanations for this disorder have been proposed, to date, there is no known single cause of SM. SM is not as prevalent as other disorders of childhood; however, it is critical that parents, teachers, caregivers, and health professionals learn about the common signs and symptoms of this disorder so that assessment and treatment can occur in a timely manner. Furthermore, while there are numerous treatment options for children with SM, it is important to note that treatment response often varies according to each child's unique situation. However, the research has provided promising results for the use of SSRIs in the treatment of SM for children who are otherwise unresponsive to psychosocial and behavioral interventions (Carlson et al., 2008). Continued research is vital in order to advance our current understanding of this disorder so that children suffering from SM can be assessed and treated in the most efficacious manner. It is likely that, with continued commitment from researchers and clinicians, our ability to understand, diagnose, and treat this disorder will continue to improve over time.

References

American Psychiatric Association. (2000). *Diagnostic and statistical manual of mental disorders* (4th ed. text revision). Washington, DC: Author.

Anstendig, K. D. (1998). Selective mutism: A review of the treatment literature by modality from 1980–1996. *Psychotherapy: Theory, Research, Practice, Training, 35*(3), 381–391.

Anstendig, K. D. (1999). Is selective mutism an anxiety disorder? rethinking its DSM-IV classification. *Journal of Anxiety Disorders, 13*(4), 417–434.

Beare, P., Torgerson, C., & Creviston, C. (2008). Increasing verbal behavior of a student who is selectively mute. *Journal of Emotional and Behavioral Disorders, 16*(4), 248–255.

Bergman, R. L., Piacentini, J., & McCracken, J. T. (2002). Prevalence and description of selective mutism in a school-based sample. *Journal of the American Academy of Child and Adolescent Psychiatry, 41*(8), 938–946.

Black, B., & Uhde, T. W. (1994). Treatment of elective mutism with fluoxetine: A double-blind, placebo-controlled study. *Journal of the American Academy of Child and Adolescent Psychiatry, 33*(7), 1000–1006.

Black, B., & Uhde, T. W. (1995). Psychiatric characteristics of children with selective mutism: A pilot study. *Journal of the American Academy of Child and Adolescent Psychiatry, 34*(7), 847–856.

Blum, N. J., Kell, R. S., Starr, H. L., Lender, W. L., BradleyKlug, K. L., Osborne, M. L., et al. (1998). Case study: Audio feedforward treatment of selective mutism. *Journal of the American Academy of Child and Adolescent Psychiatry, 37*(1), 40–43.

Boon, F. (1994). The selective mutism controversy (continued). *Journal of the American Academy of Child and Adolescent Psychiatry, 33*(2), 283.

Bradley, S., & Sloman, L. (1975). Elective mutism in immigrant families. *Journal of the American Academy of Child and Adolescent Psychiatry, 14*, 510–514.

Brix Andersson, C., & Hove Thomsen, P. (1998). Electively mute children: An analysis of 37 Danish cases. *Nordic Journal of Psychiatry, 52*(3), 231–238.

Carlson, J. S., Mitchell, A. D., & Segool, N. (2008). The current state of empirical support for the pharmacological treatment of selective mutism. *School Psychology Quarterly, 23*(3), 354–372.

Chavira, D. A., ShiponBlum, E., Hitchcock, C., Cohan, S., & Stein, M. B. (2007). Selective mutism and social anxiety disorder: All in the family? *Journal of the American Academy of Child and Adolescent Psychiatry, 46*(11), 1464–1472.

Cleator, H., & Hand, L. (2001). Selective mutism: How a successful speech and language assessment really is possible. *International Journal of Language & Communication Disorders, 36*(Suppl), 126–131.

Cline, T., & Baldwin, S. (2004). *Selective mutism in children* (2nd ed.). London: Whurr.

Cohan, S. L., Chavira, D. A., ShiponBlum, E., Hitchcock, C., Roesch, S. C., & Stein, M. B. (2008). Refining the classification of children with selective mutism: A latent profile analysis. *Journal of Clinical Child and Adolescent Psychology, 37*(4), 770–784.

Cohan, S. L., Chavira, D. A., & Stein, M. B. (2006). Practitioner review: Psychosocial interventions for children with selective mutism: A critical evaluation of the literature from 1990–2005. *Journal of Child Psychology and Psychiatry, 47*(11), 1085–1097.

Cohan, S. L., Price, J. M., & Stein, M. B. (2006). Suffering in silence: Why a developmental psychopathology perspective on selective mutism is needed. *Journal of Developmental and Behavioral Pediatrics, 27*(4), 341–355.

Compton, S. N., March, J. S., Brent, D., Albano, A. M., Weersing, V. R., & Curry, J. (2004). Cognitive-behavioral psychotherapy for anxiety and depressive disorders in children and adolescents: An evidence-based medicine review. *Journal of the American Academy of Child and Adolescent Psychiatry, 43*(8), 930–959.

Costa, P. T., Jr., & McCrae, R. R. (1985). *The NEO personality inventory manual*. Odessa, FL: Psychological Assessment Resources.

Cunningham, C. E., McHolm, A. E., & Boyle, M. H. (2006). Social phobia, anxiety, oppositional behavior, social skills, and self-concept in children with specific selective mutism, generalized selective mutism, and community controls. *European Child & Adolescent Psychiatry, 15*(5), 245–255.

Cunningham, C. E., McHolm, A., Boyle, M. H., & Patel, S. (2004). Behavioral and emotional adjustment, family functioning, academic performance, and social relationships in children with selective mutism. *Journal of Child Psychology and Psychiatry, 45*(8), 1363–1372.

Dummit, E. S. I. I. I., Klein, R. G., Tancer, N. K., & Asche, B. (1996). Fluoxetine treatment of children with selective mutism: An open trial. *Journal of the American Academy of Child and Adolescent Psychiatry, 35*(5), 615–621.

Dummit. E. S., Klein, R. G., Tancer, N. K., Asche, B., Martin, J., & Fairbanks, J. M. (1997). Systematic assessment of 50 children with selective mutism. *Journal of the American Academy of Child & Adolescent Psychiatry, 36*(5), 653–660.

Dummit, E. S., Klein, R. G., Tancer, N. K., & Asche, B. (1997). Systematic assessment of 50 children with selective mutism. *Journal of the American Academy of Child and Adolescent Psychiatry, 36*(5), 653–660.

Elizur, Y., & Perednik, R. (2003). Prevalence and description of selective mutism in immigrant and native families: A controlled study. *Journal of the American Academy of Child and Adolescent Psychiatry, 42*(12), 1451–1459.

First, M. B., Spitzer, R. L., Gibbon, M., & Williams, J. B. W. (2002). *Structured clinical interview for DSM-IV-TR axis I disorders research version, patient edition with psychotic screen (SCID-I/P W/ PSY SCREEN)*. New York: Biometrics Research, New York State Psychiatric Institute.

Fisak, B. J. J., Oliveros, A., & Ehrenreich, J. T. (2006). Assessment and behavioral treatment of selective mutism. *Clinical Case Studies, 5*(5), 382–402.

Fung, D. S. S., Manassis, K., Kenny, A., & Fiksenbaum, L. (2002). Web-based CBT for selective mutism. *Journal of the American Academy of Child and Adolescent Psychiatry, 41*(2), 112–113.

Giddan, J. J., Ross, G. J., Sechler, L. L., & Becker, B. R. (1997). Selective mutism in elementary school: Multidisciplinary interventions. *Language, Speech, and Hearing Services in Schools, 28*(2), 127–133.

Golwyn, D. H., & Sevlie, C. P. (1999). Phenelzine treatment of selective mutism in four prepubertal children. *Journal of Child and Adolescent Psychopharmacology, 9*(2), 109–113.

Guna-Dumitrescu, L., & Pelletier, G. (1996). Successful multimodal treatment of a child with selective mutism: A case report. *The Canadian Journal of Psychiatry/La Revue Canadienne De Psychiatrie, 41*(6), 417.

Harvey, B. H., & Milne, M. (1998). Pharmacotherapy of selective mutism: Two case studies of severe entrenched mutism responsive to adjunctive treatment with fluoxetine. *Southern African Journal of Child and Adolescent Mental Health, 10*(1), 59–66.

Jackson, M. F., Allen, R. S., Boothe, A. B., Nava, M. L., & Coates, A. (2005). Innovative analyses and interventions in the treatment of selective mutism. *Clinical Case Studies, 4*(1), 81–112.

Jylha, P., & Isometsa, E. (2006). The relationship of neuroticism and extraversion to symptoms of anxiety and depression in the general population. *Depression and Anxiety, 23*(5), 281–289.

Kehle, T. J., Madaus, M. R., Baratta, V. S., & Bray, M. A. (1998). Augmented self-modeling as a treatment for children with selective mutism. *Journal of School Psychology, 36*(3), 247–260.

Kendall, P. C. (1994). Treating anxiety disorders in children: Results of a randomized clinical trial. *Journal of Consulting and Clinical Psychology, 62*(1), 100–110.

Kristensen, H. (2000). Selective mutism and comorbidity with developmental disorder/delay, anxiety disorder, and elimination disorder. *Journal of the American Academy of Child and Adolescent Psychiatry, 39*(2), 249–256.

Kristensen, H., & Torgersen, S. (2001). MCMI-II personality traits and symptom traits in parents of children with selective mutism: A case-control study. *Journal of Abnormal Psychology, 110*(4), 648–652.

Krysanski, V. L. (2003). A brief review of selective mutism literature. *Journal of Psychology: Interdisciplinary and Applied, 137*(1), 29–40.

Kumpulainen, K., Rasanen, E., Raaska, H., & Somppi, V. (1998). Selective mutism among second-graders in elementary school. *European Child & Adolescent Psychiatry, 7*(1), 24–29.

Manassis, K., Fung, D., Tannock, R., Sloman, L., Fiksenbaum, L., & McInnes, A. (2003). Characterizing selective mutism: Is it more than social anxiety? *Depression and Anxiety, 18*(3), 153–161.

Manassis, K., Tannock, R., Garland, E. J., Minde, K., McInnes, A., & Clark, S. (2007). The sounds of silence: Language, cognition and anxiety in selective mutism. *Journal of the American Academy of Child and Adolescent Psychiatry, 46*(9), 1187–1195.

Maskey, S. (2001). Selective mutism, social phobia and moclobemide: A case report. *Clinical Child Psychology and Psychiatry, 6*(3), 363–369.

Paul, R., & Kellogg, L. (1997). Temperament in late talkers. *Journal of Child Psychology and Psychiatry, 38*(7), 803–811.

Pionek Stone, B., Kratochwill, T. R., Sladezcek, I., & Serlin, R. C. (2002). Treatment of selective mutism: A best-evidence synthesis. *School Psychology Quarterly, 17*(2), 168–190.

Remschmidt, H., Poller, M., HerpertzDahlmann, B., Hennighausen, K., & Gutenbrunner, C. (2001). A follow-up study of 45 patients with elective mutism. *European Archives of Psychiatry and Clinical Neuroscience, 251*(6), 284–296.

Rye, M. S., & Ullman, D. (1999). The successful treatment of long-term selective mutism: A case study. *Journal of Behavior Therapy and Experimental Psychiatry, 30*(4), 313–323.

Sharp, W. G., Sherman, C., & Gross, A. M. (2007). Selective mutism and anxiety: A review of the current conceptualization of the disorder. *Journal of Anxiety Disorders, 21*(4), 568–579.

Silverman, W. K., Saavedra, L. M., & Pina, A. A. (2001). Test-retest reliability of anxiety symptoms and diagnoses with anxiety disorders interview schedule for DSM-IV: Child and parent versions. *Journal of the American Academy of Child and Adolescent Psychiatry, 40*(8), 937–944.

Spasaro, S. A., & Schaefer, C. E. (Eds.). (1999). *Refusal to speak: Treatment of selective mutism in children*. Northvale, NJ: Jason Aronson.

Standart, S., & Le Couteur, A. (2003). The quiet child: A literature review of selective mutism. *Child and Adolescent Mental Health, 8*(4), 154–160.

Steffen, R., & van Waes, H. (1999). Elective mutism: Effect of dental treatment with N_2/O_2-inhalation sedation: Review and report of case. *Journal of Dentistry for Children, 66*(1), 66–69.

Steinhausen, H. C., & Adamek, R. (1997). The family history of children with elective mutism: A research report. *European Child & Adolescent Psychiatry, 6*(2), 107–111.

Steinhausen, H. C., & Juzi, C. (1996). Elective mutism: An analysis of 100 cases. *Journal of the American Academy of Child and Adolescent Psychiatry, 35*(5), 606–614.

Steinhausen, H. C., Wachter, M., Laimbock, K., & Winkler Metzke, C. (2006). A long-term outcome study of selective mutism in childhood. *Journal of Child Psychology and Psychiatry, 47*(7), 751–756.

Toppelberg, C. O., Tabors, P., Coggins, A., Lum, K., & Burger, C. (2005). Differential diagnosis of selective mutism in bilingual children. *Journal of the American Academy of Child and Adolescent Psychiatry, 44*(6), 592–595.

Vecchio, J. L., & Kearney, C. A. (2005). Selective mutism in children: Comparison to youths with and without anxiety disorders. *Journal of Psychopathology and Behavioral Assessment, 27*(1), 31–37.

Viana, A. G., Beidel, D. C., & Rabian, B. (2009). Selective mutism: A review and integration of the last 15 years. *Clinical Psychology Review, 29*(1), 57–67.

Yeganeh, R., Beidel, D. C., & Turner, S. M. (2006). Selective mutism: More than social anxiety? *Depression and Anxiety, 23*(3), 117–123.

Chapter 9
Juvenile Sex Offender

Take heed that ye despise not one of these little ones; for I say unto you, That in heaven their angels do always behold the face of my Father...

Matthew 18:10
King James Bible (1769)

9.1 Overview and Historical Context

Accounts from history suggest that sexual abuse has been around since the dawn of civilization. The practice of pederasty in Ancient Greek society where an older man engages in a sexual relationship with a teenage boy would clearly be considered pedophilia by contemporary standards. Giacoma Casanova, the eighteenth century Italian writer and adventurer may be recognized by history as the world's greatest lover, but he also deserves the title pedophile. In his writings, Casanova boasted about his conquests with girls as young as 11. It was not until the late eighteenth century that societies in western Europe recognized that practices such as those of Casanova or those within Ancient Greek society could severely adversely impact children. The first western society to vehemently protest childhood prostitution and codify a law about age of consent was England. In 1885, W.T. Stead of London decried the prevalence of prostitution wherein he featured the account of a 13-year-old child being bought for five pounds. As a result of this publication, the age of consent in England was raised from 13 to 16 years as public horror intensified over child prostitution. By this time, both the lay and psychiatric community recognized the adverse impact of childhood sexual abuse with a further suspicion that sexual abuse victimization leads to sexual perpetration (i.e., recognition that sexual predators are made, not born).

S.C. Dombrowski et al., *Assessing and Treating Low Incidence/High Severity Psychological Disorders of Childhood*, DOI 10.1007/978-1-4419-9970-2_9, © Springer Science+Business Media, LLC 2011

It is now widely accepted that juvenile sex offending is a significant societal problem. Research indicates that juveniles commit upwards of 30% of documented rapes and anywhere from 30 to 60% of child molestation (Hunter, 1999; Weinrott, 1996). Even more startling, retrospective studies regarding adult perpetrators indicate that about half began their perpetration during adolescence (Abel & Rouleau, 1990; Barbaree, Hudson, & Seto, 1993; Bischof, Stith, & Whitney, 1995; Ertl & McNamara, 1997). This research suggests critical need for prevention and intervention to stop the cycle of sexual abuse.

9.2   Description and Classification

The National Adolescent Perpetrator's Network defines a juvenile sex offender as a youngster ranging from puberty to the legal age of majority (Lakey, 1994), although prepubescent juveniles have also committed sexual offenses as young as age 10 (Wieckowski, Hartsoe, Mayer, & Shortz, 1998). Wieckowski et al. report that juveniles in their study, at the time of their apprehension, committed an average of 69.5 offenses on an average of 16.5 victims. The majority of the offenders use force, threats, or violence. Barbaree, Hudson, et al. (1993) report that adolescents commit up to 50% of all child molestations in the USA and nearly one-fifth of all rapes. In 1995, approximately 16,000 adolescents were arrested for sexual offenses excluding rape and childhood prostitution (Sickmund, Snyder, & Poe-Yamagata, 1997).

The DSM-IV TR does not contain a specific diagnostic category for juvenile sexual predators. Youth who commit sexual offenses would likely have DSM-IV TR classification of conduct disorder since one of the criterion of CD – violation of the rights of others – is a central feature of the juvenile sexual offender who often uses coercion, threats, or violence to commit their offenses (Wieckowski et al., 1998). In fact, the cluster of poor impulse control and antisocial behavior also indicates that juvenile sexual offending has been associated with attention–deficit/ hyperactivity disorder (Nelson, 2007). Becker (1998) suggests that juvenile sexual offenders may also experience a high degree of depression, substance abuse, adjustment disorder, and social phobia.

9.3   Etiology

There are numerous factors that are thought to contribute sexual perpetration among juveniles. These include the sexual assault cycle, prior history of sexual abuse, individual characteristics, precocious pornography exposure, and cultural context.

9.3.1 Sexual Assault Cycle

One etiological explanation for juvenile sexual offending is the sexual assault cycle (Becker, 1994; Cashwell & Caruso, 1997). Based upon learning theory, the cycle starts when the youth is sexually abused in childhood and subsequently experiences a negative self-image and distorted cognitions about the world. This leads to maladaptive coping strategies, the anticipation of negative reactions from others, and a defensive response where the youth socially isolates and withdraws. To compensate for this sense of powerlessness, the youth fantasizes about situations where the youth is in control. This fantasization leads to victimization of another child, subsequent feelings of negative self-image, and a perpetuation of the sexual assault cycle (Becker, 1994). Ryan, Miyoshi, Metzner, Krugman, and Fryer (1996) conducted a study on 1,600 juvenile sex offenders and found that predatory behavior progressed and escalated from childhood through adolescence and beyond.

9.3.2 Prior History of Sexual Abuse

It is well-known within the child maltreatment and family systems literature that sexual abuse victimization may beget sexual abuse perpetration in some children. The rate of sexual victimization among juvenile offenders ranges from 30 to 70% in some studies (Eisenman & Kristsonis, 1995; Vizard, Monck, & Misch, 1995) and from 40 to 80% in others (Hunter & Becker, 1998). Several studies indicate that a family history of sexual abuse is a risk factor for the development of perpetration (Cooper, Murphy, & Haynes, 1996; Graham, 1996; Spaccarelli, Bowden, Coatsworth, & Kim, 1997). Although many adolescents who commit sexual offenses have experienced victimization, the majority of youth who are victimized do not go on to become sex offenders (Becker & Murphy, 1998). Multiple factors, and not solely sexual victimization as a child, are associated with sexual predatory behavior.

9.3.3 Family Dysfunction

A chaotic and dysfunctional family environment often lies at the foundation of the psychopathology (Mash & Barkley, 2003). It is not different from juvenile sex offending. Predatory sexual behavior in juveniles is sometimes directly or indirectly linked to domestic violence including child maltreatment and/or partner abuse (Becker & Hunter, 1997). Several studies indicate that family instability, violence, disorganization, and sexual/physical abuse is associated with juvenile sexual offenses (Barbaree, Hudson, et al., 1993; Bischof et al., 1995).

The theme of violence in the family is common in juvenile sexual predators, including experience of or exposure to physical abuse, sexual abuse, and violence in the home.

9.3.4 Individual Characteristics

Juvenile sexual perpetrators have noted deficits in social and interpersonal skills and have been described as lonely and socially isolated from their peers (Barbaree, Hudson, et al., 1993). Other studies indicate a preference for the company of children, rather than age-typical peers and a naivete in both interpersonal style and sexual knowledge (Nelson, 2007). Juvenile predators have also experienced loss, rejection, and a lack of empathy and warmth from parental figures that contribute to a distorted sense of attachment security. Youngsters with poor attachment security are less popular with their peers and struggle with expression in intimate relationships (Marshall & Eccles, 1993). Marshall (1996) reported on young males and found that a significant number had few social contacts and close friends and absent, detached, or rejecting parents. It was hypothesized that a fear of intimacy contributed to initial sexual offending. Dombrowski, Ahia, and McQuillan (2003) and others (e.g., Browne & Finkelhor, 1986) suggest that the child abuse leads to a host of long-term psychological and behavioral sequelae including fear, anxiety, depression, anger, inappropriate sexual behavior, low self-esteem, difficulty with intimate relationships, and substance use. Other studies suggest that more chronic juvenile offenders suffer from a personality disorder (Reiss, Grubin, & Meux, 1996) as well as impaired behavioral and peer functioning (Hunter & Figueredo, 2000; van Wijk et al., 2006).

9.3.5 Pornography Exposure

Because exposure to pornography can distort a youngster's understanding of positive sexual relationships, Dworkin (1981) indicates that pornography has been linked to sexual offending, especially when the pornography contains violent themes where the victim is portrayed as enjoying the sadistic sexual acts perpetrated upon the victim (Emerick & Dutton, 1993). It seems that juvenile sex offenders use and fantasize about an offense via pornography (Zgourides, Monto, & Harris, 1997). And, juvenile sex offenders generally have been exposed to sexually explicit materials within their home as young children (Wieckowski et al., 1998). Pornography has been identified as a causative factor in sexual crimes. In research on adult offenders, Dworkin and MacKinnon (1988) found that pornography is commonly used by sex offenders, both during and after perpetration of the crime.

Hanser and Mire (2008) indicate that many youthful offenders obtain knowledge about and socialization into sexual offending not only through direct experience (e.g., victimization), but also through vicarious learning (e.g., viewing of pornographic material). The Internet is now a powerful medium for access to pornography. This makes it essential that sexual predators do not have unmonitored access to the Internet, which could only serve to hamper intervention efforts and lead to continued perpetration (Dombrowski, Gischlar, & Durst, 2007; Dombrowski, LeMasney, Ahia, & Dickson, 2004). Pornography is a powerful reinforcing mechanism for the sexual offender especially when used to augment fantasies that reinforce predatory behavior. Also, the Internet promotes early exposure to pornography or other erotic material which contributes to precocious sexual knowledge which has been linked to a variety of childhood sexual experimentation (Hanser & Mire, 2008). Also, the type of pornographic material can lay the groundwork for sexual offending, particularly if the pornography involves sadistic acts showing the victim enjoying the sexual abuse. Juvenile sex offenders have exposure to pornography at a younger age.

9.3.6 Substance Use

Substance use is not a causal factor in sexual offending, although it has been demonstrated to be associated with other antisocial behavior (Harris & Staunton, 2000). There is no apparent link between substance abuse and child sexual abuse except in situations where sexual abuse was used to fund drugs and alcohol (Wolfers, 1992). In this circumstance, the willing victim of sexual victimization might become an abuser himself. Davis and Leitenberg (1987) contend that intoxication at the time of offense is uncommon and claims of such may be used as a way of avoiding responsibility. There seems to be a schism between clinical perception of the association between substance use (e.g., Abracen, Looman, & Langton, 2008) and sexual perpetration and empirical evidence which suggests that the association with sexual predation is limited. Thus, there is no strong empirical evidence to suggest substance use is linked to sexual perpetration in young children. On the other hand, some recent adolescent research with entering college women suggests that increasing drinking combined with psychological issues increases risk for victimization (Parks, Romosz, Bradizza, & Hsieh, 2008).

9.3.7 Cultural Context

Western culture generally emphasizes sexual prowess in men and the capacity of women to use their sexuality for secondary gain. Women's bodies are objectified by western businesses to sell products. Soft pornography is now prevalent and directed toward men. Adolescent males grow up in an era of mixed messages in which attitudes toward women are ambivalent. Given the noted social-cognitive processing deficits in youth who engage in antisocial acts, this can often lead to or reinforce distorted perceptions of sexuality.

From a feminist perspective, Cossins (2000) and others (e.g., Purvis & Ward, 2006) contend that male sex offenders victimize children when there are real or perceived threats to the perpetrator's sense of power. Perpetration might occur when a male feels inadequate around other males or when an accomplished, high-status male wants to preserve his status in a group of other powerful men who perhaps represent a constant threat to the position and experience of power. Although Cossin's feminist perspective on child victimization is written about adult perpetration, the perspective can easily be extended to male, adolescent youth who feel a sense of powerlessness in either their home or social milieu (i.e., school).

9.4   Assessment

The evaluation of juvenile sexual predators should be comprehensive and include an assessment of cognitive, academic, behavioral, and social–emotional functioning. The assessment should also focus on narrow issues related to the offending. Both informal and structured interview methods and more objective psychological assessment should be used for assessment. Through both interview techniques and rating forms, the clinician may ascertain information about an offender's deviant fantasies. For instance, the youth should be asked how old he was the first time he fantasized about a specific sexual behavior and the first time he actually engaged in that behavior. Assessment for the presence of a paraphilia is also critical. Paraphilias, according to the DSM-IV TR, are recurrent, intense sexually arousing fantasies, sexual urges, or behaviors generally involving (1) nonhuman objects, (2) the suffering or humiliation of oneself or one's partner, or (3) children or other nonconsenting persons that occur over a periods of at least 6 months. Paraphilias can contribute to highly reinforced paired associations that are very resistant to change. Juvenile sex offenders that develop paraphilias have a very poor prognosis for treatment and a high rate of recidivism. The presence of a paraphilia is one of the best indicators of future sex offenses. Thus, it is crucial for clinicians to identify youth with paraphilias and develop individualized counter-conditioning exercises. In addition to paraphilias, a recent research study indicated that two additional factors – impulsivity and antisocial traits – increased risk of recidivism (Parks & Bard, 2006).

9.4.1   Self-Report Instruments

One instrument that is used to evaluate the cognitive distortions of juveniles is the Adolescent Cognitions Scale (ACS). Psychometric limitations (e.g., low test–retest reliability and internal consistency ratings) hamper utility of the instrument. Scores on the instrument may be influenced by factors other than the youth's belief/cognitions suggesting that the instrument is measuring a construct other than deviant sexual beliefs. Hunter, Becker, Kaplan, and Goodwin (1991) found no differences on the raw scores of the ACS between a sample of juvenile sex offenders and a group of community adolescents who were not in mental health treatment and who had no history of either victimization or perpetration. In combination, the ACS should not be deemed a reliable measure for the assessment of juvenile sex offenders.

The Adolescent Sexual Interest Cardsort (ASIC) is a self-report instrument that contains 64 vignettes which are rated by the respondent on a five-point scale reflecting sexual interest (i.e., arousal to the vignettes; Hunter, Becker, & Kaplan, 1995). The instrument contains adequate reliability, but limited concurrent validity as assessed by correlations with plethysmography. Due to poor validity evidence, Hunter et al. indicate that the ACS may only be useful with juveniles who are highly disclosing. One other limiting factor is the lack of normative base of community juveniles to ascertain normal from deviant. Thus, psychometric limitations significantly hamper this instrument as well.

9.4.2 Objective Assessment Instruments

The Abel Assessment for Sexual Interest (AASI) is designed to measure sexual interest in a less intrusive way than plethysmography. The AASI measures time spent viewing categories of pictures as a measure of sexual interest. Participants are not aware that their time spent viewing cards is being measured. Smith and Fischer (1999) conducted a study using the AASI and found problematic reliability and validity. Smith and Fischer reported no significant difference in time viewing between a group of sex offenders and nonsexual offenders. Abel et al. (2004) conducted a larger-scale study using receiver operating characteristic (ROC) analysis and found that the AASI does not discriminate between offenders who had molested children and those who had not. Because of poor psychometrics, the AASI should not be viewed as a valid and reliable measure of juvenile sex offending.

Although there are numerous instruments available for use in the assessment of risk of reoffending of adult offenders (e.g., Statis-99, Hanson & Thorton, 2000; SVR-20, Boer, Hart, Kropp, & Webster, 1997; sex offender risk appraisal guide, Quinsey, Harris, Rice, & Cormier, 1998), there are only two assessment instruments that assess risk of recidivism in juveniles. These two instruments – the Juveniles Sex Offender Assessment Protocol-II (J-SOAP-II; Prentky & Righthand, 2003) and the Estimate of Risk of Adolescent Sexual Offense Recidivism (ERASOR; Worling & Curwen, 2001) – have an empirical basis for use with juvenile offenders. Factor analytic research by the test authors generally confirm the facture structure posited in the technical manual of the J-SOAP-II (Righthand et al., 2005). Several scales on the J-SOAP-II also correlated highly with the Youth Level of Service/Case Management Inventory, establishing a degree of concurrent validation of the instrument (Righthand et al.). Similarly, test–retest reliability and internal consistency studies demonstrate adequate to good reliability scores. The available psychometric evidence regarding the J-SOAP-II suggests that it is a reliable instrument for assessing populations of juvenile offenders *at risk* for reoffending.

The ERASOR (Worling & Curwen, 2001) is another instrument with empirical support for use with juvenile offenders. Research evidence indicates both validity and reliability evidence. Validity evidence was established via ROC analysis where the total score and clinical rating of risk were found to be better than chance at identifying juvenile recidivism (Worling, 2004). Inter-rater reliability estimates for the ERASOR were good at 0.92. Internal consistency was adequate on all items (except for four items). Although the ERASOR demonstrated capacity to identify those juveniles who committed a sexual offense after having already been caught for a prior sexual assault, Fanniff and Becker (2006a) indicate that a high score does not necessarily reflect the same construct as recidivism.

There is need for additional research into instruments with capacity to predict future recidivism. Still, the two assessment instrument discussed above do show adequate psychometric properties but will need additional validity evidence before being able to predict recidivism. These instruments should be considered useful to clinicians conducting a comprehensive evaluation of repeat sex offender risk, but should not be relied upon as a source to determine risk of first time perpetration. The field lacks a psychometric instrument for such purposes.

9.4.2.1   Plethysmography

Penile plethysmography is one assessment approach that has been discussed in the literature. Plethysmography should not at this point be considered a valid approach to the assessment of deviant sexual arousal because it is possible that adolescents may be able to suppress arousal. Because of empirical and ethical limitations, Fanniff and Becker (2006a) contend that pletysmography does not seem to be an appropriate assessment of juveniles sex offenders.

9.4.2.2   Polygraph

Considerable controversy yet an even more considerable research base regarding the utility of the polygraphy is available. The National Research Council of the National Academies (2003) indicates that the polygraph is able to detect lying at rates greater than chance but far less than perfection. The only available research study regarding the use of polygraphs with juvenile sex offenders suggest that juveniles disclose more fully during polygraph exams than clinical interviews or through collateral sources (Emerick & Dutton, 1993). Regardless of increased disclosure via polygraph, there is insufficient evidence to recommend its use as part of a standard assessment battery.

9.4.3   Conclusion: Assessment of Juvenile Offenders

The instruments that are available to clinicians to predict first time offending in youth generally lack appropriate psychometric properties including sufficient normative properties, reliability, and validity. The instruments do not include in the normative sample an assessment of youth who do not offend. Therefore, the field lacks instruments that can differentiate normative adolescent sexual behavior from pathological. The two instruments available that assess risk of juvenile's reoffending have improved psychometric properties, but require additional predictive validity evidence. Both the plethysmograph and polygraph should generally be avoided for clinical assessment purposes given problems with accuracy, although some research contends that the plethysmograph might be useful in the clinical evaluation for older adolescents who have targeted male child victims (Fanniff & Becker, 2006a). Still, ethical concerns remain regarding their use (Association for the Treatment of Sexual Abusers, 1997).

9.5   Prevention and Intervention

The sexual abuse of youth is a pernicious crime. As a result, prevention/intervention activities are vitally important. Nelson (2007) comments that a primary goal of intervention is to prevent recidivism. Regardless of treatment style, confronting a youth's denial about the harmfulness and inappropriateness of sex offending is the first critical component of treatment and subsequent treatment goals cannot proceed without sex offender admission of offense and recognition of its adverse impact on the victim (Cashwell & Caruso, 1997; Ertl & McNamara, 1997). To aide in case conceptualization and treatment planning, the clinician is encouraged to assess sex offender motivation, emotional responses, offense patterns, and other factors that trigger sex offending (Fanniff & Becker, 2006b).

9.6   Treatment Modalities

9.6.1   Cognitive-Behavioral Therapy

The treatment of sexual offending youth through a cognitive-behavioral modality has several goals. These include eliminating or decreasing deviant sexual thoughts, changing maladaptive belief systems, increasing the understanding that perpetration harms the victim, learning how to control sexually inappropriate urges and behaviors, increasing social skills, and increasing understanding of sex and sex values (Becker, 1994). Several cognitive-behavioral techniques are used with juvenile sex offenders including role-playing to confront cognitive distortions, covert desensitization, verbal and masturbatory satiation training, imaginal systematic desensitization, and cognitive restructuring (Cashwell & Caruso, 1997; Ertl & McNamara, 1997; Nelson, 2007).

9.6.1.1   Satiation

Satiation therapy instructs offenders to use deviant cognitions through mantra-like repetition to satiate themselves with those same thoughts that previously were found arousing (Becker, 1990). Becker and Becker and Murphy (1988) used verbal satiation whereby offenders repeated statements to the point of boredom. McGrath, Hoke, and Vojtisek (1998) utilized verbal satiation following masturbation to orgasm by requiring perpetrators to repeatedly verbalize deviant sexual fantasies until they become less sexually arousing. Rosenberg (2002) used masturbatory satiation where the client and clinician attempted to shape client's masturbatory practices toward more appropriate sexual stimuli. Hunter and Santos (1990) allowed juvenile offenders to choose masturbatory or verbal satiation. An investigation of verbal satiation's effectiveness on deviant sexual arousal suggested that verbal satiation was able to reduce deviant sexual arousal in juvenile sex offenders (Hunter & Goodwin, 1992; Kaplan, Morales, & Becker, 1993). However, no statistical analyses were performed and comparison to a control group was lacking. These studies further indicated that offenders with a more extensive history of offending may be more difficult to reduce deviant sexual arousal.

9.6.1.2   Covert Sensitization

In another cognitive-behavioral intervention, McGrath et al. (1998) used covert sensitization whereby clients were asked to imagine events that led up to their sexual perpetration and to interrupt these chain of events by imagining an aversive consequence (e.g., being caught committing one of these offenses and being sent to a youth detention center). de Silva (1999) discussed a type of systematic desensitization called masturbatory reconditioning where the client switches to a conventional sexual stimuli just prior to orgasm. The hypothesis is that this type of pairing will replace deviant sexual fantasies with conventional ones. Weinrottt, Riggan, and Frothingham (1997) used vicarious sensitization, similar to covert sensitization, where offenders listened to crime scenarios, individualized to their offense and fantasies, and were subsequently exposed to video vignettes depicting aversive consequences that could result from sexually abusive behavior. Follow-up reports using the Adolescent Sexual Interest Cardsort, parent report, and reduced arousal as measures by plethysmography suggested reduced deviant arousal. Although these studies suggested improvement, Aylwin, Reddon, and Burke (2005) found that convert sensitization was not different from no treatment at 12 months follow-up. This suggests that additional research is necessary before concluding that covert sensitization is an empirically effective treatment for juvenile sex offenders.

9.6.1.3   Cognitive Restructuring

Lockhart, Saunders, and Cleveland (1988) indicate that cognitive restructuring is a useful technique for working with juvenile sex offenders. Cognitive restructuring (e.g., Becker, 1990; Becker, Kaplan, & Kavoussi, 1988) involves client's examination of distorted thoughts and beliefs that underlie sexually deviant behavior with subsequent clinician challenging of distorted thoughts and beliefs. For instance, the therapist will confront rationalizations and permission-giving statement used by offenders. Fanniff and Becker (2006b) report a dearth of empirical validation of cognitive restructuring with juvenile sex offenders. Becker (1994) reports an 8% recidivism rate following cognitive-behavioral therapy.

9.6.1.4   Combined Cognitive-Behavioral Approaches

Becker et al. (1988) analyzed a multicomponent cognitive-behavioral intervention which included satiation, cognitive restructuring, covert sensitization, social-skills training, sex education, and relapse prevention. Becker et al. found that juvenile offenders decreased their arousal to deviant stimuli posttreatment, with offenders targeting males experiencing a greater decrease than offenders targeting females. A similar analysis of a multicomponent cognitive-behavioral treatment approach was conducted by Hunter and Santos (1990). Adolescent sex offenders received satiation therapy, covert sensitization, insight-oriented group and individual psychotherapy, and family therapy. Results of this treatment indicated a decrease in deviant arousal to child victims.

9.6.1.5   Conclusion: Cognitive-Behavioral Therapy

Cognitive-behavioral therapy is a promising approach to the treatment of juvenile sex offenders. There is a modest amount of empirical support, but effectiveness determination is hampered by research that lacks comparison groups, random assignment, and has small sample sizes. Future research should include longer-term outcome assessment to determine whether cognitive-behavioral treatment reduces recidivism.

9.6.2   Multisystemic Therapy

Multisystemic therapy is an integrative, ecological approach to treatment that targets and uses individual, family, and neighborhood/school/community factors (Borduin,

Henggeler, Blaske, & Stein, 1990). Multisystemic therapy attempts to facilitate change in the youth offender's naturalistic environment using strengths at various spheres of treatment (e.g., family, peers, school, neighborhood). Borduin et al., 1990 compared MST with individual therapy with 16 juvenile sex abusers and found that MST had lower re-arrest rates for sexual offenses (12.5%) compared with 75% with offenders in individual therapy.

9.6.3 Relapse Prevention Model

Adapted from the substance abuse treatment literature, the relapse prevention model emphasizes the need for ongoing treatment, supervision, and support services for sex offenders, particularly after the offender has been released from custody (Becker, 1994). Punishment and loss of privileges are applied following inappropriate behavior such as possession of pornography our use of illicit substances. One of the initial steps of the relapse prevention model is to teach the offender to identify situations that have a high probability of relapse. The next step is to teach the offender how to deal with high-risk situations. As part of this model, self-monitoring strategies are delineated in a contract with family members where the offender agrees to avoid high-risk situations. Ertl and McNamara (1997) also recommend weekly meetings with a counselor to review treatment progress.

9.6.4 Group Therapy

Research (e.g., Lakey, 1994; Marshall, Anderson, & Fernandez, 1999) suggests that group therapy is a highly effective treatment modality for adolescent sexual predators. Group counseling can be effective in enhancing self-esteem and developing interpersonal skills. The group process also permits other group members to challenge the offender's denials and minimizations (Ertl & McNamara, 1997). The group can also be used for psychoeducational purposes where sex education and appropriate sex roles are taught. The group can also furnish the offender a support system, providing relief from feelings of isolation (Cashwell & Caruso, 1997). Other treatment issues that have been addressed during group therapy include enhancing self-esteem, increasing empathy and remorse toward victims, and facilitating stress management (Barbaree et al., 1993). Within group therapy, treatment might come in the form of lectures, discussion, exercises, instructional videos, movies, journal writing, assignments, and role playing. To develop empathy for victims, some treatment programs require offenders to read letters, poems, and drawings (Ertl & McNamara). Other anecdotal accounts used to foster empathy might include the sharing of testimonials from child victims and the lifelong pain experienced by the victim and their families (Lakey, 1994).

9.6.5   *Issues for Therapists*

The treatment of juvenile sex offenders is not an easy task and is not for the garden variety clinician. It takes a special therapist who can navigate the myriad therapeutic issues involved in working with juvenile predators. If a therapist feels that he or she cannot work with a particular client (or this entire population), then it is best to determine this immediately so that the therapist can transfer the client to another counselor with expertise in working with juvenile sex offenders. When working with juvenile sexual predators, it will be incumbent upon the therapist to inform the client of the limits to confidentiality including notification that the therapist is both legally and ethically required to inform the proper authorities upon learning that the client has victimized another youth (Dombrowski et al., 2003). This disclosure should occur at the onset of therapy. In any therapeutic relationship, therapeutic trust is an essential ingredient for successful treatment. Disclosure of the limits of a therapists' confidentiality is an essential element in fostering that trust. Clinicians with little experience in working with juvenile offenders might overlook serious behavior and instead think it may be sexual experimentation when in fact it may be sexual predation. Other potential issues include grouping together all juvenile sex offenders instead of individualizing treatment approaches. Perhaps even counselor/ therapist training programs do an insufficient job of training future clinicians to work with juvenile sex offenders? There are facilities (e.g., UC Davis Medical Center) that provide specialized training at the pre- and postdoctoral level, but these facilities tend to be rare.

9.7   Conclusion and Future Directions

The sexual abuse of children is a pernicious crime and significant social malady. Because of its long-term adverse impact on many domains of functioning, sexual abuse is often considered soul murder (Dombrowski et al., 2004), whether perpetrated by a juvenile or an adult. Appropriate and thorough assessment along with subsequent treatment and close monitoring of treatment progress are vitally important. The treatment approaches that are available in the literature have adequate empirical evidence although they suffer from small sample sizes and a lack of long-term follow-up. Future research should investigate the long-term effects of treatment and whether the effects can be sustained. Nontraditional assessment such as plethysmography and polygraphy contain insufficient validity evidence and pose ethical dilemmas, so their use should be curtailed. It is important to recognize that treatment for juvenile sexual offending should occur not only at the level of the individual, but also at a cultural level. Western culture must more fully recognize the adverse impact of marginalizing sexuality for commercial gain. Even worse is the pervasive availability of sadistic pornography. Juvenile sexual predators typically have noted social-cognitive processing deficits, so any exposure to pornography that displays sexual abuse victimization with the victim actually enjoying the abuse can furnish a model for acceptance of and continued participation in sexual perpetration. Society and mental health practitioners need to increase recognition that juvenile sexual offenders commit a large percentage of sexual offenses and that the deleterious impact of such offenses are just as devastating as those perpetrated by adult offenders. The research literature shows promise for documenting that juvenile sexual offenders respond to treatment. Only a small percentage of juveniles who receive treatment go on to re-offend (Abracen et al., 2008). Regardless of recidivism, working with youth who commit sexual offenses is complex and requires specialized education and training.

References

Abel, G. G., Jordan, A., Rouleau, J. L., Emerick, R., Barboza-Whitehead, S., & Osborn, C. (2004). Use of visual reaction time to assess male adolescents who molest children. *Sexual Abuse: A Journal of Research and Treatment, 16*, 255–265.

Abel, G. G., & Rouleau, J. L. (1990). The nature and extent of sexual assault. In W. L. Marshall, D. R. Laws, & H. E. Barbaree (Eds.), *Handbook of sexual assault* (pp. 9–21). New York, NY: Plenum Press.

Abracen, J., Looman, J., & Langton, C. M. (2008). Treatment of sexual offenders with psychopathic traits: Recent research developments and clinical implications. *Trauma Violence Abuse, 3*, 144–166.

Association for the Treatment of Sexual Abusers. (1997). *Ethical standards and principles for the management of sexual abusers*. Beaverton, OR: Author.

Aylwin, A., Reddon, J., & Burke, A. (2005). Sexual fantasies of adolescent male sex offenders in residential treatment: A descriptive study. *Archives of Sexual Behavior, 34*(2), 231–239.

Barbaree, H. E., Hudson, S. M., & Seto, M. C. (1993). Sexual assault in society: The role of the juvenile offender. In H. E. Barbaree, W. L. Marshall, & S. M. Hudson (Eds.), *The juvenile sex offender* (pp. 1–24). New York: Guilford Press.

Becker, J. V. (1990). Treating adolescent sex offenders. *Professional Psychology: Research and Practice, 21*, 362–365.

Becker, J. V. (1994). Offenders: Characteristics and treatment. *The Future of Children, 4*(2), 176–197.

Becker, J. V. (1998). What we know about the characteristics and treatment of adolescents who have committed sexual offenses. *Child Maltreatment, 3*, 317–329.

Becker, J. V., & Hunter, J. A. (1997). Understanding and treating child and adolescent sexual offenders. *Advances in Clinical Child Psychology, 19*, 177–197.

Becker, J. V., Kaplan, M. S., & Kavoussi, R. (1988). Measuring the effectiveness of treatment for the aggressive adolescent sexual offender. *Annals of the New York Academy of Sciences, 528*, 215–222.

Becker, J., & Murphy, W. (1998). What we know and don't know about assessing and treating sex offenders. *Psychology, Public Policy and Law, 4*, 116–137.

Bischof, G. P., Stith, S. M., & Whitney, M. L. (1995). Family environments of adolescent sex offenders and other juvenile delinquents. *Adolescence, 30*(117), 157–171.

Boer, D. P., Hart, S. D., Kropp, P. R., & Webster, C. D. (1997). *Manual for the Sexual Violence Risk-20: Professional guidelines for assessing risk of sexual violence*. Burnaby, BC: The British Columbia Institute Against Family Violence.

Borduin, C. M., Henggeler, S. W., Blaske, D. M., & Stein, R. (1990). Multisystemic treatment of adolescent sexual offenders. *International Journal of Offender Therapy and Comparative Criminology, 35*, 105–114.

Browne, A., & Finkelhor, D. (1986). Impact of child sexual abuse: A review of the research. *Psychological Bulletin, 99*, 66–77.

Cashwell, C. S., & Caruso, M. E. (1997). Adolescent sex offenders: Identification and intervention strategies. *Journal of Mental Health Counseling, 19*(4), 336–348.

Cooper, C. L., Murphy, W. D., & Haynes, M. R. (1996). Characteristics of abused and nonabused adolescent sex offenders. *Sexual Abuse: A Journal of Research and Treatment, 8*, 105–119.

Cossins, A. (2000). *Masculinities, sexualities and child sexual abuse*. The Hague, Netherlands: Kluwer Law International.

Davis, G. E., & Leitenberg, H. (1987). Adolescent sexual offenders. *Psychological Bulletin, 101*, 417–427.

De Silva, W. (1999). Public attitudes toward the treatment of sex offenders. *Legal and Criminological Psychology, 4*, 239–252.

Dombrowski, S. C., Ahia, C. E., & McQuillan, K. (2003). Protecting children through mandated child abuse reporting. *The Educational Forum, 67*(2), 76–85.

Dombrowski, S. C., Gischlar, K., & Durst, T. (2007). Safeguarding youth from cyber pornography and cyber sexual predation: A major dilemma of the Internet. *Child Abuse Review, 16*(3), 153–170.

Dombrowski, S. C., LeMasney, J. W., Ahia, C. E., & Dickson, S. A. (2004). Protecting children from online sexual predators: Technological, legal, and psychoeducational considerations. *Professional Psychology: Research and Practice, 35*(1), 65–73.

Dworkin, A. (1981). *Pornography: Men possessing women*. New York: Perigree Books.

Dworkin, A., & MacKinnon, C. A. (1988). *Pornography and civil rights: A new day for women's equality*. Minneapolis: Organizing Against Pornography.

Eisenman, R., & Kristsonis, W. (1995). How children learn to become sex offenders. *Psychology, 32*(1), 25.

Emerick, R. L., & Dutton, W. A. (1993). The effect of polygraphy on the self-report of adolescent sex offenders: Implications for risk assessment. *Annals of Sex Research, 6*, 83–103.

Ertl, M., & McNamara, J. (1997). Treatment of juvenile sex offenders: A review of the literature. *Child and Adolescent Social Work Journal, 14*(3), 199–221.

Fanniff, A. M., & Becker, J. V. (2006a). Specialized assessment and treatment of adolescent sex offenders. *Aggression and Violent Behavior, 11*, 265–282.

Fanniff, A. M., & Becker, J. V. (2006b). Developmental considerations in working with juvenile sex offenders. In R. Longo & D. Prescott (Eds.), *Current perspectives on working with sexually aggressive youth and youth with sexual behavior problems* (pp. 119–141). Holyoke, MA: NEARI Press.

Graham, K. R. (1996). The childhood victimisation of sex offenders: An underestimated issue. *International Journal of Offender Therapy and Comparative Criminology, 36*(3), 192–203.

Hanser, R., & Mire, S. (2008). Juvenile sex offenders in the United States and Australia: A comparison. *International Review of Law Computers and Technology, 22*, 101–114.

Hanson, R., & Bussiere, M. (1998). Predicting relapse: A meta-analysis of sexual offender recidivism studies. *Journal of Consulting and Clinical Psychology, 66*, 348–364.

Hanson, R. K., & Thorton, D. (2000). Improving risk assessment for sex offenders: A comparison of three actuarial scales. *Law and Human Behavior, 24*(1), 119–136.

Harris, V., & Staunton, C. (2000). *The atecedents of young make offenders*. London: Whurr.

Hunter, J. (1999). *Understanding juvenile sexual offending behavior: Emerging research, treatment approaches, and management practices*. Washington, DC: Center for Sex Offender Management. Available from http://www.csom.org. Accessed January 20, 2011.

Hunter, J., & Becker, J. (1998). Motivators of adolescent sex offenders and treatment perspectives. In J. Shaw (Ed.), *Sexual aggression*. Washington, DC: American Psychiatric Press Inc.

Hunter, J. A., Becker, J. V., & Kaplan, M. S. (1995). The Adolescent Sexual Interest Card Sort: Test-retest reliability and concurrent validity in relation to phallometric assessment. *Archives of Sexual Behavior, 24*, 255–261.

Hunter, J. A., Becker, J. V., Kaplan, M., & Goodwin, D. W. (1991). Reliability and discriminative validity of the Adolescent Cognitions Scale for juvenile offenders. *Annals of Sex Research, 4*, 281–286.

Hunter, J. A., & Figueredo, A. J. (2000). The influence of personality and history of sexual victim-ization in the prediction of juvenile perpetrated child molestation. *Behavior Modification, 24*, 241–263.

Hunter, J. A., & Goodwin, D. W. (1992). The clinical utility of satiation therapy with juvenile sexual offenders: Variations and efficacy. *Annals of Sex Research, 5*, 71–80.

Hunter, J., & Santos, D. (1990). The use of specialized cognitive-behavioral therapies in the treat-ment of adolescent sexual offenders. *International Journal of Offender Therapy and Comparative Criminology, 34*, 239–247.

Kaplan, M. S., Morales, M., & Becker, J. V. (1993). The impact of verbal satiation on adolescent sex offenders: A preliminary report. *Journal of Child Sexual Abuse, 2*, 81–88.

Lakey, J. F. (1994). The profile and treatment of male adolescent sex offenders. *Adolescence, 29*(116), 755–61.

Lockhart, L., Saunders, B., & Cleveland, P. (1988). Adult male sexual offenders: An overview of treatment techniques. *Journal of Social Work and Human Sexuality, 7*, 1–31.

Marshall, W. L. (1996). Assessment, treatment, and theorizing about sex offenders: Developments during past twenty years and future directions. *Criminal Justice and Behavior, 23*(1), 162–199.

Marshall, W. L., Anderson, D., & Fernandez, Y. M. (1999). *Cognitive behavioural treatment of sexual offenders*. Chichester: Wiley.

Marshall, W. L., & Eccles, A. (1993). Pavolvian conditioning processes in adolescent sex offenders. In H. E. Barbaree, W. L. Marshall, & S. M. Hudson (Eds.), *The juvenile sex offender* (pp. 118–142). New York: The Guilford Press.

Mash, E. J., & Barkley, R. A. (2003). *Child psychopathology*. New York: Gilford Press.

McGrath, R. J., Hoke, S. E., & Vojtisek, J. E. (1998). Cognitive-behavioral treatment of sex offend-ers: A treatment comparison and long-term follow-up study. *Criminal Justice and Behavior, 25*(2), 203–225.

National Research Council of the National Academies. (2003). *The polygraph and lie detection*. Washington, DC: The National Academies Press.

Nelson, M. (2007). Characteristics, treatment and practictioner's perceptions of juvenile sex offenders. *Journal for Juvenile Services, 21*, 7–16.

Parks, G. A., & Bard, D. E. (2006). Risk factors for adolescent sex offender recidivism: Evaluation of predictive factors and comparison of three groups based upon victim type. *Sex Abuse, 18*(4), 319–342.

Parks, K. A., Romosz, A. M., Bradizza, C. M., & Hsieh, Y. P. (2008). A dangerous transition: Women's drinking and related victimization from high school to the first year at college. *Journal of Studies on Alcohol and Drugs, 69*(1), 65–74.

Prentky, R., & Righthand, S. (2003). *Juvenile Sex Offender Assessment Protocol – II (JSOAP – II)*. Washington, DC: Center for Sex Offender Management Available from http://www.csom.org. Accessed January 20, 2011.

Purvis, M., & Ward, T. (2006). The role of culture in understanding child sexual offending: Examining feminist perspectives. *Aggression and Violent Behavior, 11*(3), 298–312.

Quinsey, V. L., Harris, G. T., Rice, M. E., & Cormier, C. A. (1998). *Violent offenders: Appraising and managing risk*. Washington, D.C.: American Psychological Association.

Reiss, D., Grubin, D., & Meux, C. (1996). Young 'psychopaths' in special hospital: treatment and outcome. *The British Journal of Psychiatry, 168*, 99–104.

Righthand, S., Prentky, R., Knight, R., Carpenter, E., Hecker, J. E., & Nangle, D. (2005). Factor structure and validation of the Juvenile Sex Offender Assessment Protocol (J-SOAP). *Sexual Abuse: A Journal of Research and Treatment, 17*, 13–30.

Rosenberg, M. (2002). Treatment considerations for pedophilia: Recent headlines aside, this dis-order has long confronted the behavioral healthcare community with difficult challenges. *Behavioral Health Management, 22*, 38–42.

Ryan, G., Miyoshi, T., Metzner, J., Krugman, R., & Fryer, G. (1996). Trends in a national sample of sexually abusive youths. *Journal of the American Academy of Child and Adolescent Psychiatry, 35*(1), 17–25.

Sickmund, M., Snyder, H. N., & Poe-Yamagata, E. (1997). *Juvenile offenders and victims: 1997 update on violence.* Washington, DC: Office of Juvenile Justice and Delinquency Prevention.

Smith, G., & Fischer, L. (1999). Assessment of juvenile sexual offenders: Reliability and validity of the Abel Assessment for Interest in Paraphilias. *Sexual Abuse: A Journal of Research and Treatment, 11*, 207–216.

Spaccarelli, S., Bowden, B., Coatsworth, J. D., & Kim, S. (1997). Psychosocial correlates of male sexual aggression in a chronic delinquent sample. *Criminal Justice and Behavior, 24*(1), 71–95.

Van Wijk, A., Vermeiren, R., Loeber, R., 't Hart-Kerkhoffs, L., Doreleijers, T., & Bullens, R. (2006). Juvenile sex offenders compared to non-sex offenders: A review of the literature 1995–2005. *Trauma Violence Abuse, 7*, 227–243.

Vizard, E., Monck, E., & Misch, P. (1995). Child and adolescent sex abuse perpetrators: A review of the research literature. *Journal of Child Psychology and Psychiatry, 36*, 731–756.

Weinrott, M. R. (1996). *Juvenile sexual aggression: A critical review.* Boulder, CO: Center for the Study and Prevention of Violence.

Weinrottt, M. R., Riggan, M., & Frothingham, S. (1997). Reducing deviant arousal in juvenile sex offenders using vicarious sensitization. *Journal of Interpersonal Violence, 12*, 704–728.

Wieckowski, E., Hartsoe, P., Mayer, A., & Shortz, J. (1998). Deviant sexual behavior in children and young adolescents: Frequency and patterns. *Sexual Abuse: A Journal of Research and Treatment, 10*(4), 293–303.

Wolfers, O. (1992). Same abuse, different parent. *Social Work Today, 23*(26), 16–22.

Worling, J. R. (2004). The Estimate of Risk of Adolescent Sexual Offense Recidivism (ERASOR): Preliminary psychometric data. *Sexual Abuse: A Journal of Research and Treatment, 16*, 235–254.

Worling, J. R., & Curwen, T. (2001). *The "ERASOR": Estimate of risk of juvenile sexual offense recidivism version 2.0. SAFE-T program.* Toronto, ON: Thistletown Regional Center.

Zgourides, G., Monto, M., & Harris, R. (1997). Correlates of adolescent male sexual offense: Prior adult sexual contact, sexual attitudes, and use of sexually explicit materials. *International Journal of Offender Therapy and Comparative Criminology, 41*(3), 272–283.

Chapter 10
Childhood Onset Schizophrenia

If you talk to God, you are praying; If God talks to you, you have schizophrenia.

–Thomas Szasz, Psychiatrist and Social Critic

10.1 Overview

Typically, the onset of schizophrenia occurs during late adolescence or early adulthood. Childhood onset schizophrenia (COS) is relatively rare, but is thought to represent a particularly severe and chronic form of the illness (Asarnow, Tompson, & Goldstein, 1994; Jacobsen & Rapoport, 1998). Children with COS present with a variety of symptoms, including hallucinations, delusions, disordered thought, and difficulty distinguishing psychotic symptoms from normal experience. The disorder can be debilitating because it impacts every aspect of a child's life (Foster, Swartz, & de Jager, 2006). Currently, children are diagnosed with schizophrenia using the same *Diagnostic and Statistical Manual of Mental Disorders-IV Text Revision* [DSM-IV TR; American Psychiatric Association (APA), 2000] criteria that are used for adult diagnosis (Asarnow, 1994; Gonthier & Lyon, 2004; Werry, 1992). COS, like other psychotic disorders, appears to be continuous with the adult-onset type, but developmental differences have been noted (McClellan & McCurry, 1999). For example, in children, psychosis develops rather gradually, without the sudden psychotic break that often is observed in the adult population. Furthermore, the poor functioning that is observed in children with COS may be attributable to failure to acquire skills, rather than deterioration, as is found in adults with schizophrenia (Gonthier & Lyon, 2004). Despite these developmental differences, Eggers, Bunk, and Krause (2000) suggest that COS can be reliably diagnosed in children using adult criteria and that use of comparable criteria facilitates analysis of the progression of symptoms.

S.C. Dombrowski et al., *Assessing and Treating Low Incidence/High Severity Psychological Disorders of Childhood*, DOI 10.1007/978-1-4419-9970-2_10,
© Springer Science+Business Media, LLC 2011

In recent years, myriad studies have been conducted with children with COS. Results of this research indicate three major findings that: (a) COS exists and can be reliably diagnosed; (b) there are similarities between COS and schizophrenia that develops later in life; and (c) the majority of children diagnosed with COS will continue to present with a schizophrenia-spectrum disorder in adulthood (Asarnow, Tompson, & McGrath, 2004). However, despite these advances into understanding of the disease, there continues to be a need for research into the treatment of schizophrenia in children (Asarnow et al.). This chapter provides an overview of the studies that have been conducted into the etiology and symptomatology of COS, including biological and genetic research. Along with discussion of symptoms, included are sections on assessment and intervention. Finally, the chapter ends with suggestions for future research that will enhance our understanding of COS and effective treatment modalities.

10.2   Historical Context

10.2.1   The Late 1800s and Early 1900s

The first book on child psychiatry, written by Emminghaus (1887), listed symptoms of childhood psychosis that included reduction in cognitive abilities, mood changes, and sleep disturbances. Further, Emminghaus posited that the etiology of psychosis arose from disturbances to the blood vessels of the cortex. Perhaps most importantly, his seminal work suggested that childhood psychosis should be studied from a developmental perspective and that the task of psychiatry was to distinguish typical from pathological processes at each stage of development (Remschmidt, Schulz, Martin, Warnke, & Trott, 1994).

Following the work of Emminghaus, Kraepelin (1896) who is considered to be the architect of the modern psychiatric diagnostic system, described "dementia paranoides," a condition in which the patient rapidly develops "nonsensical and incoherent persecutory and grandiose delusions." Kraepelin developed subgroups among people affected with this disorder, including dementia praecox and manic-depressive psychoses (Kendler & Tsuang, 1981; Remschmidt et al., 1994). In the early 1900s, Bleuler (1911) introduced the term "schizophrenia" and suggested that there were different forms of the disease that needed to be distinguished from one another. Further, Bleuler stated that there were no differences in the presentation of schizophrenia in children and adults, but did note that diagnosis in childhood was more difficult (Remschmidt, 2001).

A decade later, Homburger (1926) delineated the negative symptoms of COS – withdrawal, negativism, and strange and unexpected behavior. He indicated that delusions in young children were rare and listed premorbid characteristics of schizophrenia. According to Homburger, a child can generally be placed into one of the three groups: (a) children developing normally, with good intellectual functioning and no character anomalies; (b) children with mental retardations; and (c) children with normal intellectual functioning, but who display character anomalies and/or strange behaviors. Homburger's work suggested that schizophrenia in children took one of the two major forms: the slow retarded hebephrenic form with cognitive deterioration and the acute catatonic form (Remschmidt et al., 1994).

During the same time period, Karl Menninger (1928a, 1928b) discussed a possible association between influenza during pregnancy and schizophrenia in offspring. Menninger made his observation following the 1918–1919 influenza pandemic, the most virulent epidemic during that century. He suggested that the virus may have adversely impacted the developing brain of the fetus, who later was identified with schizophrenic symptoms (Dombrowski & Martin, 2009). Menninger (1928a, 1928b) initially believed that approximately one-third of those exposed to influenza in utero had characteristics of schizophrenia. As a result, he suggested that schizophrenia might be caused by the virus.

10.2.2   The Mid-1900s

Research with psychotic children continued and in the 1940s, Bender and colleagues, who observed more than 100 children diagnosed with COS at Bellevue Hospital, developed positive diagnostic criteria. Specifically, the group suggested that to be diagnosed with schizophrenia, the child must not be mentally defective, postencephalitic, or psychopathic (Bender, 1941). Further, these researchers deemed schizophrenia as a "total psychobiological disorder" (Bender, 1958). Twenty years later, a British Working Party led by Creak (1964) proposed nine diagnostic criteria for schizophrenia in children: (a) gross and sustained impairment in emotional relationships; (b) unawareness of personal identity relative to expectations for developmental level; (c) preoccupation with objects or parts of objects, without regard to function; (d) resistance to change in the environment; (e) excessive or unexpected response to sensory stimuli; (f) acute and excessive anxiety; (g) speech that has been lost or never acquired; (h) distorted motility patterns; and (i) mental retardation, accompanied by normal or exceptional functioning in isolated areas.

10.2.3   More Recent Developments in Research

Leonhard (1986), proposed some new ideas regarding the diagnosis of COS in the mid-1980s. First, he suggested that "schizophrenia" is a constellation of disorders that does not have a single etiology. Second, Leonhard did not subscribe to the traditional subcategories of schizophrenia: hebephrenic, paranoid, catatonic, and so forth. Rather, he categorized schizophrenia as being either unsystematic or systematic. The two categories that Leonhard described differ in symptoms, course, and prognosis. Unsystematic schizophrenia is characterized by affective symptoms, including anxiety, delusions, and hallucinations. The symptoms are acute and periodic and chance for remission is favorable. Systematic schizophrenia, on the other hand, is characterized by cognitive dysfunction and disturbances of voluntary functions. The course is chronic and the prognosis is poor and Leonhard posited that the etiology lies within the cerebral systems. He also suggested a form of COS, early infantile catatonia, with symptoms that included absence of language or poorly developed language skills, motor symptoms, intellectual impairment, and negativism (Remschmidt et al., 1994).

Although research in the area has spanned more than 100 years, the etiology of schizophrenia and the degree to which early behavioral deviance predicts adult diagnosis have not been conclusively determined (Bearden et al., 2000). Research has shown that some children display increased adjustment problems, including withdrawal, anxiety and aggression, and cognitive and motor dysfunction prior to diagnosis in early adulthood. However, the severity and nature of these precursors vary greatly from person to person and some have a relatively typical developmental course prior to the prodromal phase of the illness (Neumann, Grimes, Walker, & Baum, 1995). There is some evidence to suggest that poorer premorbid functioning is associated with more debilitating symptoms and poorer prognosis (Jahshan, Heaton, Golshan, & Cadenhead, 2010; Neumann et al.). However, Auther, Gillett, and Cornblatt (2008) caution that diagnosable illness will not necessarily be the case for all individuals. These findings beg more research in the area to determine the best evaluative and early intervention methods.

10.3   Description, Diagnosis, and Prevalence

10.3.1   DSM Diagnostic Criteria

The DSM-IV TR (APA, 2000) lists the following symptoms as characteristic of schizophrenia: (a) delusions; (b) hallucinations; (c) disorganized speech; (d) grossly disorganized or catatonic behavior; and (e) negative symptoms that include flat affect, alogia, or avolition. In addition to these symptoms, diagnostic criteria include social/occupational dysfunction with continuous signs of disturbance for at least a 6-month period, including at least a 1-month period of active-phase symptoms (or less if successful treatment has been administered). Schizoaffective and mood disorders, medical conditions, and substance abuse must be ruled out before a diagnosis of schizophrenia is made (APA). These criteria are used to diagnosis both adults and children (Gonthier & Lyon, 2004).

The diagnosis of a subtype of the disorder is made based on the predominant symptomatology at the time of evaluation (APA, 2000). There are five subtypes of schizophrenia:

- Paranoid
- Disorganized

- Catatonic
- Undifferentiated
- Residual (APA, 2000).

To be diagnosed with the paranoid subtype, an individual must exhibit preoccupation with one or more delusions or frequent auditory hallucinations. With this subtype, none of the following are prominent – disorganized speech, disorganized or catatonic behavior, or flat or inappropriate affect. The second subtype, disorganized type, on the other hand, has as criteria disorganized speech, disorganized behavior, and flat or inappropriate affect. Catatonic, the third subtype, is characterized by at least two of the following criteria: (a) motoric immobility or stupor; (b) excessive motor activity that appears to be purposeless; (c) extreme negativism; (d) peculiarities of voluntary movement including posturing, stereotyped movements, or prominent mannerisms or grimacing; and (e) echolalia or echopraxia. The undifferentiated subtype of schizophrenia is diagnosed when characteristic symptoms are present (see above), but criteria for the paranoid, disorganized, or catatonic subtypes are not met. Finally, the residual subtype is assigned when there has been at least one episode of schizophrenia, but the current clinical picture does not present psychotic symptoms, such as delusions, hallucinations, or disorganized speech and behavior. The individual with this diagnosis continues to present negative symptoms, including flat affect or avolition and attenuated positive symptoms, such as eccentric behavior or odd beliefs (APA, 2000).

10.3.2 Prevalence

According to the DSM-IV TR (APA, 2000), schizophrenia prevalence among the worldwide adult population is within the range of 0.5–1.5%, with annual diagnoses occurring at a rate of 0.5–5.0 per 10,000. It should be noted that numerous studies have documented the increased prevalence in first-degree relatives of patients with schizophrenia. In fact, data from family studies suggest that the prevalence rate for first-degree relatives is between 10 and 15% (Hans, Auerbach, Styr, & Marcus, 2004). Further, these same studies report that first-degree relatives of persons with schizophrenia also have a higher prevalence of personality disorders, specifically schizotypal and paranoid personality disorders. These data may suggest that schizophrenia is a spectrum disorder, although this theory remains open to investigation (Hans et al.).

10.3.2.1 Age at Onset

The median age for onset is in the early to mid-20s for males and late 20s for females (APA, 2000). Schizophrenia in children is much rarer, with rates of approximately two in one million children below the age of 13 years meeting criteria for diagnosis. During adolescence, the prevalence rate increases and symptomatology becomes similar to that found in the adult population (Remschmidt, 2008). The diagnosis of schizophrenia in children is decided with the same criteria as for adults, but the process is more difficult. At early ages, false-positive diagnoses frequently occur (Remschmidt). Although the DSM-IV-TR (APA, 2000) delineates differences between schizophrenia, schizoaffective disorder, and mood disorders, symptoms may be difficult to differentiate and, thus, diagnoses may change over the course of an individual's lifetime. Further, although numerous studies of psychosis with the adult population have been undertaken, limited studies into the clinical features and evolution of psychotic disorders in children have been conducted (Ledda, Fratta, Pintor, Zuddas, & Cianchetti, 2009).

10.3.2.2   Gender Differences

COS is diagnosed more frequently in males than females, with ratios estimated from 2:1 to 5:1 (Asarnow & Asarnow, 2003; Green, Padron-Gayol, Hardesty, & Bassiri, 1992). The ratio of males to females diagnosed with schizophrenia in adolescence is not as great. Although the exact reason for the higher prevalence among young males is not known, it has been suggested that they are more biologically vulnerable. Similar patterns are seen with neurological disorders (Asarnow & Asarnow, 2003). There appears to be no gender differences in the age of onset, however (Eggers & Bunk, 1997).

10.4   Etiological Hypotheses and Theoretical Frameworks

Commonly, schizophrenia is a recurrent disorder that has poor to moderate outcomes for most afflicted individuals (Gaebel & Frommann, 2000). Although there is no one definitive cause of schizophrenia, research has begun to unravel some of the mystery surrounding the disorder and its symptoms. Preliminary results have suggested that serious mental health disorders, including schizophrenia and bipolar disorder, may involve subtle interactions between susceptibility genes and the environment (Husted, Greenwood, & Bassett, 2006; Kestenbaum, 1980). Given that some children may be predisposed to developing schizophrenia (Husted et al.), it would be prudent to identify the early features of the disorder in designing assessment, intervention, and, ultimately, prevention tools.

Evidence is mounting that suggests that there is some degree of social and cognitive impairments present in adolescents, and perhaps even children, that are precursors to the development of adult schizophrenia (Tarbox & Pogue-Geile, 2008). It is important to study these early deficits in functioning because, although there is a known link between genes and the environment, the pathological processes that lead to psychosis and the point at which these pathologies emerge in development remains unknown. Identification of early deficits, or symptoms, may offer insight into the specific genetic and environmental correlates that cause a person to be susceptible to schizophrenia. Further, research has suggested that early pharmacological and psychotherapeutic interventions may improve long-term outcomes and, perhaps, even delay the onset of the first full psychotic episode (Tarbox & Pogue-Geile).

10.4.1   Premorbid Behavioral Indicators

In a review of the extant literature, Tarbox and Pogue-Geile (2008) suggested that poor social functioning may be the most important prepsychosis deficit in individuals with schizophrenia. Results of their review indicated that poor undifferentiated social functioning is a moderately sensitive predictor of schizophrenia in children among the general population beginning around age 7–8 years, but that it is not a good predictor with younger children. However, in families at high risk (i.e., one or both parents have a diagnosis), poor social functioning may be a good predictor of schizophrenia in children as young as 5–6 years of age. In addition, antisocial-externalizing behaviors have been demonstrated as sensitive predictors among the general population for ages 5–12 years, when compared with nonpsychotic disorders, including depression, anxiety, and neurosis. Antisocial-externalizing behaviors lose sensitivity as predictors with children older than 12 in the general population, but remain sensitive predictors among the high-risk group. Finally, social withdrawal-internalizing behaviors appear to be a moderately sensitive predictor of schizophrenia among the general population at around age 11, but the same level of sensitivity has not been observed among the high-risk group (Tarbox & Pogue-Geile). In sum, studies have demonstrated that the persistent and individual differences in social functioning associated with the disorder are among the most stable and are predictive of course and outcomes. The level of the affected individual's social functioning prior to the onset of psychosis appears to be a predictor of postonset symptom severity, cognitive deficits, and overall functioning (Tarbox & Pogue-Geile).

10.4.2   Brain Structural Differences

In addition to behavioral differences observed in children with COS, research has suggested that structural brain abnormalities may be related to the psychotic symptoms and neurocognitive deficits found within this population (Sowell, Toga, & Asarnow, 2000). In a review of the extant literature in magnetic resonance imaging (MRI) studies of children with COS, Sowell et al. found that results have consistently evidenced increased ventricular volume, reduced cerebral gray matter, and increased caudate volume in the brains of these children. In addition, although findings were inconsistent across studies, there was some indication that children with COS have reduced total brain volume. These results are similar to those found in MRI studies of the adult-onset population (Sowell et al.).

More recently, magnetic resonance spectroscopy (MRS) has been used to examine the brain chemistry of people with schizophrenia (Asarnow & Asarnow, 2003). When Thomas et al. (1998) and Bertolino et al. (1998) conducted MRS on patients with schizophrenia, they found a decrease in the ratio of *N*-acetylaspartase to creatine in the frontal gray matter, which may indicate decreased density of neurons. Results of MRI and MRS studies suggest that COS may be associated with reductions in brain gray matter, but not white matter (Asarnow & Asarnow, 2003). The neuronal circuits that appear to be compromised in children with COS include the subcortical and cortical components. These findings suggest that deviations in brain development occur during the fetal period (Asarnow & Asarnow). Continued research in this area could lead to very early identification of children at-risk for developing COS and could inform early intervention and prevention efforts.

10.4.3   Dopamine Hypothesis

It has been hypothesized that dopamine plays a role in the pathogenesis of schizophrenia (Asarnow & Asarnow, 2003) because of the powerful antipsychotic action of dopamine antagonists (Gaspar, Bustamante, Silva, & Aboitiz, 2009). Meisenzahl, Schmitt, Scheuerecker, and Möller (2007) reported that the positive symptoms of schizophrenia appear to be related to an excess of dopamine. Indeed, brain imaging studies have shown a clear dysregulation of the dopaminergic system in studies with patients experiencing clinical exacerbation of the disease (Meisenzahl et al.). However, recent studies (e.g., Carlsson, 2006; Winterer, 2006) have proposed that differences in dopamine production in individuals with schizophrenia may only be part of a broader pathological process. Dopamine antagonists do not appear to relieve the negative symptoms associated with schizophrenia, suggesting that other processes are occurring. Furthermore, there are other factors, including movement, arousal, stress, and smoking, which are associated with dopamine release that have been rarely considered in studies (Moncrieff, 2009). Dopamine stabilizers, such as clozapine, can cause serious motor and mental side effects (Carlsson, Carlsson, & Nilsson, 2004), so should be prescribed and monitored carefully. Certainly, more research on the neurobiological basis of schizophrenia needs to be conducted to identify the processes and inform the development of new medications and treatments.

10.4.4   Genetic Indicators

Harrison and Weinberger (2005) suggested that heritability estimates for schizophrenia may be as high as 85% and, thus, the examination of risk genes may be of value. Addington and colleagues (2007) explored the association between neuregulin 1 (NRG1) and schizophrenia, a link first reported by Stefansson et al. in

2002 (as cited in Addington et al.) and replicated numerous times. The neuregulins are at least four genes that together affect growth and differentiation factors for glia and neurons. The genetic research indicates particular risk genes and the work completed by Addington et al. demonstrated that one identified risk allele, NRG1, was associated with poorer premorbid social functioning in children with schizophrenia. Further, when the group with COS was compared to healthy controls who also had this risk allele, different trajectories of changes in the brain were found. The children with schizophrenia had greater total gray and white matter volume in childhood, with a steeper rate of subsequent decline in volume as they matured and reached adolescence. The controls, on the other hand, had decline in the frontal lobes only, which suggested mediating effects on NRG1 influence on brain development (Addington et al.). With advances in genetic research, it may be possible one day to identify children at-risk for developing schizophrenia at an early age and intervene to ameliorate the effects, or even impede development of the disease.

10.4.5   Prenatal Exposures

10.4.5.1   Diabetes

A review by Van Lieshout and Voruganti (2008) examined the association between maternal diabetes during pregnancy and the development of schizophrenia in offspring. Within the review, the authors considered a neurodevelopmental hypothesis for explaining the etiology of the disease. This theory assumes an interaction between multiple susceptibility genes and one or more environmental insults during pre- and/or perinatal development. Van Lieshout and Voruganti (2008) suggested that maternal diabetes might increase the risk for schizophrenia in the child because elevated insulin levels increase oxygen consumption and metabolism in the fetus and the placenta is unable to meet the increasing demand for oxygen delivery. This state of hypoxia can affect neurodevelopment by altering myelination and cortical connectivity and causing cell death. Furthermore, maternal diabetes has been shown to deplete antioxidants, increasing oxidative stress in the mother; cord blood taken from infants of mothers with diabetes has demonstrated that this milieu is shared with the fetus. Oxidative stress has been implicated in the etiology of schizophrenia (Van Lieshout & Voruganti). Although further research in this area is needed, this review indicates another risk factor that may be helpful in early identification of children at-risk for developing schizophrenia.

10.4.5.2   Influenza

For over 200 years, it has been speculated that prenatal influenza infection may produce adverse developmental outcomes for offspring (see Martin & Dombrowski, 2008 and Dombrowski & Martin, 2009 for an in-depth discussion).

In 1787, William Perfect wondered whether a particularly virulent influenza epidemic during that year was responsible for an increase in insanity among those gestationally exposed. In 1845, Esquirol commented that insanity is more prevalent during epidemic years and this increase seems to be independent of moral causes. At the beginning of the twentieth century, Emil Kraeplin (1919) commented that "infections in the years of development might have a causal significance" for dementia praecox (p. 240). Following the 1918–1919 influenza pandemic, which killed more people than World War I, Karl Menninger (1928a, 1928b) speculated that influenza infection may be causally related to schizophrenia.

Over the past 20 years, more than three dozen studies have suggested a link between maternal infection with influenza during the second and third trimester of pregnancy and the development of schizophrenia in offspring (Brown et al., 2004; McGrath & Castle, 1995; Machon, Mednick, & Huttenen, 1997; Mednick, Machon, Huttenen, & Bonnett, 1988; Dombrowski & Martin, 2009; Martin & Dombrowski, 2008). This gestational influenza-schizophrenia association has been explained as part of a neurodevelopmental hypothesis of brain perturbation. The neurodevelopmental hypothesis suggests that an insult to brain development at an earlier stage (second trimester) contributes to a vulnerability to psychopathology at a later stage of development (Dombrowski & Martin, 2007; Waddington et al., 1999). There are several biologically plausible mechanisms that might contribute to alterations of fetal brain development. The first involves the impact of fever, produced in response to influenza infection (Dombrowski & Martin, 2009; Dombrowski, Martin, & Huttenen, 2003). Maternal fever in the mother is thought to either directly or indirectly disrupt the development of the fetal central nervous system at the cellular, rather than structural, level as the mother's immune system is mobilized to fight foreign bodies. Barr, Mednick, and Munk-Jorgensen (1990) indicate that the developing nervous system is especially vulnerable to the direct impact of hyperthermia (i.e., fever) which can either alter or inhibit cellular generation. More indirectly, maternally generated cytokines, a type of protein, produced in response to infection are thought to cross the placental barrier and disrupt the developing fetal nervous system. Cytokines are known to regulate brain development and they have been observed in the central nervous systems of individuals diagnosed with psychiatric disorders in childhood (Dombrowski & Martin, 2009; Martin & Dombrowski, 2008). The disruption from gestational exposure to influenza is subtle, not observable at birth, and usually remains clinically silent until later in the child's life. Interestingly, female offspring may be more susceptible to the effects of maternal influenza than males, which differs from overall prevalence rates (Martin & Dombrowski). The prenatal exposures research suggests that it is of vital importance for pregnant women to protect themselves from infection, particularly influenza, which often can be avoided through taking proper precautions, such as obtaining a flu shot, washing hands, and avoiding others who are infected (Dombrowski et al., 2003; Cordero, 2003).

10.4.6 Environmental Risk Factors

In addition to genetic risk factors, environmental risk factors, such as child abuse (Read, van Os, Morrison, & Ross, 2005) and prenatal stress, (King, Laplante, & Joober, 2005) also may predispose a child to schizophrenia. A study by Bikmaz (2007) examined the relationship between childhood trauma and the disease. Fifty-seven patients with first-episode schizophrenia were evaluated at admission with the Brief Psychiatric Research Scale, the Scale for the Assessment of Positive Symptoms, and the Scale for the Assessment of Negative Symptoms. The group also was assessed for childhood trauma at discharge with the Childhood Abuse Questionnaire and Childhood Trauma Questionnaire. Findings indicated that 29.8% of participants reported childhood sexual abuse; 40.9% reported childhood emotional abuse; 13.6% reported childhood physical abuse; 29.5% reported childhood emotional neglect; and 20.5% reported childhood physical neglect. Patients who had reported sexual abuse had higher scores on the Scale for the Assessment of Positive Symptoms at admission and also had attempted suicide more frequently than the other groups prior to admission. The patients who had reported emotional abuse experienced more hallucinations and delusions. Bikmaz concluded that these findings suggested a high prevalence of childhood trauma among those diagnosed with schizophrenia and that the severity of the trauma correlated with the severity of positive symptoms, but was not associated with negative symptoms.

Although the Bikmaz (2007) study had several limitations, including use of self-report measures of trauma, lack of a control group, and little examination of potential confounding variables, the findings beg further research in this area. When one considers this line of research together with the genetic literature base, findings suggest that there may be myriad factors that predict and influence development of the disease and severity of symptoms. For example, a child with both the risk gene and an abusive home life may be a greater risk for onset of schizophrenia than a child who had one or the other factor present. Greater research into combinations of predictive factors certainly is warranted.

10.5 Assessment

There is little research that examines the diagnosis of psychotic disorders, including schizophrenia, in youth. Symptoms in children appear to be continuous with those in adults, with possible developmental variations (McClellan & McCurry, 1999) and, thus, COS is diagnosed using the same criteria as for adult diagnosis (McClellan, Werry, & The Workgroup on Quality Issues, 2001), the DSM-IV TR (APA, 2000) or *International Classification of Diseases* (ICD-10; World Health Organization, 1992) diagnostic criteria (McDonnell & McClellan, 2007). The initial assessment should include psychiatric, physical, and psychological evaluations. During the psychiatric evaluation, the examiner should conduct interviews with the child and family, when possible, and a review of past records. Specific issues that should be addressed during the interviews and review include the presenting symptoms, the course of the illness, any pertinent factors, such as developmental problems or substance abuse, family psychiatric history, and the Mental Status Exam, with a focus on psychotic symptoms (McClellan et al.).

In addition to the psychiatric evaluation, an assessment of the child's physical status should be conducted to rule out general medical causes of the psychotic symptoms. Conditions such as intoxication, central nervous system lesions, tumors, and infections could evoke symptoms. It may be necessary to complete tests and procedures, such as blood work, neuroimaging, and electroencephalographs to rule out these conditions (McClellan et al.). Finally, a psychological assessment may be necessary to evaluate cognitive functioning, which would aid in eventual treatment planning. Although there are no specific neuropsychological profiles, there is research to indicate that children with COS have global impairments across tasks that require information processing, which suggests that assessment of such may be important to the intervention process (McDonnell & McClellan, 2007). Other psychological testing, including personality and projective measures, are not indicated in the diagnosis of COS and, therefore, are not necessary to administer. A diagnosis is made when the prerequisite criteria for the disorder have been met (i.e., the DSM-IV-TR or ICD-10 criteria) and other disorders and diseases have been ruled out as the cause of the presenting symptoms (McClellan et al.).

10.5.1 Behavioral History

It is important to note that the majority of children who have COS typically have premorbid developmental and/or behavioral difficulties. In fact, some reports indicate that as many as 90% of children display some level of abnormality in the years prior to diagnosis (McDonnell & McClellan, 2007). Commonly, children with schizophrenia have language, communication, and global cognitive deficits and these differences in functioning may affect the range and quality of the premorbid symptoms. Prior to diagnosis, children may present with bizarre preoccupations and behaviors, social withdrawal, academic difficulties, behavior problems, and speech and language disorders (McDonnell & McClellan). In a study by McClellan and McCurry (1998), it was suggested that social withdrawal and poor peer relations differentiated the premorbid histories of children receiving an eventual diagnosis of schizophrenia from those diagnosed with bipolar disorder. A second study by Hollis (2003) indicated that impairments in premorbid social functioning are a key indicator in differentiating children with COS from those with other psychotic disorders. Findings from these studies emphasize the importance of the psychiatric history as an evaluation tool.

In the prodromal phase of the disease, the child experiences a significant decline in social, cognitive, and or academic behaviors from baseline or premorbid functioning. Generally, symptoms during this phase include the development of odd beliefs, worsening school performance, social isolation, and worsening personal hygiene (McDonnell & McClellan, 2007). The prodromal phase varies from acute change that occurs within days or weeks to chronic impairment that occurs over the course of months or years. There is research to indicate that chronic onset is predictive of a more severe course of illness, than is acute onset (McClellan & McCurry, 1998; McClellan, Werry, & Ham, 1993; Werry, McClellan, & Chard, 1991).

10.5.2   Assessment of Symptoms

Generally, schizophrenia is characterized by the presentation of two broad sets of symptom clusters, positive and negative (McClellan et al., 2001). Positive symptoms include hallucinations, delusions, and disordered thought and negative symptoms include flat affect, diminished energy, and paucity of speech and thought. Research has demonstrated that hallucinations, thought disorder, and flat affect are commonly found symptoms in children with COS, while delusions and catatonic behavior are less common. In a study by Bettes and Walker (1987), it was found that positive symptoms of schizophrenia increased linearly with age, with negative symptoms found most frequently in early childhood and late adolescence. Results of this study also indicated that children with high intelligence quotient (IQ) standard scores presented with greater positive and fewer negative symptoms than did children with lower IQ standard scores (Bettes & Walker, 1987). Findings from all of these studies suggest important avenues to explore in the diagnosis of children with schizophrenia. The disorder is rare in children and often times can be difficult to diagnosis.

10.5.3   Standardized Measures

In diagnosing COS, accuracy may be enhanced through the use of structured interviews (McDonnell & McClellan, 2007). There are a variety of instruments available that contain either screening items for psychosis in children or complete diagnostic criteria for schizophrenia. Examples include the *Diagnostic Interview Schedule for Children-Version IV* (*DISC*), the *Schedule for Affective Disorders and Schizophrenia for School-Age Children* (*K-SADS*), and the *Structured Clinical Interview for DSM-IV, Childhood Diagnoses* (*KID SCID*), among others (Doss, 2005). However, as McDonnell & McClellan stated, the clinician using a structured interview should be familiar with both COS and developmental psychopathology in children. Clinician-based interviews, such as the *K-SADS* and the *KID SCID* are recommended for use because they allow the clinician to probe and to reword items (McDonnell & McClellan), which may help to increase diagnostic validity.

10.5.4   Stability of Diagnosis Over Time

Misdiagnosis of schizophrenia in children commonly occurs, given the overlap of symptoms with other disorders. McClellan and McCurry (1999) examined the diagnostic stability of early onset psychotic disorders in a 2-year longitudinal prospective study that included children diagnosed with schizophrenia ($n=18$), bipolar disorder ($n=14$), schizoaffective disorder ($n=7$), organic psychosis ($n=1$), and psychosis not otherwise specified ($n=11$). Standardized diagnostic assessments were administered at baseline and at 1- and 2-year follow-up. Of the 51 participants who began the study, 39 were reassessed at year 1 and 24 at year 2. For 50% of the participants, the study diagnosis was the same as the onset diagnosis that was given prior to entrance to the study. Over the course of 2 years, the initial study diagnosis remained the same for more than 90% of the participants. Results indicated that children diagnosed with schizophrenia had higher rates of premorbid social withdrawal and poorer peer relationships than those with bipolar disorder, and also had higher rates of delusions and bizarre behavior at 1-year follow-up. The children diagnosed with bipolar disorder presented with cyclical symptom courses, while those with schizophrenia tended to be more chronically impaired. McClellan & McCurry concluded that the findings suggested that early onset psychotic disorders can be reliably diagnosed when standardized, valid tools are used, and are generally stable over time. These results suggest the importance of the use of appropriate diagnostic tools because accurate diagnosis can inform early intervention that has the potential to ameliorate symptoms.

10.6   Treatment and Intervention

According to the American Academy of Child and Adolescent Psychiatry's Work Group on Quality Issues (McClellanet al., 2001), treatment of schizophrenia in children is twofold, including strategies that are both specific and general. Specific treatments are aimed at the symptomatology and general interventions are related to the psychological, social, educational, and cultural needs of the child and family. Most children will require multiple interventions to address symptoms of schizophrenia and may also require treatment for comorbid disorders, such as substance abuse. The types and intensity of the interventions depend on patient characteristics and the phase of the disorder and can include outpatient and community programs, medication, psychotherapeutic and psychoeducational services, family support, vocational assistance, and medical services (McClellan et al.).

10.6.1   Pharmacological Intervention

Typically, children diagnosed with schizophrenia are administered medications, including antipsychotic drugs, which reduce psychotic symptoms and improve overall functioning (McClellan et al., 2001). However, only a few randomized studies have been conducted that demonstrate the efficacy of typical and atypical antipsychotics for children with schizophrenia and, thus, treatment practices are largely informed by clinical experience, case reports, and studies conducted with the adult population (McDonnell & McClellan, 2007). Masi, Mucci, and Pari (2006) reviewed studies in which children with COS were treated with typical and atypical antipsychotic medications. Studies reviewed included controlled and open studies and case reports on the use of pharmacotherapy in children less than 12 years of age diagnosed with schizophrenia. It should be noted that only one double-blind, placebo-controlled study of typical antipsychotics was found in the search up to and inclusive of 2006. Results indicated the efficacy of risperidone and olanzapine with this population and also suggested that clozapine is an effective option in treatment-refractory cases. However, at the time of the review, there were less data to support the use of atypical antipsychotic medications, including quetiapine, ziprasidone, and aripiprazole. In fact, limited studies with these drugs suggested that they cause adverse side effects, such as weight gain, hyperprolactinaemia, seizures, neuroleptic malignant syndrome, and cardiovascular problems, which may contraindicate their use with the pediatric population (Masi et al.).

In another review and meta-analysis of 15 studies conducted in the use of antipsychotic medications in children ages 5–18 years diagnosed with COS, Armenteros and Davies (2006) compared typical antipsychotics to atypical ones. Although measurement of drug side effects was not standardized across the studies included in the meta-analysis, differences were found between the two classes in weight gain, extrapyramidal syndrome (EPS), and sedation. EPS was defined as the presence of any of the following symptoms: tremor, drooling, dystonia, parkinsonian syndrome, akathissia, and dyskinesia. When weight gain was considered, the participants taking typical antipsychotics gained an average of 3.1 pounds, whereas those treated with atypical drugs gained an average 9.9 pounds. Although the rate of EPS was similar for the two groups (i.e., typical antipsychotics = 57.4% of participants affected and atypical = 56.5% affected), there was a difference between the groups in rates of sedation. Sedation occurred in 38.3% of those participants treated with a typical medication, whereas it occurred in 53.0% of those treated with an atypical (Armenteros & Davies). The authors caution that EPS data were missing in some studies and that prior treatment with typical antipsychotics in some participants may have artificially increased the rate for the atypical drugs. Furthermore, the authors were unable to analyze results for variables including age and gender because many of the studies were missing these data (Armenteros & Davies). Because antipsychotic medications typically are prescribed for youngsters with COS, more research in this area certainly is warranted to identify the most effective class of drugs.

Clozapine is an antipsychotic that is commonly prescribed for adults with schizophrenia because of its documented effectiveness. Remschmidt, Fleischhaker, Hennighausen, and Schulz (2000) reported that clozapine also has been found effective for children and adolescents with schizophrenia and that the advantages of using it with youngsters include its high efficacy during acute episodes, the marked improvements seen in those with a high number of negative symptoms, and the presence of fewer extrapyramidal adverse effects. However, in reviewing studies where clozapine was administered to children, Remschmidt et al. found that administration resulted in adverse effects on the hematopoietic, cardiovascular, and central nervous systems and on liver functioning. In addition, hypersalivation and weight gain (Toren, Ratner, Laor, & Weizman, 2004) were found in some participants. The authors concluded that these adverse effects should rule out clozapine as a first-line antipsychotic medication with children (Remschmidt et al., 2000); it should be used only when the patient becomes resistant to other psychotropic medications. Reviews such as this are important in considering the benefit to risk ratio of administering antipsychotics to children, especially those commonly prescribed in the adult population.

Because ethnicity has been suggested as a factor in symptom expression in schizophrenia, a study was conducted to examine differences between African American ($n = 38$), Caucasian ($n = 30$), and Hispanic ($n = 37$) youths who had been diagnosed with a schizophrenia-spectrum disorder and who were taking risperidone, another commonly prescribed drug for individuals with psychosis (Patel et al., 2006). In previous studies of youngsters with COS, Caucasian individuals reported more negative symptoms than African Americans, and more behavioral problems than African Americans and Hispanics. In addition, one study reported that Caucasians exhibited more severe excitement symptom scores on a measure for schizophrenia that may indicate an increased risk for aggressive behavior (Patel et al.). It should be noted that differences in reporting could have been affected by cultural differences in sociocentric and expressed emotion constructs, religious beliefs, and family factors. However, given that ethnicity has been indicated as a potential factor in symptomatology, it is important to explore medication effects across ethnic groups.

Participants in Patel et al.'s (2006) study were evaluated with the Child Behavior Checklist (CBCL) at baseline and at 2-year follow-up while being treated with risperidone. Results indicated that all three groups showed significant improvement in CBCL total scores over the 2 years from baseline to follow-up, but that there were differences among the ethnic groups. For example, the African American participants demonstrated significant average improvement from baseline to follow-up for total and internalizing CBCL scores, but not for externalizing scores. The Hispanic participants showed significant improvement in internalizing CBCL scores over the 2-year period, but no significant improvements were found for the Caucasian group. Analyses were controlled for gender (Patel et al.). The findings suggested not only ethnic differences in symptom presentation and reporting, but that there may be a difference in responses to risperidone, a commonly prescribed drug for children with psychotic symptoms. More research in this area needs to be conducted to examine both ethnic and gender differences to identify the most efficacious course of treatment for particular young patients diagnosed with schizophrenia.

Armenteros and Mikhail (2002) raised the question of whether it is necessary to use placebos in the evaluation of new drugs for youth diagnosed with COS. The authors cited the ethical debate over the use of placebos that has been around for decades. The debate centers on the intrinsic risks to the patient when a placebo is administered rather than a medication and Armenteros & Mikhail suggested that concern is accentuated with the pediatric population. Schizophrenia is an illness that could potentially disturb cognitive functions, which leaves the patient vulnerable and in need of immediate treatment (Armenteros & Mikhail).

At the time of their review, Armenteros and Mikhail (2002) discovered only two methodologically sound placebo-controlled trials with children and adolescents with schizophrenia. The first study reviewed the use of neuroleptics (e.g., haloperidol and loxapine) and the second examined the use of haloperidol in children diagnosed with schizophrenia. The results of the two studies did not establish the medications as best practice treatments because of lack of proven effectiveness over placebos. Armenteros & Mikhail did report that studies with adults have suggested that the placebo response does have weight and, thus, concluded that the true efficacy of psychotropic agents in children with schizophrenia is best demonstrated through comparison with placebo treatment. Even comparison to a standard drug may not be enough to demonstrate medication effectiveness (Armenteros & Mikhail).

10.6.2 Psychotherapeutic Treatment

Although administration of antipsychotic medications is standard treatment practice for individuals diagnosed with schizophrenia, a multidisciplinary approach, including psychosocial interventions, generally is needed to address the complexity of symptoms (McDonnell & McClellan, 2007). McClellan et al. (2001) recommended that in addition to treatment with medication, the child diagnosed with schizophrenia also should receive psychosocial interventions. These interventions include therapy for the patient, which encompasses education about the illness, treatment options, social skills training, relapse prevention measures, life skills training, and problem-solving skills and strategies. Specific training in communication skills, self-advocacy skills, coping strategies, and self-care skills, including hygiene, should be a part of the package (Dulmus & Smyth, 2000).Depending on the severity of the cognitive and functional deficits, the child also might benefit from specialized educational and vocational training, or placement in a day treatment or residential facility. In addition, the child or adolescent may require interventions or services for comorbid disorders, such as substance abuse, depression, and suicidality. Finally, psychoeducational therapy for the family of the child is indicated. This therapy should focus on helping the family to understand the illness and its treatment and also aid them in developing strategies to cope with the child's symptoms (McClellan et al.). The limited studies that have explored family educational programs to date have suggested that these treatment packages, when used in conjunction with individual treatment and psychopharmacology, consistently result in lower relapse rates, greater treatment adherence, and improvements in family problem-solving skills (Asarnow et al., 2004). These findings suggest that treatment should be multidimensional, including interventions that target overall family functioning. The primary goal of any treatment package should be to return the child to his/her premorbid level of functioning, while also promoting the development and mastery of age-appropriate skills and tasks. Treatment should be focused on the individual needs of the child, and not on those needs generally specific to a diagnosis of schizophrenia. Although most of the treatment literature has been conducted with adults, it is reasonable to expect that the cognitive-behavioral strategies and social skills training that have proven effective with adults would also be beneficial for use with youth. Social skills training is directed at improving the patient's strategies for dealing with conflict, identifying the content of social exchange, and enhancing socialization and vocational skills (Hall & Bean, 2008; McClellan et al., 2001). Because these skills are necessary for daily functioning, any treatment package should include these specific training areas, in addition to drug therapies. Given the dearth of studies examining psychosocial interventions with children with COS, more research in this area is needed to determine if therapies used with adults are, in fact, effective with the childhood population.

10.6.3 Educational Intervention

Because most children with COS have difficulties in school (Helling, Öhman, & Hultman, 2003), this population generally qualifies for special education services under the Individuals with Disabilities Education Act (IDEA; Gonthier & Lyon, 2004). Eligibility entitles children with COS to special services, including smaller classes sizes and teachers with specialized training in working with children with psychiatric disorders. Furthermore, modifications to schoolwork can be made to accommodate the cognitive dysfunction and poor attention skills often observed in children with COS. Children with more severe symptoms may need to receive educational services in day treatment or residential facilities (Gonthier & Lyon). Any education program designed for a child should involve his family and medical care providers to ensure an optimal service delivery model.

10.7 Outcome and Prognostic Factors

According to the DSM-IV TR (APA, 2000), the variable course of schizophrenia makes an accurate prognosis of long-term outcomes impossible. Complete remission of the disorder is not common and for those individuals who remain ill, some stay relatively stable while others become progressively disabled. There is some indication that positive symptoms are responsive to treatment and, thus, diminish while negative symptoms persist. Despite the variable course of schizophrenia, a number of studies have identified factors that are associated with a better prognosis including: (a) good premorbid adjustment; (b) acute onset; (c) later age at onset; (d) being female; (e) treatment with antipsychotic medications shortly after diagnosis; (f) consistent medication compliance; (g) brief duration of active-phase symptoms; (h) minimal residual symptoms; (i) absence of structural brain abnormalities; (j) normal neurological functioning; and (k) no family history of schizophrenia (APA).

In a review conducted by Remschmidt et al. (1994), it was reported that few studies dealing with the prognosis of children and adolescents with schizophrenia have been conducted and a decade and a half later, this seems to be the case. The early review suggested that schizophrenia diagnosed in pre-puberty or adolescence had a less favorable course than schizophrenia with a first manifestation in adulthood, with the poorest prognosis observed when the diagnosis was made before the age of 10 years (Remschmidt et al.).

10.8   Future Directions

Certainly, an interesting avenue for future research is to continue to examine the genetic and structural brain differences in children identified with COS. The early identification of physical differences would enable both careful monitoring of the environment for risk factors and enable early intervention services. The research has identified some possible early factors, such as social behavior differences, abuse, and trauma that may interact with genetic vulnerability to evoke symptoms. Early physical identification could suggest environmental factors to be identified, monitored, and intervened upon to alter the course of the disease, or even prevent manifestation. Along these lines, careful consideration should be given to the proposed inclusion of the "Attenuated Psychotic Symptoms Syndrome" in the upcoming DSM-V (APA, 2010). Longitudinal research should be conducted to determine whether inclusion of this diagnostic category would be beneficial or detrimental to children considered to be at-risk for the development of schizophrenia. Although early identification certainly has its benefits, a risk/benefits analysis should be undertaken across time to decide whether this category would be beneficial to include.

Other research should be focused on treatment for children diagnosed with schizophrenia. Antipsychotic medications are generally prescribed, but there is research to suggest that medication should not be the sole treatment. A comprehensive package should include education about the illness, treatment options, social skills training, relapse prevention measures, life skills training, and problem-solving skills and strategies. Also, for the child whose academic skills are being affected by the disease, it is important to address these skill deficits. Although the scant research that exists regarding these treatment options has been conducted with adults, it stands to reason that these components would be just as necessary for the pediatric patient.

Finally, more research with typical and atypical antipsychotic medications should be conducted with children. There are few randomized, controlled double-blind studies conducted with children. Armenteros and Mikhail (2002) suggested that a placebo effect has been demonstrated in the adult population with schizophrenia and, thus, it is vital to study this effect in children. Given the oft time serious side effects of antipsychotic medications (e.g., weight gain, sedation, effects on the cardiovascular system, dystonia, and dyskinesia, to name a few), it is important to study effects specifically in children. It may be that medications would have even further detrimental effects on a developing brain and nervous system. These risks beg longitudinal research that incorporates the comparison of medications to placebo and also one another.

COS is rare with rates of approximately two in one million children below the age of 13 years meeting criteria for diagnosis (APA, 2000). However, it is a lifelong illness that has pervasive detrimental effects. Given the devastating nature of schizophrenia, more research needs to be conducted into its etiology, diagnosis, and treatment in an effort to ameliorate effects.

References

Addington, A. M., Gornick, M. C., Shaw, P., Seal, J., Gogtay, N., Greenstein, D., et al. (2007). Neuregulin 1 (8p12) and childhood-onset schizophrenia: Susceptibility haplotypes for diagnosis and brain developmental trajectories. *Molecular Psychiatry, 12*, 195–205.

American Psychiatric Association. (2000). *Diagnostic and statistical manual of mental disorders* (4th ed., rev.). Washington, DC: Author.

American Psychiatric Association. (2010). DSM-5 development: Attenuated psychotic symptoms syndrome. Retrieved August 24, 2010, from http://www.dsm5.org/ProposedRevisions/Pages/proposedrevision.aspx?rid=412.

Armenteros, J. L., & Davies, M. (2006). Antipsychotics in early onset schizophrenia: Systematic review and meta-analysis. *European Child and Adolescent Psychiatry, 15*, 141–148.

Armenteros, J. L., & Mikhail, A. G. (2002). Do we need placebos to evaluate new drugs in children with schizophrenia? *Psychopharmacology, 159*, 117–124.

Asarnow, J. R. (1994). Childhood-onset schizophrenia. *Journal of Child Psychology and Psychiatry, 35*, 1345–1371.

Asarnow, J. R., & Asarnow, R. F. (2003). Childhood-onset schizophrenia. In E. J. Mash & R. A. Barkley (Eds.), *Child Psychopathology* (2nd ed., pp. 455–485). New York, NY: The Guilford Press.

Asarnow, J. R., Tompson, M. C., & Goldstein, M. J. (1994). Childhood-onset schizophrenia: A followup study. *Schizophrenia Bulletin, 20*, 599–617.

Asarnow, J. R., Tompson, M. C., & McGrath, E. P. (2004). Childhood-onset schizophrenia: Clinical and treatment issues. *Journal of Child Psychology and Psychiatry, 45*, 180–194.

Auther, A. M., Gillett, D. A., & Cornblatt, B. A. (2008). Expanding the boundaries of early intervention for psychosis: Intervening during the prodrome. *Psychiatric Annals, 38*, 528–537.

Barr, C. E., Mednick, S. A., & Munk-Jorgensen, P. (1990). Exposure to influenza epidemics during gestation and adult schizophrenia. *Archives of General Psychiatry, 47*, 869–874.

Bearden, C. E., Rosso, I. M., Hollister, J. M., Sanchez, L. E., Hadley, T., & Cannon, T. D. (2000). A prospective cohort study of childhood behavioral deviance and language abnormalities as predictors of adult schizophrenia. *Schizophrenia Bulletin, 26*, 395–410.

Bender, L. (1941). Childhood schizophrenia. *Nervous Child, 1*, 138–140.

Bender, L. (1958). Psychiatric problems of childhood. *Medical Clinics of North America, 42*, 755–767.

Bertolino, A., Kumra, S., Callicott, J. H., Mattay, V. S., Lestz, R. M., Jacobsen, L., et al. (1998). Common pattern of cortical pathology in childhood-onset and adult-onset schizophrenia as identified by proton magnetic resonance spectroscopic imaging. *American Journal of Psychiatry, 155*, 1376–1383.

Bettes, B., & Walker, E. (1987). Positive and negative symptoms in psychotic and other psychiatrically disturbed children. *Journal of Child Psychology and Psychiatry, 28*, 555–567.

Bikmaz, A. U. S. (2007). The effects of childhood trauma in patients with first-episode schizophrenia. *Acta Psychiatrica Scandinavica, 116*, 371–377.

Bleuler, E. (1911). *Dementia praecox oder die Gruppe der Schizophrenien*. Handbuch der Psychiatrie, Halfte 1. Leipzig: Deuticke.

Brown, A. S., Begg, M. D., Gravenstein, S., Schaefer, C. A., Wyatt, R. J., Bresnahan, M. A., et al. (2004). Serological evidence for prenatal influenza in the etiology of schizophrenia. *Archives of General Psychiatry, 61*, 774–780.

Carlsson, A. (2006). The neurochemical circuitry of schizophrenia. *Pharmacopsychiatry, 39*, 10–14.

Carlsson, M. L., Carlsson, A., & Nilsson, M. (2004). Schizophrenia: From dopamine to glutamate and back. *Current Medicinal Chemistry, 11*, 267–277.

Cordero, J. F. (2003). A new look at behavioral outcomes and teratogens: A commentary. *Birth Defects Research (Part A): Clinical and Molecular Teratology, 67*(11), 900–902.

Creak, M. (1964). Schizophrenia syndrome in childhood: Further progress report of a working party. *Developmental Medicine and Child Neurology, 6*, 530–535.

Dombrowski, S. C., & Martin, R. P. (2007). Pre and perinatal exposures in later psychological, behavioral, and cognitive disability. *School Psychology Quarterly, 22*, 1–7.

Dombrowski, S. C., & Martin, R. P. (2009). *Maternal fever during pregnancy: Association with temperament, behavior and academic outcomes in children*. Saarbrucken, Germany: VDM Verlag.

Dombrowski, S. C., Martin, R. P., & Huttenen, M. O. (2003). Association between maternal fever and psychological/behavioral outcomes: An hypothesis. *Birth Defects Research (Part A): Clinical and Molecular Teratology, 67*, 905–910.

Doss, A. J. (2005). Evidence-based diagnosis: Incorporating diagnostic instruments into clinical practice. *Journal of the American Academy of Child and Adolescent Psychiatry, 44*, 947–952.

Dulmus, C. N., & Smyth, N. J. (2000). Early-onset schizophrenia: A literature review of empirically based interventions. *Child and Adolescent Social Work Journal, 17*, 55–69.

Eggers, C., & Bunk, D. (1997). The long-term course of childhood-onset schizophrenia: A 42-year follow up. *Schizophrenia Bulletin, 23*, 105–117.

Eggers, C., Bunk, D., & Krause, D. (2000). Schizophrenia with onset before the age of eleven: Clinical characteristics of onset and course. *Journal of Autism and Developmental Disorders, 30*, 29–38.

Emminghaus, H. (1887). *Die psychischen Storungen des Kindesalters*. Tubingen: Laupp.

Foster, K. A., Swartz, L., & de Jager, W. (2006). The clinical presentation of childhood-onset schizophrenia: A literature review. *South African Journal of Psychology, 36*, 299–318.

Gaebel, W., & Frommann, N. (2000). Long-term course in schizophrenia: Concepts, methods and research strategies. *Acta Psychiatrica Scandinavica, 102*, 49–53.

Gaspar, P. A., Bustamante, M. L., Silva, H., & Aboitiz, F. (2009). Molecular mechanisms underlying glutamatergic dysfunction in schizophrenia: Therapeutic implications. *Journal of Neurochemistry, 111*, 891–900.

Gonthier, M., & Lyon, M. A. (2004). Childhood-onset schizophrenia: An overview. *Psychology in the Schools, 41*, 803–811.

Green, W., Padron-Gayol, M., Hardesty, A. S., & Bassiri, M. (1992). Schizophrenia with childhood onset: A phenomenological study of 38 cases. *Journal of the American Academy of Child and Adolescent Psychiatry, 35*, 968–976.

Hall, S. D., & Bean, R. A. (2008). Family therapy and childhood-onset schizophrenia: Pursuing clinical and bio/psycho/social competence. *Contemporary Family Therapy, 30*, 61–74.

Hans, S. L., Auerbach, J. G., Styr, B., & Marcus, J. (2004). Offspring of parents with schizophrenia: Mental disorders during childhood and adolescence. *Schizophrenia Bulletin, 30*, 303–315.

Harrison, P. J., & Weinberger, D. R. (2005). Schizophrenia genes, gene expression, and neuropathology: On the matter of their convergence. *Molecular Psychiatry, 10*, 40–68.

Helling, I., Öhman, A., & Hultman, C. M. (2003). School achievements and schizophrenia: A case-control study. *Acta Psychiatrica Scandinavica, 108*, 381–386.

Hollis, C. (2003). Developmental precursors of child- and adolescent-onset schizophrenia and affective psychoses: Diagnostic specificity and continuity with symptom dimensions. *British Journal of Psychiatry, 182*, 37–44.

Homburger, A. (1926). *Vorlesungen uber psychopathologie des kindesalters*. Berlin: Springer.

Husted, J. A., Greenwood, C. M. T., & Bassett, A. S. (2006). Heritability of schizophrenia and major affective disorder as a function of age, in the presence of strong cohort effects. *European Archives of Psychiatry and Clinical Neuroscience, 256*, 222–229.

Jacobsen, L. K., & Rapoport, J. L. (1998). Research update: Childhood-onset schizophrenia: Implications of clinical and neurobiological research. *Journal of Child Psychology and Psychiatry, 39*, 101–113.

Jahshan, C., Heaton, R. K., Golshan, S., & Cadenhead, K. S. (2010). Course of neurocognitive deficits in the prodrome and first episode of schizophrenia. *Neuropsychology, 24*, 109–120.

Kendler, K. S., & Tsuang, M. T. (1981). Nosology of paranoid schizophrenia and other paranoid psychoses. *Schizophrenia Bulletin, 7*, 594–610.

Kestenbaum, C. J. (1980). Children at risk for schizophrenia. *American Journal of Psychotherapy, 2*, 164–177.

King, S., Laplante, D., & Joober, R. (2005). Understanding putative risk factors for schizophrenia: Retrospective and prospective studies. *Review of Psychiatric Neuroscience, 30*, 342–348.

Kraepelin, E. (1896). *Psychiatrie: Ein Lehrbuch fur Studirende und Aerzte*. Leipzig, East Germany: Ambrosius Barth.

Kraepelin, E. (1919). *Dementia Praecox and Paraphrenia*. Edinburgh: E&S Livingstone.

Ledda, M. G., Fratta, A. L., Pintor, M., Zuddas, A., & Cianchetti, C. (2009). Early on-set psychoses: Comparison of clinical features and adult outcome in 3 diagnostic groups. *Child Psychiatry and Human Development, 40*, 421–437.

Leonhard, K. (1986). *Aufteilung der endogenen Psychosen und ihre differenzierte Ätiologie* (2nd ed.). Berlin, Germany: Akademie-Verlag.

Machon, R. A., Mednick, S. A., & Huttenen, M. O. (1997). Adult major affective disorder after prenatal exposure to an influenza epidemic. *Archives of General Psychiatry, 54*, 322–328.

Martin, R. P., & Dombrowski, S. C. (2008). *Prenatal exposures: Psychological and educational consequences for children*. New York, NY: Springer.

Masi, G., Mucci, M., & Pari, C. (2006). Children with schizophrenia: Clinical picture and pharmacological treatment. *CNS Drugs, 20*, 841–866.

McClellan, J., & McCurry, C. (1998). Neurocognitive pathways in the development of schizophrenia. *Seminars in Clinical Neuropsychiatry, 3*, 320–332.

McClellan, J., & McCurry, C. (1999). Early onset psychotic disorders: Diagnostic stability and clinical characteristics. *European Child and Adolescent Psychiatry, 8*(Suppl. 1), I/13–I/19.

McClellan, J. M., Werry, J. S., & Ham, M. (1993). A follow-up study of early onset psychosis: Comparison between outcome diagnoses of schizophrenia, mood disorders and personality disorders. *Journal of Autism and Developmental Disorders, 23*, 243–262.

McClellan, J., Werry, J., & The Workgroup on Quality Issues. (2001). Practice parameter for the assessment and treatment of children and adolescents with schizophrenia. *Journal of the American Academy of Child and Adolescent, 40*(7), 4S–23S.

McDonnell, M. G., & McClellan, J. M. (2007). Early-onset schizophrenia. In E. J. Mash & R. A. Barkely (Eds.), *Assessment of childhood disorders* (4th ed., pp. 526–550). New York, NY: The Guilford Press.

McGrath, J., & Castle, D. (1995). Does influenza cause schizophrenia? A five year review. *Australian and New Zealand Journal of Psychiatry, 29*, 23–31.

Mednick, S. A., Machon, R. A., Huttenen, M. O., & Bonnett, D. (1988). Adult schizophrenia following prenatal exposure to an influenza epidemic. *Archives of General Psychiatry, 45*, 189–192.

Meisenzahl, E. M., Schmitt, G. J., Scheuerecker, J., & Möller, H. J. (2007). The role of dopamine for the pathophysiology of schizophrenia. *International Review of Psychiatry, 19*, 337–345.

Menninger, K. A. (1928a). Medicolegal proposals of the American Psychiatric Association. *Journal of the American Institute of Criminal Law and Criminology, 19*(3), 367–377.

Menninger, K. A. (1928b). The schizophrenic syndromes as a product of acute infectious disease. *Archives of Neurology and Psychiatry, 20*, 464–481.

Moncrieff, J. (2009). A critique of the dopamine hypothesis of schizophrenia and psychosis. *Harvard Review of Psychiatry, 17*, 214–225.

Neumann, C. S., Grimes, K., Walker, E. F., & Baum, K. (1995). Developmental pathways to schizophrenia: Behavioral subtypes. *Journal of Abnormal Psychology, 104*, 558–566.

Patel, N. C., Crismon, M. L., Shafer, A., DeLeon, A., Lopez, M., & Lane, D. C. (2006). Ethnic variation in symptoms and response to risperidone in youths with schizophrenia-spectrum disorders. *Social Psychiatry and Psychiatric Epidemiology, 41*, 341–346.

Read, J., van Os, J., Morrison, A. P., & Ross, C. A. (2005). Childhood trauma, psychosis, and schizophrenia: A literature review with theoretical and clinical implications. *Acta Psychiatrica Scandinavica, 112*, 330–350.

Remschmidt, H. E. (2001). *Schizophrenia in children and adolescents.* Cambridge: Cambridge University Press.

Remschmidt, H. (2008). Schizophrenia in children and adolescents. In T. Banaschewski & L. A. Rohde (Eds.), *Biological child psychiatry: Recent trends and developments.* Basel, Switzerland: Karger.

Remschmidt, H., Fleischhaker, C., Hennighausen, K., & Schulz, E. (2000). Management of schizophrenia in children and adolescents: The role of clozapine. *Paediatric Drugs, 2*(4), 253–262.

Remschmidt, H. E., Schulz, E., Martin, M., Warnke, A., & Trott, G. (1994). Childhood-onset schizophrenia: History of the concept and recent studies. *Schizophrenia Bulletin, 20*, 727–745.

Sowell, E. R., Toga, A. W., & Asarnow, R. (2000). Brain abnormalities observed in childhood-onset schizophrenia: A review of the structural magnetic resonance imaging literature. *Mental Retardation and Developmental Disabilities Research Reviews, 6*, 180–185.

Tarbox, S. I., & Pogue-Geile, M. F. (2008). Development of social functioning in preschizophrenic children and adolescents: A systematic review. *Psychological Bulletin, 134*(4), 561–583.

Thomas, M. A., Yong, K., Levitt, J., Caplan, R., Curran, J., Asarnow, R., et al. (1998). Preliminary study of frontal lobe [^{1}H] MR spectroscopy in childhood-onset schizophrenia. *Journal of Magnetic Resonance Imaging, 8*, 841–846.

Toren, P., Ratner, S., Laor, N., & Weizman, A. (2004). Benefit-risk assessment of atypical antipsychotics in the treatment of schizophrenia and comorbid disorders in children and adolescents. *Drug Safety, 27*, 1135–1156.

Van Lieshout, R. J., & Voruganti, L. P. (2008). Diabetes mellitus during pregnancy and increased risk of schizophrenia in offspring: A review of the evidence and putative mechanisms. *Journal of Psychiatry and Neuroscience, 33*, 395–404.

Waddington, J. L., O'Callaghan, E., Youssef, H. A., Buckley, P., Lane, A., Cotter, D., et al. (1999). Schizophrenia: Evidence for a "cascade" process with neurodevelopmental origins. In E. S. Susser, A. S. Brown, & J. M. Gorman (Eds.), *Prenatal exposure in schizophrenia* (pp. 3–34). Washington, DC: American Psychiatric Press.

Werry, J. S. (1992). Child and adolescent (early onset) schizophrenia: A review in light of DSM-III-R. *Journal of Autism and Developmental Disorders, 22*, 601–624.

Werry, J. S., McClellan, J., & Chard, L. (1991). Early onset schizophrenia, bipolar and schizoaffective disorders: A clinical follow-up study. *Journal of the American Academy of Child and Adolescent Psychiatry, 30*, 457–465.

Winterer, G. (2006). Cortical microcircuits in schizophrenia: The dopamine hypothesis revisited. *Pharmacopsychiatry, 39*, 68–71.

World Health Organization (WHO). (1992). *The ICD-10 classification of mental health and behavioral disorders: Clinical descriptions and diagnostic guidelines.* Geneva: Author.

Chapter 11
Self-Injurious Behavior

I hurt myself today
To see if I still feel.
I focus on the pain
The only thing that's real.
The needle tears a hole
The old familiar sting.
Try to kill it all away
But I remember everything

–Nine Inch Nails, Hurt (1994)

11.1   Overview

Self-injurious behavior, more technically referred to as nonsuicidal self-injury (NSSI), is the purposeful and repetitive destruction or alteration of one's own body tissue without intent to die (Cloutier, Martin, Kennedy, Nixon, & Muehlenkamp, 2009; Nock & Mendes, 2008). The injuries occur outside the context of socially and medically sanctioned procedures, such as piercing and circumcision (Nock & Mendes), and include behaviors like cutting, hair pulling, banging, burning, and needle sticking (Klonsky & Olino, 2008). At one time, NSSI was thought to occur only among individuals who had suffered early life trauma, or who had serious mental disorders, including borderline personality disorder, posttraumatic stress disorder, and major depression. However, current research has suggested that NSSI occurs among a wide variety of people within the general population, who have no psychiatric history at all (Walsh, 2007). Although the behavior occurs among adults, the greatest prevalence of NSSI is found within the adolescent population (Nock & Prinstein, 2005), with onset typically around age 12 or 13 years (Klonsky & Muehlenkamp, 2007; Nock, Teper, & Hollander, 2007). Despite the prevalence and dangerous nature of the behavior, research into the causes of and treatments for NSSI is in its infancy. Several factors have inhibited research in these areas, including practical constraints (e.g., recruitment of participants and the collection of reliable

S.C. Dombrowski et al., *Assessing and Treating Low Incidence/High Severity Psychological Disorders of Childhood*, DOI 10.1007/978-1-4419-9970-2_11,
© Springer Science+Business Media, LLC 2011

data), reliance on clinical case reports and surveys, and failure to incorporate context and theories regarding the factors that elicit and maintain NSSI (Nock & Prinstein).

The purpose of this chapter is to review the studies that have been conducted into the etiology, assessment, intervention, and prevention of NSSI in the adolescent population and to suggest future research. Furthermore, there is discussion of the relationship between NSSI and suicidal ideation and the debate as to whether these are two distinct constructs, or whether they exist on a continuum of self-harm behaviors (Cloutier et al., 2009). It should be noted that throughout this chapter, the term *nonsuicidal self-injury* is used, but various terms are found in the extant literature base, including *self-injurious behavior*, *self-harm*, *parasuicide*, and *self-mutilation*.

11.2 Historical Aspects

One of the earliest references to the term "self-mutilation" appeared in a study by Emerson in 1913. He posited that individuals used self-cutting symbolically as a substitution for masturbation. Two decades later, the term reappeared in an article and a book by Menninger (1935, 1938) wherein he differentiated self-mutilation from suicidal behaviors. In these seminal works, Menninger described self-mutilation as a meaningful act that could be categorized along several dimensions, including the severity and type of psychological or physical dysfunction resulting from the injury, the meaning of the injury within the given culture, and the functions of the behavior (Menninger 1935, 1938; Yates, 2004). Menninger coined the term "partial suicide" to describe acts that he believed were nonfatal expressions of an attenuated death wish and developed a classification system for these injuries:

- Neurotic, including nail biters and skin pickers.
- Psychotic, such as limb removal and genital self-mutilation.
- Religious, specifically those who self-flagellate.
- Organic, including brain diseases that result in repetitive head banging, hand biting, or eye removal (Menninger, 1938).

Despite this early work, NSSI did not receive close attention in the literature until the late 1970s, when Ross and McKay (1979) introduced a classification system. These researchers proposed two categories of NSSI. The first included direct behaviors (e.g., cutting, biting, burning, hitting, etc.) and the second category included indirect self-injurious behaviors (e.g., overeating, substance abuse, and refusal of medical treatment). In the mid-1980s, Favazza (1987) made the distinction between NSSI that is performed within the context of a ritual or a group and that which is pathological in nature. Rituals, such as piercing, tattooing, and branding are considered rites of passage that enable the adolescent to mark him/herself as "different" from the mainstream culture (Yates, 2004). These types of body modifications are planned, decorative, and socially acceptable in a way that pathological NSSI is not. The key difference between the two behaviors is that in ritualistic body modification, the individual feels a sense of pride or defiance, whereas in NSSI, the individual feels shame for having engaged in a secretive, taboo act

(Favazza; Yates). Since these early references to NSSI in the literature, the research base has greatly evolved. The following section discusses more contemporary terminology and classification systems.

11.3 Description, Diagnosis, and Prevalence

11.3.1 Description

NSSI is the deliberate destruction of one's own body tissue without lethal intent. It is distinguished from suicidal behaviors and other behaviors in which there might be harmful, unintended consequences, such as smoking, which can cause cancer (Nock, 2009). Although NSSI most often involves cutting or carving the skin (Nock), there are other behaviors an adolescent may use to injure herself:

- Banging or hitting
- Hair pulling
- Pinching
- Biting
- Wound picking
- Deep scratching
- Rubbing skin against rough surfaces
- Burning
- Needle sticking
- Swallowing chemicals (Klonsky & Olino, 2008)

It is noted that at least one researcher, Favazza (1998), excluded swallowing chemicals or objects from his definition of NSSI because these behaviors do not directly affect body tissue. Many individuals who engage in NSSI behaviors use multiple methods, but most only self-injure once, or a few times; a minority of individuals engages in the behavior chronically (Klonsky & Muehlenkamp, 2007). Any body part can be affected, but a study by Whitlock, Eckenrode, and Silverman (2006) indicated that the most common location for injury is the arm (47.3% of injuries), followed by the hands, wrists, thighs, stomach, calves, head, and fingers.

It also should be noted that in at least one study (i.e., Laye-Gindhu & Schonert-Reichl, 2005), adolescents identified both direct and indirect behaviors as NSSI. Direct behaviors included cutting, hitting, biting, and bone-breaking, behaviors that have been reported throughout the literature as methods for self-injury. However, the adolescents in this study also included behaviors such as disordered eating and drug abuse in their definition of NSSI. Although these findings are limited to the 424 school-based youth included in the study, there are important implications for practice. In treating the adolescent who engages in NSSI, the practitioner may need to expand his view beyond the parameters of research to include the actual experiences and perceptions of his client (Laye-Gindhu & Schonert-Reichl).

11.3.1.1 Common Misperceptions

There are common misperceptions surrounding adolescents who engage in NSSI behaviors. First is the belief that children who hurt themselves are suicidal (Kanan, Finger, & Plog, 2008). Although there is debate surrounding whether NSSI and suicidal behaviors are two distinct entities or whether they belong to the same class, it is not true that all youngsters who injure themselves intend to die. Second is the misperception that all adolescents who engage in NSSI have been abused either sexually or physically at some point in their lives (Kanan et al.). Some self-injurers have been abused, but there are also large numbers who have no maltreatment in their histories. In fact, Klonsky and Moyer (2008) completed a meta-analysis of 45 articles in which the association between childhood sexual abuse and NSSI was examined and found that the relationship between the two was relatively small; childhood sexual abuse accounted for less than 5% of the variance in the development of NSSI. A third misperception is that adolescents who hurt themselves are diagnosable with borderline personality disorder (Kanan et al.). To the contrary, there are many adolescents who engage in NSSI who do not meet criteria for any psychiatric diagnosis (Walsh, 2007). Finally, is the mistaken belief that an adolescent who is hurting herself must be hospitalized. School attendance provides a routine and structure wherein a student can access supportive services. An adolescent should only be admitted to the hospital when her injuries need immediate attention, or when she is thinking about suicide (Kanan et al.).

11.3.2 Diagnosis/Classification

In 2001, Simeon and Favazza proposed a classification system that included four categories of NSSI behaviors: stereotypic, major, compulsive, and impulsive. Individuals with pervasive developmental disorders, such as autism and mental retardation, sometimes engage in behaviors that can be classified as stereotypic NSSI, the first category in this system. These behaviors generally are performed in a repetitive, rhythmic fashion and are devoid of affective content (Simeon & Favazza; Yates, 2004). The second category proposed by Simeon and Favazza, major NSSI, includes severe instances of self-mutilation, such as self-castration, that usually occur during the course of a psychotic episode. Major instances of NSSI result in permanent damage to the body (Simeon & Favazza; Yates). A third category in this taxonomy is compulsive NSSI, which includes ritualistic behaviors, such as hair pulling and scratching. These behaviors occur many times per day and are often referred to as impulse control disorders (e.g., trichotillomania). Finally, the fourth category, impulsive, includes intermittent NSSI behaviors, such as cutting, burning, and hitting, that result in the release of stress and mood elevation. With time, impulsive behaviors may become repetitive and addictive as the individual becomes preoccupied with injuring herself (Simeon & Favazza; Yates).

Table 11.1 APA's proposed diagnostic criteria for NSSI

(a) In the last year, the individual has, on 5 or more days, engaged in intentional self-inflicted damage to the surface of his or her body, of a sort likely to induce bleeding or bruising or pain (e.g., cutting, burning, stabbing, hitting, excessive rubbing), for purposes not socially sanctioned (e.g., body piercing, tattooing, etc.), but performed with the expectation that the injury will lead to only minor or moderate physical harm. The absence of suicidal intent is either reported by the patient or can be inferred by frequent use of methods that the patient knows, by experience, not to have lethal potential (when uncertain, code with NOS 2). The behavior is not of a common and trivial nature, such as picking at a wound or nail biting

(b) The intentional injury is associated with at least two of the following:

Negative feelings or thoughts, such as depression, anxiety, tension, anger, generalized distress, or self-criticism, occurring in the period immediately prior to the self-injurious act

Prior to engaging in the act, a period of preoccupation with the intended behavior that is difficult to resist

The urge to engage in self-injury occurs frequently, although it might not be acted upon

The activity is engaged in with a purpose; this might be relief from a negative feeling/cognitive state or interpersonal difficulty or induction of a positive feeling state. The patient anticipates these will occur either during or immediately following the self-injury

(c) The behavior and its consequences cause clinically significant distress or impairment in interpersonal, academic, or other important areas of functioning

(d) The behavior does not occur exclusively during states of psychosis, delirium, or intoxication. In individuals with a developmental disorder, the behavior is not part of a pattern of repetitive stereotopies. The behavior cannot be accounted for by another mental or medical disorder (i.e., psychotic disorder, pervasive developmental disorder, mental retardation, Lesch–Nyhan Syndrome; APA, 2010)

Currently, NSSI itself is not recognized as a diagnosable disorder. The *Diagnostic and Statistical Manual of Mental Disorders-IV Text Revision* [DSM-IV TR; American Psychiatric Association (APA), 2000] refers to self-injury only once throughout the text. The fifth criterion for borderline personality disorder states that the individual engages in "recurrent suicidal behavior, gestures, or thoughts or self-mutilating behavior" (APA). There is myriad evidence that demonstrates that individuals who engage in self-injurious behaviors display more symptoms of borderline personality disorder than individuals in the general population (Klonsky, Oltmanns, & Turkheimer, 2003), but the presence of NSSI does not always warrant a diagnosis of borderline personality disorder. Other diagnoses that may increase the likelihood of NSSI behavior are depression, anxiety, eating disorders, and substance abuse (Klonsky & Muehlenkamp, 2007).

11.3.2.1 DSM-V: Proposed Changes

Because identification of NSSI as a distinct disorder may improve identification and treatment, it has been proposed as a diagnostic category in the upcoming DSM-V (APA, 2010). The criteria for identification is proposed to include the following (Table 11.1).

The rationale for including NSSI in the upcoming DSM-V involves six key points (APA, 2010). First, the behavior currently is only represented in the DSM as a criterion for borderline personality disorder. Research with the adolescent and adult populations across inpatient and outpatient settings has demonstrated that NSSI occurs with a variety of diagnoses and many who engage in the behavior do not warrant a diagnosis of borderline personality disorder (APA). Because NSSI can be dangerous to the individual, it should be recognized as a diagnosis warranting intervention.

Second, in the current criterion for borderline personality in which NSSI is mentioned, it is linked to suicidal ideation and behaviors. This may promote the view that self-injury with a sharp object is an attempt at suicide. This conclusion may erroneously lead to unnecessarily restrictive, expensive, and burdensome treatments, including inpatient hospitalization and extensive psychotherapies. This point is reinforced by data from the National Center for Injury Prevention and Control that indicate that between 10 and 30% of individuals who seek treatment at a hospital for self-injury are admitted as inpatients (APA, 2010).

A third reason for including NSSI in the forthcoming edition of the DSM is to distinguish the behaviors from attempted suicide (APA, 2010). The APA cited research which demonstrates that cutting with a sharp object infrequently leads to death. In fact, in 2005, cutting accounted for only 0.4% of suicides in the under-age-24 population. Furthermore, in studies where adolescents who engage in superficial injury were compared to those who had taken an overdose and survived, it was found that those who self-injured were less likely to wish to die, as were their counterparts who had overdosed. In the APA's definition of NSSI, a requirement for diagnosis is that injuries are superficial and frequently repeated, which suggests that adolescents who engage are aware of the nonlife-threatening nature of their behaviors (APA).

A fourth reason for including NSSI as a distinct diagnosis centers on public health impact. Because key benchmark and prevalence surveys do not currently differentiate between NSSI and suicidal behaviors, reports of suicide attempts in adolescents may be inflated. Current statistics demonstrate that between 9 and 11% of high school students have attempted suicide during the course of their lifetimes (APA, 2010). These numbers may decline if NSSI is reported as a separate and distinct behavior, which could impact prevention efforts and treatment regimens.

As its fifth point, APA (2010) lists the impact that including diagnostic criteria for NSSI would have on research. Identifying NSSI as a separate behavior class from suicide attempt may act as a stimulus for innovative studies (APA). Nock and Prinstein (2005) have clearly identified the inhibitors to research into the causes of and treatments for NSSI. The development of diagnostic criteria should help to eliminate these pitfalls by distinguishing NSSI as a separate entity from suicidal behaviors. Individuals who engage in NSSI would be more clearly identified which would enhance data collection and the study of valid prevention and treatment options within this population.

Finally, the sixth reason indicated by the APA (2010) for the inclusion of NSSI in the DSM is the distinct clinical features associated with the behavior, including prevalence, impairment, and history. One difficulty in measuring prevalence is that reports have failed to discriminate between *any incident* and *repeated incidents* of NSSI. As indicated by Klonsky and Muehlenkamp (2007), there are greater numbers of adolescents who engage in NSSI one time, as compared to those who engage chronically. If the distinction is not made in prevalence reporting, numbers could be considerably inflated. Another clinical feature is that of impairment. Although NSSI may temporarily bring feelings of relief to the adolescent, in the long term she may feel embarrassment or shame, which could cause her to withdraw from social interaction. Furthermore, medical complications can arise as a result of NSSI, including infection at the site of the wound. Finally, historical studies have indicated that NSSI usually commences around puberty, peaks in mid-adolescence, and decreases in adulthood, independent of other symptoms (APA, 2010). Development of diagnostic criteria would aid in determining actual numbers of cases, which would then inform intervention and preventive efforts.

11.3.3 Prevalence

As stated in the APA's (2010) rationale for developing criteria, actual prevalence rates of NSSI, as distinct from suicidal behaviors, are unknown. According to Nock (2009), approximately 1–4% of adults and 13–23% of adolescents report having self-injured at some point in their lives. The considerably higher rate among teens suggests one of two reasons – the rate of NSSI has increased in recent years, or adults may be less apt to report NSSI behaviors than adolescents are. When they examined NSSI in sixth, seventh, and eighth graders ($n = 508$), Hilt, Nock, Lloyd-Richardson, and Prinstein (2008) found that 7.5% reported having engaged in the behavior. No significant differences were revealed across genders, ethnicities, or grade levels, but there were differences among groups in reported health-risk behaviors. Results indicated that those participants who reported NSSI engaged in hard drug and nicotine use at higher rates than their peers who did not self-injure. Furthermore, adolescents in the NSSI group were more likely to describe themselves as overweight and to have reported binge eating in the previous year (Hilt et al.). A study by Ross, Heath, and Toste (2009) also found a strong association between disordered eating and NSSI, which may suggest that this population is particularly vulnerable to self-injury.

Although Hilt et al. (2008) reported no significant differences between genders in their study, Goldston and Compton (2007) reported that females engage in higher rates of NSSI behaviors than males, but that males are the more likely of the two genders to die by suicide. These gender differences appear to be especially evident in clinical samples (Goldston and Compton). Hilt et al. also reported no differences across ethnic groups, but there are few studies that have examined NSSI across races and these have yielded mixed results. One study (i.e., Nock, Joiner, Gordon, Lloyd-Richardson, & Prinstein, 2006) suggested that it may occur more frequently in Caucasians, whereas others have found similar rates across racial groups (Lloyd-Richardson, 2008). Although there are disparities among studies regarding gender and racial differences in NSSI, the correlated behaviors should indicate to professionals working with youth red flag behaviors, such as drug use and binge eating.

Research has also indicated that NSSI co-occurs with other disorders and that prevalence within the psychiatric population is greater than general prevalence (Langbehn & Pfohl, 1993). In one study adolescents who had attempted suicide were divided into two groups, those with a history of NSSI and those without. Results indicated that the group who had reported engaging in NSSI behaviors was significantly more likely to be diagnosed with oppositional defiant disorder, major depression, and dysthymia than their counterparts (Guertin, Lloyd-Richardson, Spirito, Donaldson, & Boergers, 2001). Research also has suggested that NSSI behaviors and attempted suicide occur frequently among individuals with eating disorders (Lacey, 1993; Wildman, Lilenfeld, & Marcus, 2004). The association between self-harm and eating disorders may lie in the fact that both have been linked to traumatic experiences, specifically sexual and/or physical abuse (Paul, Schroeter, Dahme, & Nutzinger, 2002; van der Kolk, Perry, & Herman, 1991). Finally, NSSI has been found to be more prevalent in gay, lesbian, and bisexual youth (DeLiberto & Nock, 2008; Whitlock et al., 2006). There is no clear indication for the increase of self-harm behaviors among this population, but it may be related to the social stigma, marginalization, and identity confusion that these young people often experience (Serras, Saules, Cranford, & Eisenberg, 2010). These comorbid disorders and behaviors may not predict NSSI in adolescents, but they should cause increased awareness in the practitioner.

11.4 Etiological Hypotheses and Theoretical Frameworks

Currently, the literature base regarding NSSI lacks research that provides a clear understanding of why adolescents engage in self-harm behaviors. There is some theoretical and empirical evidence to suggest that behaviors may be goal directed (Hilt et al., 2008). Nock and Prinstein (2004) made a distinction between studies into the causes of NSSI that take a syndromal approach and those that take a functional approach. A syndromal approach focuses on the classification and treatment of self-injurious behaviors by topographical characteristics, such as signs and symptoms. In contrast, a functional approach to studying the etiology of NSSI classifies and treats behaviors according to the functional processes that elicit and maintain them, including antecedent and consequent conditions. Although application of a functional approach has led to advances in conceptualization, assessment, and treatment of other disorders, this approach has not been applied with regularity in understanding NSSI in adolescents (Nock and Prinstein).

11.4.1   Functional Approach to Classification

In her examination, Suyemoto (1998) proposed four major functional categories – environmental, drive, affect regulation, and interpersonal. These four classifications are interrelated and more than one can apply to an individual at any given time. The first category, the environmental model, focuses on the adolescent who engages in NSSI and her environment. This model incorporates theory from both behavioral and systemic developmental perspectives and purports that NSSI behaviors begin through (a) family modeling of abuse that leads the adolescent to link pain and care, or (b) through modeling and learning about the reinforcement of self-injury. Once the adolescent begins to self-injure, she is reinforced either internally through the feeling of relief associated with harming herself, or environmentally through the attention of and control over others (Suyemoto). Nock (2009) also proposed that social learning plays a role in the adolescent's decision to self-injure because many who engage in NSSI report first learning about the behavior from friends, family, and the media. Indeed, the contagion effect has been noted in school settings (Carlson, DeGeer, Deur, & Fenton, 2005).

The second major category, the drive model, is rooted primarily in psychoanalytic theory which suggest that NSSI is an expression or repression of life, death, and/or sexual drives (Suyemoto, 1998). Within the drive model is the belief that self-injury is a compromise between life and death because the adolescent avoids complete destruction by channeling suicidal impulses into self-mutilation, which is viewed as an active coping mechanism in averting death. The drive functional category also includes the sexual model. This model suggests a link between NSSI and sexual development because self-injury behaviors rarely occur in children prior to puberty. The self-injurious behaviors are viewed as a way to obtain sexual gratification, to punish oneself for engaging in sexual thoughts or actions, or as an attempt to control sexual maturation. NSSI is an attempt to destroy or purify the body, or to take control of impulses, in the sexual model (Suyemoto). Nock (2009) also suggested that NSSI can be motivated by the need to self-punish, but indicated that the behaviors are learned through repeated punishment and criticism by others.

Affect regulation, the third major category examined by Suyemoto (1998), is viewed by many researchers to be the primary function of NSSI. In this model, self-harm behaviors are viewed as a method for expressing emotions. Injuring herself enables the adolescent to achieve a sense of control over emotions that may overwhelm her or to dissociate. NSSI provides a method for the individual to externalize what she is feeling internally. The emotion may be anger that is redirected onto self for fear of hurting the other or emotional pain that is the result of perceived abandonment or rejection. Self-injury in this model is conceptualized as the need to feel physical pain, as opposed to emotional pain. NSSI produces physical evidence of the emotions that validates or justifies what the adolescent is feeling (Suyemoto). Furthermore, NSSI can enable the adolescent to dissociate as the injury distracts her from aversive, stressful, or unmanageable thoughts or feelings (Nock, 2009), or can serve to end dissociation (Brown, Houck, Grossman, Lescano,

& Frenkel, 2002). It remains unclear how NSSI may help to end dissociation, but the blood that usually appears after injury may be a possible agent, as it shocks the individual. The scars that are left may serve to create continuity of existence for the adolescent, as episodes of dissociation are integrated into her sense of identity (Suyemoto, 1998).

The final category discussed by Suyemoto (1998) was an interpersonal model. This model focuses on the adolescent's need to affirm the boundaries of self. The individual perceives a sense of loss or abandonment and her lack of boundaries leads her to experience the loss of other as loss of self. To combat these feelings, the adolescent self-injures to define boundaries because the skin is the primary boundary between self and others. The resultant blood and scars create a distinct and separate self and provide the adolescent with a unique identity (Suyemoto).

Nock and Prinstein (2004) also proposed a functional model for classifying NSSI behaviors. Their model includes four primary functions that differ along dichotomous dimensions. The two dimensions include contingencies that are automatic vs. social and reinforcement that is negative vs. positive. *Automatic-negative reinforcement* refers to the adolescent's use of NSSI to reduce tension or other negative affect states. Events that precipitate the negative feeling state include conflict, rejection, separation, and abandonment; these circumstances may be real, imagined, or threatened (Haines, Williams, Brain, & Wilson, 1995). A number of studies in which individuals reported negative feelings prior to self-injuring endorse this function (e.g., Gardner & Gardner, 1975; Haines et al., 1995; Rosenthal, Rinzler, Walsh, & Klausner, 1972) and in theoretical accounts, it is the most commonly cited (Nock & Prinstein). Biological research has implicated the endogenous opioid system in both the etiology and maintenance of NSSI. Regardless of the mode of injury, it is often self-reported to be accompanied by partial or full analgesia (Yates, 2004). Along the same dimension are NSSI behaviors whose primary function is *automatic-positive reinforcement*. The adolescent self-injures to create a desirable psychological state, in which she feels something, even if it is physical pain (Nock & Prinstein).

In contrast, the second dimension includes social reinforcement functions for NSSI that enable the adolescent to modify or regulate her environment (Nock & Prinstein, 2004). Although the existence of *social-negative reinforcement* as a function has not been strongly endorsed in the literature, it is possible that an adolescent may receive negative reinforcement for injuring herself. For example, NSSI may enable her to avoid an unpleasant task or punishment from others (Nock & Prinstein). Finally, *social-positive reinforcement* involves gaining attention from others or gaining access to a desired object within the environment. This function has been widely discussed in the theoretical literature, but as with the social-negative function, there is little empirical evidence supporting its existence (Nock & Prinstein). Certainly, more research needs to be done into the social aspects that may be reinforcing NSSI. This area is especially important to explore, given that some authors have proposed a contagion effect through which adolescents observe others being reinforced for NSSI and then imitate the behavior (Simpson, 1975; Suyemoto, 1998).

To explore the proposed functions within their model, Nock and Prinstein (2004) assessed data from 108 adolescents (32 boys and 76 girls) who had been admitted to an inpatient care unit. Of the overall sample, 82.4% of participants reported at least one incident of NSSI in the previous 12-month period. Only 7% of those who self-injured reported one incident; 50.6% reported 19 or more incidents of NSSI in the previous year. When a confirmatory factor analysis was conducted to examine the proposed functions, the theoretically derived four-function model was deemed to be the best fit (Nock & Prinstein). This study demonstrated that adolescents engage in NSSI for a variety of reasons. The key to providing treatment rests in determining the function for an individual and teaching alternative replacement behaviors that meet the function, but that are less harmful and more socially acceptable.

11.4.2 Pain Pathways

Some research also exists to suggest that adolescents who self-injure may process pain differently than their peers who do not engage in NSSI. There are data to indicate that the neural pathways of physical and emotional pain within the NSSI adolescent population overlap (Brown, Houck, Grossman, Lescano, & Frenkel, 2008). Correlational data suggest that an early traumatic event, such as sexual abuse, may disrupt the development of central nervous system pathways. This biological difference may cause certain adolescents to experience physical pain differently than others (Brown et al.). Because disruptive family factors (e.g., child abuse, family substance abuse, and family violence) have been associated with the occurrence of NSSI in adolescents (Guertin et al., 2001), it may prove beneficial to monitor children who have been exposed to these types of risk factors and to provide intensive treatment early in an effort to prevent self-injurious behaviors.

11.4.3 Conclusions: Syndromal vs. Functional Approaches

NSSI has been conceptualized through both a syndromal approach and a functional approach in the literature (Nock, 2009). The syndromal approach associates self-injurious behavior with psychiatric disorders, as a symptom. However, Nock argues that because NSSI occurs across many disorders and is not symptomatic of any one, it may be more appropriate to take a functional approach. A functional approach assumes that behaviors are directly related to immediate antecedents and consequences (Nock). Assessing and determining function (i.e., to gain positive reinforcement or to escape undesired feelings) aids in intervention design because it allows for the development of alternative, less harmful behaviors that meet the same function, or purpose, for the adolescent. The next sections discuss assessment and treatment from a functional approach, including a school-based component.

11.5   Assessment

In 1995, Rosen and Heard reported a variety of terms from the literature that had been used historically to describe self-harm behaviors. Among the terms included were *self-mutilation*, *attempted suicide*, *partial suicide*, *focal suicide*, *parasuicide*, *wrist cutting*, and *deliberate self-harm*. According to these authors, past research had grouped all self-harm behaviors from the extremely mild to the disfiguring, without regard for severity or location on the body. These are important aspects to consider because the severity of the wound dictates the level of treatment that follows. Categorizing behavior would allow clinicians and researchers to report behavior in a standardized way, target treatment, and provide new avenues for study (Rosen & Heard). Rosen and Heard examined 32 adolescents with 128 reported self-injuries and proposed the following model of categorization:

- Level 1, composed of superficial injuries, resulting in damage to only the first layer of skin, and requiring no medical treatment.
- Level 2, including injuries that break the skin, bleed, and require a bandage.
- Level 3, which encompasses injuries that bleed significantly and require medical treatment, such as stitches or another sterile closure device.
- Level 4, which includes serious wounds that require multiple stitches and that are potentially disfiguring or life-threatening (Rosen & Heard, 1995).

Rosen and Heard (1995) contend that this method of assessment is efficient and reliable and allows for a standardized method of reporting injuries. Although a clear understanding of the severity of the behavior is important to the intervention process, this type of categorization provides little insight into the motivation or reason for the behavior. Determining the function is key to designing an intervention package because it enables the practitioner to focus treatment. For example, if an adolescent is engaging in NSSI behaviors as a way to cope with negative emotions, treatment should focus on emotion regulation skills. Assessing function may also help the clinician to identify the adolescent who is at-risk for a psychological disorder or suicidal behavior (Klonsky & Muehlenkamp, 2007). Within the general population, function may be evaluated through interview or self-report scales, but within the population with developmental disabilities or cognitive impairment, it may be necessary to determine the function through direct observational techniques (Iwata, Dorsey, Slifer, Bauman, & Richman, 1994; Iwata et al., 1994).

Walsh (2007) suggested a function-based assessment that included two aspects – the informal response and the details of self-injury. The informal response focuses on the professional's reaction to the client who discloses NSSI behaviors. Walsh advises that the service provider should attempt to respond in a low-key dispassionate demeanor when the client first shares that she is hurting herself. A response of shock or disgust could cause the adolescent to avoid revealing additional information. Likewise, effusive expressions of support should be avoided upon disclosure because such may inadvertently reinforce the behavior, depending on the function. The professional should also avoid jumping directly to a "contract for safety" because forbidding the adolescent to engage in NSSI behaviors can be invalidating and unrealistic at the start. Rather, in this early stage, the professional should proceed with respectful curiosity, asking such questions as "What does self-injury do for you?" This type of questioning during assessment can open the door for direct and open communication about the function of the NSSI behaviors (Walsh).

Once the tone has been set, the practitioner can begin a more detailed assessment of the NSSI behavior (Walsh, 2007). First, the history of the behavior should be determined. History includes details pertaining to the age of onset, types of NSSI (e.g., cutting or burning), duration and frequency of the behavior, and the level of physical damage. Generally, the longer the problem has existed, the greater the challenge will be in alleviating it (Walsh). Once a history has been established, the clinician should begin to assess the current problem by asking questions about the extent of damage, the location of injury on the body, and the antecedent and consequent conditions. To assess the level of physical damage, Walsh suggests using the *Suicide Attempt Self-Injury Interview* (SASII; Linehan, Comtois, Brown, Heards, & Wagner, 2006a) and observing wounds directly, with the client's permission and within the bounds of modesty because self-report may not be accurate. Further, the location on the body may signal that the adolescent needs referral for an immediate mental health assessment. NSSI typically occurs on the abdomen or extremities. If injuries are observed on face, eyes, breasts in girls, or genitals, the adolescent may be experiencing a psychotic decompensation or trauma-related behavior. To assess antecedent and consequent conditions, the practitioner may encourage the client to keep a log, in which she records events or feelings directly prior to and after the NSSI incident (Walsh).

11.5.1   Standardized Measures

There are several standardized instruments that can be used during the NSSI assessment process to determine suicide intent and risk. However, Prinstein, Nock, Spirito, and Grapentine (2001) cautioned that the agreement between different evaluative instruments and methods is not always strong and, thus, it is important to obtain information through multiple methods (Goldston & Compton, 2007). A scale should not be the only source of data collection, but should be used as one piece of information in a comprehensive assessment. Different classes of standardized instruments include those designed as detection instruments, as predictors of suicidality, and as assessment of clinical characteristics of self-harm behaviors (Goldston & Compton). Detection instruments assess current suicidal ideation and/or NSSI through interviews, self-report questionnaires, or behavior checklists. Two structured interviews that can be used for detection purposes are the Schedule for Affective Disorders and Schizophrenia for School-Age Children – Epidemiological Version (K-SADS-E) and the Diagnostic Interview Schedule for Children (DISC), although the DISC does not contain questions regarding nonsuicidal behaviors. In addition to the scales, depression scales also can be used as screeners for suicidal ideation (Goldston & Compton).

11.5.2   Critical Need: Evaluation for Suicidality

Assessment should also include risk for future suicidal behavior. Risk assessment instruments generally include self-report questionnaires that survey cognitive states associated with suicide (Goldston & Compton, 2007). One such scale is the Beck Hopelessness Scale (BHS), which includes a child version, the Hopelessness Scale for Children (HSC) for ages 6 through 13 years. Studies have documented the association between scores on the BHS and the HSC with depression and fewer reasons for living. However, there are mixed data pertaining to whether the HSC actually predicts future suicide attempts (Goldston & Compton), so the scale should be used with caution and in conjunction with other data collection methods. Another suicide risk measure, the Columbia Suicide Screen, can be administered in a group setting. However, this measure can produce false positives, so it is recommended that the DISC, or a similar scale, be used as a second stage screener to identify at-risk youth appropriately (Goldston & Compton). A number of other scales also are available for suicidality screening purposes. An example of an instrument that can be used to assess the clinical characteristics of suicidal behaviors is the Beck Suicide Intent Scale (SIS). The SIS assesses the objective and subjective intent of a suicide attempt. The objective intent focuses on behaviors that can be observed, such as precautions taken against discovery and the amount of planning. Subjective intent includes questions regarding the client's perceived seriousness of the attempt (Goldston & Compton).

Another scale that can be used for assessment purposes is the Deliberate Self-Harm Inventory (DSHI; Gratz, 2001). The DSHI is a behaviorally based, self-report questionnaire that is composed of 17 items that assess direct destruction or alteration of body tissue in which there is no conscious wish to die. Gratz selected the term *self-harm* to describe behaviors that are episodic and repetitive and that result in injuries that are superficial to moderate. These behaviors are deliberate, as opposed to indirect self-harm behaviors, such as reckless driving and substance abuse. Questions on the DSHI pertain to history and nature of the self-harm behaviors. Sample questions include: (a) "Have you ever intentionally (i.e., on purpose) cut your wrist, arms, or other area(s) of your body (without intending to kill yourself)?" (b) "How old were you when you first did this?" The measure questions a variety of self-harm behaviors, such as burning and carving, in addition to cutting. Preliminary data suggested that the DSHI demonstrated high internal consistency and adequate validity. However, the original sample included 150 undergraduate students, whose ages ranged from 18 to 64 ($m = 23.19$, SD $= 7.13$) (Gratz). Thus, the scale should be interpreted with caution when used with adolescents or younger children, but may provide a good starting point in obtaining information regarding the history and nature of NSSI.

11.5.3   Standardized Measures of NSSI

One promising measure that has been recently examined is the inventory of statements about self-injury (ISAS; Klonsky & Glenn, 2008). The ISAS was designed to assess the function and lifetime history of NSSI behaviors. Thirteen functions are included in the measure: (a) affect regulation; (b) antidissociation; (c) antisuicide; (d) marking distress; (e) self-punishment; (f) autonomy; (g) interpersonal boundaries; (h) interpersonal influence; (i) peer bonding; (j) revenge; (k) self-care; (l) sensation seeking; and (m) toughness. These functions comprised two factors representing interpersonal and intrapersonal functions. When the ISAS was administered to 235 young adults, it demonstrated both reliability and validity (Klonsky & Glenn), suggesting that it may be a useful tool in assessment of the adolescent who engages in NSSI.

Although a few other measures have been developed to assess NSSI, they are either unpublished (e.g., Self-Harm Behavior Survey), contain limited questions regarding NSSI within the context of risk behaviors (e.g., Chronic Self-Destructiveness Scale; Beasley & Dolin, 1998), or were developed for use with persons with developmental disabilities (e.g., Timed Self-Injurious Behavior Scale; Brasic et al., 1997). Certainly, more research into the development of tools that assess the history and function of NSSI are needed to inform intervention packages. However, it should be kept in mind that a scale should only be one component of a multidimensional assessment system. As noted, other means for assessment include interviews, logs that document antecedent and consequent conditions, and direct observation of wounds, when possible. Data should be collected in an on-going fashion to enable the practitioner to operationalize the behavior and design appropriate treatment.

11.6   Treatment and Intervention

When the functional model of NSSI is considered, the implication is that different learning experiences both elicit and maintain the behavior across individuals (Nock & Prinstein, 2004). Thus, treatment should be diverse and individualized, with the goal of replacing NSSI with functionally equivalent behaviors. For example, if an adolescent's NSSI is maintained through social reinforcement, an approach that teaches more adaptive interpersonal communication skills would be appropriate. Likewise, if the function of an adolescent's NSSI behavior is automatic reinforcement (i.e., escape from emotional pain), treatment should focus on teaching alternative affect-regulation skills (Nock & Prinstein). Claes and Vandereycken (2007) stated that before jumping to general etiological models of NSSI, the practitioner should start with an analysis of the functions, or motives, of the behavior for the adolescent. A functional approach, with insight into the situation–behavior relations and the antecedent and consequent cognitive and affective processes that elicit and maintain them, should become the cornerstone for development of the treatment package (Claes & Vandereycken).

11.6.1 Dialectical Behavior Therapy

Some research (e.g., Linehan et al., 2006b; Linehan, Armstrong, Suarez, Allmon, & Heard, 1991; Suyemoto, 1998) suggests that dialectical behavior therapy (DBT), which combines behavioral, cognitive, and supportive interventions, may be a treatment option for adolescents who engage in NSSI. DBT consists of behavioral techniques, including contingency management and exposure to emotional cues, that are balanced with supportive techniques, such as reflection, empathy, and acceptance (Linehan et al., 1991). Linehan et al. (2006b) stated that the goals of this type of therapy are to (a) increase behavioral capabilities; (b) improve motivation for skillful behavior through contingency management; (c) assure generalization of new behaviors to the daily environment; (d) structure the environment so that it reinforces functional, rather than dysfunctional behaviors; and (e) enhance the therapist's capabilities to treat the individual with NSSI behaviors effectively. Within this individualized treatment framework, adolescents also attend group therapy sessions that focus on the development of interpersonal and emotional regulation skills (Suyemoto, 1998).

11.6.2 Psychodynamic Therapy

Another treatment for NSSI that has received attention in the literature is psychodynamic therapy. This type of therapy has generally been used with patients with borderline personality disorder, but many times it is the NSSI behaviors that are a target of the treatment. Therapeutic elements include (a) processing the past relationships and building new positive interpersonal relationships; (b) increasing self-awareness and expression of affect; and (c) developing a positive self-image (Klonsky & Muehlenkamp, 2007). Although no studies to date have identified the mechanisms of therapeutic change in individuals with NSSI, research has demonstrated significant improvements in interpersonal relationships, general distress, and self-injurious behaviors that were maintained over time (Klonsky & Muehlenkamp). Research findings suggest that psychodynamic therapy may be beneficial for some adolescents, especially if the function for behavior is to gain attention or express negative feelings, given that therapy focuses on relationships and expression of affect.

11.6.3 Narrative Therapy

Hoffman and Kress (2008) cautioned that often individuals who engage in NSSI perceive themselves to be a burden to others. If the practitioner treats the adolescent as manipulative or attention-seeking or communicates the idea that she has a mental illness, these feelings of being a burden could be inadvertently reinforced. Thus,

Hoffman and Kress suggested using a narrative treatment approach to therapy. Narrative therapy supports the individual's motivation to change. Without the motivation component to therapy, the adolescent may be ambivalent about or resistant to disengaging from the behavior. Within this approach, the therapist and the client collaborate to identify the presenting problem. The goal of narrative therapy is for the therapist to aid the adolescent in re-authoring her problem story to incorporate positive, empowering aspects of herself and to realize that NSSI is not the result of a personality flaw. Ultimately, the practitioner helps the adolescent to realize that the NSSI behaviors are separate and external from her. Techniques employed include naming the problem and writing a letter to or drawing the problem. Hoffman and Kress concluded that externalizing the behavior can potentially reduce the feelings of blame, guilt, and shame that often accompany NSSI.

The literature (e.g., Selekamn, 2010; Yip, 2006) also has suggested that therapy with the adolescent who engages in NSSI should be strengths-based. This approach focuses on the wellness of the adolescent and her family, rather than what is wrong with them. Family members take the lead in determining goals for treatment, setting the agenda for sessions, determining who attends, and setting the frequency of sessions. The idea behind the strengths-based approach is that if the adolescent is empowered with control over her own treatment, the likelihood of her ending prematurely or becoming resistant is greatly reduced. If the adolescent's goals are different from her family's, then the therapist can establish different goals. The therapist should meet with the adolescent and her family together and also independent of one another. This enables the parents to share past treatment attempts and to learn more effective parent management skills. When the adolescent meets without her parents, she can share her self-injury stories freely and discuss life stressors that she may want help managing. During family meeting time, the parent–child relationship is fostered (Selekamn). Although there are no data to support the use of strengths-based therapy, it may be a useful component to add to a functional approach because its focus is on wellness and not on pathology.

11.6.4 Psychopharmacology

Finally, some researchers have suggested that medication may be helpful in reducing NSSI behaviors. Favazza (1998) wrote that uncontrolled cutting can often be treated rapidly and effectively with high doses of serotonin reuptake inhibitors (SRIs), such as fluoxetine. After several weeks, the SRI should be tapered and a mood stabilizer started. However, Klonsky and Muehlenkamp (2007) caution that there has been no research conducted to date to evaluate the effectiveness of medications in reducing NSSI. Rather, there is research to document the usefulness of pharmacotherapy in reducing the symptoms of mental disorders that sometimes co-occur with NSSI, such as borderline personality disorder. Thus, the decision whether to prescribe medication should be made on an individual basis, with comorbid disorders considered.

Given that NSSI has been diagnosed both across and apart from a variety of disorders (Suyemoto, 1998), the function-based approach to assessment and treatment may be the most valid route to take. The behavior appears to be elicited and maintained across individuals for a variety of reasons. Treatment effectiveness depends on the identification of the motivation and reinforcement for the behavior in the adolescent's life. Identification of the function and the related antecedent conditions and reinforcing contingencies can aid the therapist in teaching the adolescent appropriate replacement skills to meet her needs.

11.7   Prevention

Because NSSI prevalence rates appear to be increasing among the adolescent population, the need to prevent the behavior from occurring is of importance (Muehlenkamp, Walsh, & McDade, 2009). Roberts-Dobie and Donatelle (2007) suggest that self-injury education could be incorporated into schools' existing mental health curricula. Student education should focus on the signs of mental stress, risk factors, and coping strategies. Further, students should receive training in acting as referral agents or "gatekeepers" for friends who are suspected of engaging in NSSI behaviors because peers are usually the first to notice or to be told. Any education program should avoid detailed descriptions of self-injury to limit suggestion, however (Roberts-Dobie & Donatelle).

Prevention activities can serve a dual purpose – to stop an adolescent from suffering serious physical injury and to avert a potential pathway to suicide. However, prevention activities generally are implemented on a minimal basis. As Muehlenkamp et al. (2009) note, this is concerning because recent research has indicated that adolescents believe the best ways to prevent NSSI behaviors are to have access to nonjudgmental persons at school, to provide education to teachers, parents, and peers about how to respond, and to reduce concerns about confidentiality and the stigma associated with seeking help. School provides an optimal place to offer a preventative program because adolescents spend a significant amount of their time in school (Muehlenkamp et al.). A comprehensive prevention program should include training in coping skills, interpersonal communication, goal setting, anger management, and advocacy skills for all students (Shapiro, 2008).

One such prevention program that has been examined is the Signs of Self-Injury program (SOSI). The goals of the SOSI program are to (a) increase knowledge of NSSI, including warning signs; (b) improve attitudes and capability to respond to peers who engage in NSSI; (c) increase help-seeking behaviors; and (d) decrease NSSI. The program includes two general modules – one for students and one for faculty and staff. The module for faculty includes psychoeducational material about NSSI and how to respond if a student self-discloses the behavior. The student module includes a DVD that presents information about NSSI and a series of vignettes that teaches them how to respond to peers who are engaging in NSSI. An implementation guide that contains discussion questions and answers are included with the program (Muehlenkamp et al., 2009).

When Muehlenkamp and colleagues (2009) implemented SOSI with 274 adolescents across five schools, the results of pre- and postsurveys indicated that the program increased accurate knowledge of NSSI and improved help-seeking attitudes and intentions among the student participants. Although no significant changes were found in regard to self-reported formal help-seeking actions, the survey data suggest that implementation of the program may help to increase awareness and foster positive attitudes toward seeking help. Furthermore, school personnel indicated that the program was easy to implement (Muehlenkamp et al., 2009). These preliminary data are positive and certainly suggest that more research with prevention programs, such as SOSI, needs to be conducted.

11.8 Suicidal Ideation

In the recent literature NSSI has been distinguished from suicidal behaviors, in that there is no intent to die for youth who engage in NSSI. NSSI usually involves behaviors that are considered low in lethality, such as cutting and burning, whereas the majority of deaths by suicide include behaviors such as self-inflicted gunshots, hanging, overdosing, and jumping from lethal heights (Muehlenkamp & Kerr, 2010). Despite the differences in method and intent, research has shown that NSSI is a risk factor for future suicidal behavior (Brausch & Gutierrez, 2010). An important area to examine involves the factors that predict which adolescents who engage in NSSI will go on to attempt suicide from those who do not. To date there is scant research in this area (Brausch & Gutierrez).

When Muehlenkamp and Gutierrez (2004) examined the differences between adolescents who engage in NSSI and those who attempt suicide, they found no significant differences in suicidal ideation or depressive symptoms. This may be due to the fact that both groups are experiencing high levels of distress and that the self-harm is a response to these feelings. As such, scores on suicide ideation or depression measures may not adequately identify those adolescents with a history of NSSI who are at risk for suicide. Muehlenkamp and Gutierrez posited that the difference between the groups may lie in the individual's attitude toward life, with the more positive attitude underlying the decision to engage in NSSI, rather than commit suicide (Muehlenkamp & Gutierrez, 2004).

Brausch and Gutierrez (2010) also examined the differences between adolescents who engaged in NSSI and those who had a history of NSSI in addition to a suicide attempt. These authors found that group who engaged in NSSI only had fewer depressive symptoms, lower suicidal ideation, greater self-esteem, and more parental support than their peers who had also attempted suicide. Certainly, the results of these two studies suggest that much more work is needed to identify the factors that predict which adolescents who engage in NSSI will go on to attempt suicide. However, they suggest that adolescents who have a history of NSSI should be screened for suicidal ideation and should be monitored for increasing depression and more lethal behaviors. Furthermore, findings from the second study suggest that parental support may play a role in the adolescent's behavior and thereby suggest an area that may be a protective factor in future suicidal ideation.

11.9   Conclusion and Future Directions

Although NSSI is not currently a diagnosable disorder, it can be dangerous to the individual and, thus, warrants identification and intervention. The DSM-V working group has proposed a diagnostic model for the upcoming edition of the manual. There is a growing literature base that suggests assessment of NSSI behaviors should include analysis of the function, or motivation, it serves for the individual. Future research in this area should explore the functions that have been proposed and identify related treatment procedures. Along these lines, new measures that evaluate NSSI behaviors need to be developed and validated. Currently, there are a few measures that are self-report in nature that assess NSSI, but they have been evaluated on a limited basis and a few remain unpublished. In addition, given prevalence rates and the contagion factor, prevention programs should be investigated. One program, the SOSI increased awareness and improved attitudes toward help-seeking behaviors in a sample of adolescents. This suggests that education may be a key factor in reducing rates of NSSI, especially when conducted in schools where children spend most of their time and have the opportunity to learn from each other and/or observe behaviors being reinforced. Finally, much more work is needed to identify the factors that put an adolescent who engages in NSSI at risk for future suicide attempt. Intervention for suicidal ideation can be time and resource intensive and can disrupt the adolescent's life. If clear differences between adolescents who engage solely in NSSI and those who also attempt suicide can be uncovered, intervention could be better designed and delivered. Indeed, this is an area replete with research opportunities.

References

American Psychiatric Association. (2000). *Diagnostic and statistical manual of mental disorders* (4th ed., rev.) Washington, DC: Author.
American Psychiatric Association (2010). *DSM-5 development: Non-suicidal self injury*. Retrieved November 8, 2010, from http://www.dsm5.org/ProposedRevisions/Pages/proposedrevision. aspx?rid=443#
Brausch, A. M., & Gutierrez, P. M. (2010). Differences in non-suicidal self-injury and suicide attempts in adolescents. *Journal of Youth and Adolescence, 39*, 233–242.
Beasley, T. M., & Dolin, I. H. (1998). Factor analyses of the Chronic Self-Destructiveness Scale among delinquent and non-delinquent adolescent males. *Journal of Offender Rehabilitation, 26*, 141–156.

Brasic, J. R., Barnett, J. Y., Ahn, S. C., Nadrich, R. H., Will, M. V., & Clair, A. (1997). Clinical assessment of self-injurious behavior. *Psychological Reports, 80*, 155–160.

Brown, M. Z., Comtois, K. A., & Linehan, M. M. (2002). Reasons for suicide attempts and nonsuicidal self-injury in women with borderline personality disorder. *Journal of Abnormal Psychology, 111*, 198–202.

Brown, L. K., Houck, C. D., Grossman, C. I., Lescano, C. M., & Frenkel, J. L. (2008). Frequency of adolescent self-cutting as a predictor of HIV risk. *Journal of Developmental and Behavioral Pediatrics, 29*, 161–165.

Carlson, L., DeGeer, S. M., Deur, C., & Fenton, K. (2005). Teachers' awareness of self-cutting behavior among the adolescent population. *Praxis, 5*, 22–29.

Claes, L., & Vandereycken, W. (2007). Self-injurious behavior: Differential diagnosis and functional differentiation. *Comprehensive Psychiatry, 48*, 137–144.

Cloutier, P., Martin, J., Kennedy, A., Nixon, M. K., & Muehlenkamp, J. J. (2009). Characteristics and co-occurrence of adolescent non-suicidal self-injury and suicidal behaviors in pediatric emergency crises services. *Journal of Youth and Adolescence, 39*, 259–269.

DeLiberto, T., & Nock, M. (2008). An exploratory study of correlates, onset, and offset of non-suicidal self-injury. *Archives of Suicide Research, 12*, 219–231.

Emerson, L. E. (1913). The case of Miss A: A preliminary report of a psychoanalysis study and treatment of a case of self-mutilation. *The Psychoanalytic Review: A Journal Devoted to an Understanding of Human Conduct, 1*, 41–54.

Favazza, A. R. (1987). *Bodies under siege: Self-mutilation and body modification in culture and psychiatry.* Baltimore, MD: John Hopkins University Press.

Favazza, A. R. (1998). The coming of age of self-mutilation. *Journal of Nervous and Mental disease, 186*, 259–268.

Gardner, A. R., & Gardner, A. J. (1975). Self-mutilation, obsessionality and narcissism. *British Journal of Psychiatry, 127*, 127–132.

Goldston, D. B., & Compton, J. S. (2007). Adolescent suicidal and nonsuicidal self-harm behaviors and risks. In E. J. Mash & R. A. Barkely (Eds.), *Assessment of childhood disorders* (4th ed., pp. 305–343). New York, NY: The Guilford Press.

Gratz, K. L. (2001). Measurement of deliberate self-harm: Preliminary Data on the Deliberate Self-Harm Inventory. *Journal of Psychopathology and Behavioral Assessment, 23*, 253–263.

Guertin, T., Lloyd-Richardson, E., Spirito, A., Donaldson, D., & Boergers, J. (2001). Self-mutilative behavior in adolescents who attempt suicide by overdose. *Journal of the American Academy of Child and Adolescent Psychiatry, 40*, 1062–1069.

Haines, J., Williams, C. L., Brain, K. L., & Wilson, G. V. (1995). The psychophysiology of self-mutilation. *Journal of Abnormal Psychology, 104*, 471–489.

Hilt, L. M., Nock, M. K., Lloyd-Richardson, E. E., & Prinstein, M. J. (2008). Longitudinal study of nonsuicidal self-injury among young adolescents: Rates, correlates, and preliminary test of an interpersonal model. *Journal of Early Adolescence, 28*, 455–469.

Hoffman, R. M., & Kress, V. E. (2008). Narrative therapy and non-suicidal self-injurious behavior: Externalizing the problem and internalizing personal agency. *Journal of Humanistic Counseling, Education and Development, 47*, 157–171.

Iwata, B. A., Dorsey, M. F., Slifer, K. J., Bauman, K. E., & Richman, G. S. (1994). Toward a functional analysis of self-injury. *Journal of Applied Behavior Analysis, 27*, 197–209.

Iwata, B. A., Pace, G. M., Dorsey, M. F., Zarcone, J. R., Vollmer, T. R., Smith, R. G., et al. (1994). The functions of self-injurious behavior: An experimental-epidemiological analysis. *Journal of Applied Behavior Analysis, 27*, 215–240.

Kanan, L. M., Finger, J., & Plog, A. E. (2008). Self injury and youth: Best practices for school intervention. *School Psychology Forum: Research in Practice, 2*, 67–79.

Klonsky, E. D., & Glenn, C. R. (2008). Assessing the functions of non-suicidal self-injury: Psychometric properties of the Inventory of Statements About Self-injury (ISAS). *Journal of Psychopathology & Behavioral Assessment, 31*, 215–219.

Klonsky, E. D., & Moyer, A. (2008). Childhood sexual abuse and non-suicidal self-injury: Meta-analysis. *The British Journal of Psychiatry, 192*, 166–170.

Klonsky, E. D., & Muehlenkamp, J. J. (2007). Self-injury: A research review for the practitioner. *Journal of Clinical Psychology: In Session, 63*, 1045–1056.

Klonsky, E. D., & Olino, T. M. (2008). Identifying clinically distinct subgroups of self-injurers among young adults: A latent class analysis. *Journal of Consulting and Clinical Psychology, 76*, 22–27.

Klonsky, E. D., Oltmanns, T. F., & Turkheimer, E. (2003). Deliberate self-harm in a nonclinical population: Prevalence and psychological correlates. *American Journal of Psychiatry, 160*, 1501–1508.

Lacey, J. H. (1993). Self-damaging and addictive behavior in bulimia nervosa: A catchment area study. *British Journal of Psychiatry, 163*, 190–194.

Langbehn, D. R., & Pfohl, B. (1993). Clinical correlates of self-mutilation among psychiatric inpatients. *Annals of Clinical Psychiatry, 5*, 45–51.

Laye-Gindhu, A., & Schonert-Reichl, K. A. (2005). Nonsuicidal self-harm among community adolescents: Understanding the "whats" and "whys" of self-harm. *Journal of Youth and Adolescence, 34*, 447–457.

Linehan, M. M., Comtois, K. A., Brown, M. Z., Heards, H. L., & Wagner, A. (2006). Suicide Attempt Self-injury Interview (SASII): Development, reliability, and validity of a scale to assess suicide attempts and intentional self-injury. *Psychological Assessment, 18*, 303–312.

Linehan, M. M., Comtois, K. A., Murray, A. M., Brown, M. Z., Gallop, R. J., Heard, H. L., et al. (2006). Two-year randomized control trial and follow-up of dialectical behavior therapy vs therapy by experts for suicidal behaviors and borderline personality disorder. *Archives of General Psychiatry, 63*, 757–766.

Linehan, M. M., Armstrong, H. E., Suarez, A., Allmon, D., & Heard, H. L. (1991). Cognitive-behavioral treatment of chronically parasuicidal borderline patients. *Archives of General Psychiatry, 48*, 1060–1064.

Lloyd-Richardson, E. E. (2008). Adolescent nonsuicidal self-injury: Who is doing it and why? *Journal of Development and Behavioral Pediatrics, 29*, 216–218.

Menninger, K. (1935). A psychoanalytic study of the significance of self-mutilation. *Psychoanalytic Quarterly, 4*, 408–466.

Menninger, K. (1938). Self-mutilations. In *Man against himself* (Part IV, Section II, pp. 203–249) New York: Harcourt & Brace.

Muehlenkamp, J. J., & Gutierrez, P. M. (2004). An investigation of differences between self-injurious behavior and suicide attempts in a sample of adolescents. *Suicide and Life Threatening Behavior, 34*, 12–23.

Muehlenkamp, J. J., & Kerr, P. L. (2010). Untangling a complex web: How non-suicidal self-injury and suicide attempts differ. *The Prevention Researcher, 17*, 8–10.

Muehlenkamp, J. J., Walsh, B. W., & McDade, M. (2009). Preventing non-suicidal self-injury in adolescents: The Signs of Self-injury Program. *Journal of Youth and Adolescence, 39*, 306–314.

Nock, M. K. (2009). Why do people hurt themselves? New insights into the nature and functions of self-injury. *Current Directions in Psychological Science, 18*, 78–83.

Nock, M. K., Joiner, T. E., Jr., Gordon, K. H., Lloyd-Richardson, E., & Prinstein, M. J. (2006). Non-suicidal self-injury among adolescents: Diagnostic correlates and relation to suicide attempts. *Psychiatry Research, 144*, 65–72.

Nock, M. K., & Mendes, W. B. (2008). Physiological arousal, distress tolerance, and social problem-solving deficits among adolescent self-injurers. *Journal of Consulting and Clinical Psychology, 76*, 28–38.

Nock, M. K., & Prinstein, M. J. (2004). A functional approach to the assessment of self- mutilative behavior. *Journal of Consulting and clinical Psychology, 72*, 885–890.

Nock, M. K., & Prinstein, M. J. (2005). Contextual features and behavioral functions of self-mutilation among adolescents. *Journal of Abnormal Psychology, 114*, 140–146.

Nock, M. K., Teper, R., & Hollander, M. (2007). Psychological treatment of self-injury among adolescents. *Journal of Clinical Psychology: In Session, 63*, 1081–1089.

Paul, T., Schroeter, K., Dahme, B., & Nutzinger, D. O. (2002). Self-injurious behavior in women with eating disorders. *American Journal of Psychiatry, 159*, 408–411.

Prinstein, M., Nock, M., Spirito, A., & Grapentine, W. (2001). Multimethod assessment of suicidality in adolescent psychiatric inpatients: Preliminary results. *Journal of the American Academy of Child and Adolescent Psychiatry, 40*, 1053–1061.

Roberts-Dobie, S., & Donatelle, R. J. (2007). School counselors and student self-injury. *Journal of School Health, 77*, 257–264.

Rosen, P. M., & Heard, K. V. (1995). A method for reporting self-harm according to level of injury and location on the body. *Suicide and Life Threatening Behavior, 25*, 381–385.

Rosenthal, R. J., Rinzler, C., Walsh, R., & Klausner, E. (1972). Wrist-cutting syndrome: The meaning of the gesture. *American Journal of Psychiatry, 128*, 1363–1368.

Ross, S., Heath, N. L., & Toste, J. R. (2009). Non-suicidal self-injury and eating pathology in high school students. *American Journal of Orthopsychiatry, 79*, 83–92.

Ross, R. R., & McKay, H. B. (1979). *Self-mutilation.* Lexington, MA: Lexington Books.

Selekamn, M. D. (2010). Collaborative strengths-based brief therapy with self-injuring adolescents and their families. *The Prevention Researcher, 17*, 18–20.

Serras, A., Saules, K. K., Cranford, J. A., & Eisenberg, D. (2010). Self-injury, substance abuse, and associated risk factors in a multi-campus probability sample of college students. *Psychology of Addictive Behaviors, 24*, 119–128.

Shapiro, S. (2008). Addressing self-injury in the school setting. *The Journal of School Nursing, 24*, 124–130.

Simeon, D., & Favazza, A. R. (2001). Self-injurious behaviors: Phenomenology and assessment. In D. Simeon & E. Hollander (Eds.), *Self-injurious behaviors: Assessment and treatment* (pp. 1–28). Washington, DC: American Psychiatric Publishing.

Simpson, M. A. (1975). The phenomenology of self-mutilation in a general hospital setting. *Canadian Psychiatric Association Journal, 20*, 429–434.

Suyemoto, K. L. (1998). The functions of self-mutilation. *Clinical Psychology Review, 18*, 531–554.

Van der Kolk, B. A., Perry, J. C., & Herman, J. L. (1991). Childhood origins of self-destructive behavior. *American Journal of Psychiatry, 148*, 1665–1641.

Walsh, B. (2007). Clinical assessment of self-injury: A practical guide. *Journal of Clinical Psychology: In Session, 63*, 1057–1068.

Whitlock, J., Eckenrode, J., & Silverman, D. (2006). Self-injurious behaviors in a college population. *Pediatrics, 117*, 1939–1948.

Wildman, P., Lilenfeld, L. R. R., & Marcus, M. D. (2004). Axis I comorbidity onset and parasuicide in women with eating disorders. *International Journal of Eating Disorders, 35*, 190–197.

Yates, T. M. (2004). The developmental psychopathology of self-injurious behavior: Compensatory regulation in posttraumatic adaption. *Clinical Psychology Review, 24*, 35–74.

Yip, K. (2006). A strengths perspective in working with an adolescent with self-cutting behaviors. *Child and Adolescent Social Work Journal, 23*, 134–146.

Index

S.C. Dombrowski et al., *Assessing and Treating Low Incidence/High Severity*
Psychological Disorders of Childhood, DOI 10.1007/978-1-4419-9970-2,
© Springer Science+Business Media, LLC 2011

CPSIA information can be obtained at www.ICGtesting.com
Printed in the USA
LVOW010325021111

253134LV00004B/2/P